Dedicated to the staff and campers of Camp Wee-Kan-Tu, a camp for children with epilepsy sponsored by the Massachusetts-Rhode Island Epilepsy Foundation. Children who live with seizures 24 hours a day, seven days a week, can teach us a great deal about epilepsy.

Contents

Epilepsy: Definitions and Background

I. DEFINITION OF EPILEPSY

Hippocrates recognized epilepsy as an organic process of the brain. However, many ancient writers considered seizures to be the work of supernatural forces. The word *epilepsy* comes from a Greek word meaning "to be seized by forces from without."

J. H. Jackson gave direction to the understanding of epilepsy in the late 19th century by carefully analyzing individual cases. From his observations, Jackson (15) formulated the modern definition of *epilepsy*: "An occasional, excessive, and disorderly discharge of nerve tissue." Jackson further concluded, "This discharge occurs in all degrees; it occurs with all sorts of conditions of ill health at all ages, and under innumerable circumstances." His emphasis on the clinical description of a seizure, beginning with the mode of onset, led to the concept of focal epilepsy with subsequent spread of discharging cells.

Epilepsy is a complex symptom caused by a variety of pathologic processes in the brain. It is characterized by occasional (paroxysmal), excessive, and disorderly discharging of neurons that can be detected by clinical manifestations, electroencephalographic (EEG) recording, or both. Paroxysmal discharges of neurons occur when the threshold for firing of the neuronal membranes is reduced beyond the capability of intrinsic membrane-threshold–stabilizing mechanisms to prevent firing (see section **VI**). The attack may be localized and remain restricted in its focus, or it can spread to other areas of the brain. When the size of the discharging area is sufficient, a clinical seizure occurs; otherwise, the effects may be limited to localized, asymptomatic electrical disturbances. The particular site of the brain affected determines the clinical expression of the seizure. When the synchronized discharges of a neuronal population are recorded by an EEG from the scalp, the paroxysms appear as spikes, slow waves, and spike–wave potentials.

For the patient with epilepsy, the disorder is defined in more personal terms, such as what the patient experiences or recalls about the experience, what others observe and describe, the frequency and duration of attacks, and the impact on self-image and social adjustment.

II. PARTS OF A SEIZURE

The period during which the seizure actually occurs is called the *ictus* or *ictal period*. The *aura* is the earliest portion of a seizure recognized, and the only part remembered by the patient; it may act as a warning. The time immediately after a seizure is referred to as the *postictal period*. The interval between seizures is the *interictal period*.

1

III. TYPES OF EPILEPTIC SEIZURES AND TYPES OF EPILEPSY: CLASSIFICATIONS

Two types of classifications are used for epilepsy: (a) classifications of the epileptic seizures and (b) classifications of the epilepsies. Classifications of epileptic seizures are concerned with classifying each individual seizure as a single event, based on clinical and EEG information. Classifications of the epilepsies are designed to classify syndromes in which the type or types of seizure(s) are one, but not the only, feature of the syndrome. Other features, such as etiology, age at onset, genetics, and evidence of brain pathology, are also included in classifications of the epilepsies.

The classification of epileptic seizures used throughout this book is the 1981 revision of the Clinical and Electroencephalographic Classification of Epileptic Seizures of the International League Against Epilepsy (henceforth, International Classification of Epileptic Seizures) (5). In 2001, the International League Against Epilepsy proposed a new classification of epileptic seizures (6). This proposal has not yet been accepted and is cumbersome in clinical use. The authors have elected to continue use of the approved classification.

In 2001, the International League Against Epilepsy also proposed a revised classification of epilepsies and epileptic syndromes (8) to replace the 1989 revision of the Classification of Epilepsies and Epileptic Syndromes of the International League Against Epilepsy. The 2001 revision has not been approved. However, so many new epilepsy syndromes have been described since 1989 that the authors have elected to use the 2001 classification in this volume.

A. International Classification of Epileptic Seizures

The International Classification of Epileptic Seizures is summarized in Table 1-1 and presented in detail in Table 2-1. Seizures are first classified into two broad categories: (a) partial seizures

Table 1-1.   Summary of international classification of epilepsies

I. Partial (focal, local) seizures
   A. Simple partial seizures (consciousness not impaired)
   B. Complex partial seizures (temporal lobe or psychomotor seizures; consciousness impaired)
   C. Partial seizures evolving to secondarily generalized seizures [tonic–clonic (grand mal), tonic, or clonic]
II. Generalized seizures (convulsive or nonconvulsive)
   A. Absence (petit mal) seizures
   B. Myoclonic seizures
   C. Tonic seizures
   D. Atonic seizures
   E. Clonic seizures
   F. Tonic–clonic (grand mal) seizures
III. Unclassified epileptic seizures (caused by incomplete data)

(seizure beginning in a relatively small location in the brain) and (b) generalized seizures (seizures that are bilaterally symmetric and without local onset). Seizures are then further classified depending on their exact clinical and EEG manifestations. A summary of the clinical manifestations of the principal types of epileptic seizures recognized by the International Classification of Epileptic Seizures is presented in sections III.A.1–8. For a complete description of the clinical and EEG features of each seizure type, see Chapter 2.

1. Simple Partial (Focal) Seizures

Simple partial seizures are caused by a local cortical discharge, which results in seizure symptoms appropriate to the function of the discharging area of the brain without impairment of consciousness. Simple partial seizures may consist of motor, sensory, autonomic, or psychic signs or symptoms, or combinations of these (see Chapter 2).

2. Complex Partial (Psychomotor, Temporal Lobe) Seizures

The crucial distinction between simple partial seizures and complex partial seizures is that consciousness is impaired in the latter and not in the former. *Impaired consciousness* is defined as the inability to respond normally to exogenous stimuli, owing to altered awareness or responsiveness.

At the onset of a complex partial seizure, any of the symptoms or signs (motor, sensory, autonomic, or psychic) of a simple partial seizure may occur without impairment of consciousness, providing an aura. The central feature of the complex partial seizure is impairment of consciousness, which may occur with or without a preceding simple partial aura. No other symptoms or signs may be present during the period of impaired consciousness, or automatisms may appear (i.e., unconscious acts that are "automatic" and of which the patient has no recollection). The attack characteristically ends gradually, with a period of postictal drowsiness or confusion (see Chapter 2).

3. Absence (Petit Mal) Seizures

Absence seizures consist of sudden onset and cessation of impaired responsiveness, accompanied by a unique 3-Hz spike-and-wave EEG pattern. No aura is present, and few or no postictal symptoms occur. The majority of absence seizures last 10 seconds or less and may be accompanied by mild clonic components, atonic or tonic components, automatisms, or autonomic components. Absence seizures usually first manifest between the ages of 5 and 12 years and often stop spontaneously in the teens (see Chapter 2).

4. Myoclonic Seizures

Myoclonic seizures consist of brief, sudden muscle contractions that may be generalized or localized, symmetric or asymmetric, synchronous or asynchronous. No loss of consciousness is usually detectable (see Chapter 2).

5. Tonic Seizures

Tonic seizures consist of a sudden increase in muscle tone in the axial or extremity muscles, or both, producing a number of characteristic postures. Consciousness is usually partially or completely lost. Prominent autonomic phenomena occur. Postictal alteration of consciousness is usually brief, but it may last several minutes. Tonic seizures are relatively rare and usually begin between 1 and 7 years of age (see Chapter 2).

6. Atonic Seizures

Atonic seizures consist of sudden loss of muscle tone. The loss of muscle tone may be confined to a group of muscles, such as the neck, resulting in a head drop. Alternatively, atonic seizures may involve all trunk muscles, leading to a fall to the ground (see Chapter 2).

7. Clonic Seizures

Clonic seizures occur almost exclusively in early childhood. The attack begins with loss or impairment of consciousness associated with sudden hypotonia or a brief, generalized tonic spasm. This is followed by 1 minute to several minutes of bilateral jerks, which are often asymmetric and may appear predominantly in one limb. During the attack, the amplitude, frequency, and spatial distribution of these jerks may vary greatly from moment to moment. In other children, particularly those aged 1 to 3 years, the jerks remain bilateral and synchronous throughout the attack. Postictally, recovery may be rapid, or a prolonged period of confusion or coma may ensue (see Chapter 2).

8. Tonic–Clonic (Grand Mal) Seizures

Before the tonic phase of a tonic–clonic seizure, bilateral jerks of the extremities or focal seizure activity may occur. The onset of the seizure is marked by loss of consciousness and increased muscle tone (tonic phase), which usually results in a rigid, flexed posture at first, and then a rigid, extended posture. This is followed by bilateral rhythmic jerks that become further apart (clonic phase). Prominent autonomic phenomena are observable during the tonic and clonic phases. In the postictal phase, increased muscle tone occurs first, followed by flaccidity. Incontinence may occur. The patient awakens by passing through stages of coma, confusional state, and drowsiness (see Chapter 2).

B. International Classification of Epilepsies

The International Classification of Epilepsies (Table 1-2) begins by dividing epilepsies according to overall seizure type: generalized or focal. Generalized epilepsies involve seizures with initial activation of neurons in both cerebral hemispheres, whereas focal epilepsies involve seizures with initial activation of a group of neurons within one hemisphere. Note that the terms *focal, localization-related, partial*, and *local* are often used synonymously.

Epilepsies are next divided according to etiology: idiopathic, symptomatic, or familial. *Idiopathic* means arising spontaneously

Table 1-2. An example of a classification of epilepsy syndromes

Groups of Syndromes	Specific Syndromes
Idiopathic focal epilepsies of infancy and childhood	Benign infantile seizures (nonfamilial) Benign childhood epilepsy with centrotemporal spikes Early-onset benign childhood occipital epilepsy (Panayiotopoulos type) Late-onset childhood occipital epilepsy (Gastaut type)
Familial (autosomal dominant) focal epilepsies	Benign familial neonatal seizures Benign familial infantile seizures Autosomal dominant nocturnal frontal lobe epilepsy Familial temporal lobe epilepsy Familial focal epilepsy with variable foci

Symptomatic (or probably symptomatic) focal epilepsies	Limbic epilepsies
	  Mesial temporal lobe epilepsy with hippocampal sclerosis
	  Mesial temporal lobe epilepsy defined by specific etiologies
	  Other types defined by location and etiology
	Neocortical epilepsies
	  Rasmussen syndrome
	  Hemiconvulsion–hemiplegia syndrome
	  Other types defined by location and etiology
	  Migrating partial seizures of early infancy

Idiopathic generalized epilepsies	Benign myoclonic epilepsy in infancy
	Epilepsy with myoclonic astatic seizures
	Childhood absence epilepsy
	Epilepsy with myoclonic absences
	Idiopathic generalized epilepsies with variable phenotypes
	  Juvenile absence epilepsy
	  Juvenile myoclonic epilepsy
	  Epilepsy with generalized tonic–clonic seizures only
	Generalized epilepsies with febrile seizures plus (GEFS+)

continued

Table 1-2. *Continued*

Groups of Syndromes	Specific Syndromes
Reflex epilepsies	Idiopathic photosensitive occipital lobe epilepsy Other visual-sensitive epilepsies Primary reading epilepsy Startle epilepsy
Epileptic encephalopathies (in which the epileptiform abnormalities may contribute to progressive dysfunction)	Early myoclonic encephalopathy Ohtahara syndrome West syndrome Dravet syndrome (previously known as severe myoclonic epilepsy in infancy) Myoclonic status in non-progressive encephalopathies Lennox–Gastaut syndrome Landau–Kleffner syndrome Epilepsy with continuous spike waves during slow-wave sleep
Progressive myoclonus epilepsies	See specific diseases
Seizures not necessarily requiring a diagnosis of epilepsy	Benign neonatal seizures Febrile seizures Reflex seizures Alcohol-withdrawal seizures Drug or other chemically induced seizures Immediate and early post-traumatic seizures Single seizures or isolated clusters of seizures Rarely repeated seizures (oligoepilepsy)

From Engel J Jr. A proposed diagnostic scheme for people with epileptic seizures and with epilepsy: report of the ILAE Task Force on Classification and Terminology. *Epilepsia* 2001;42:796–803, with permission.

from an obscure or unknown cause. *Symptomatic* epilepsies arise as symptoms of a known brain abnormality. *Familial* means arising from a known gene defect. Three special categories also are used: *reflex epilepsies, epileptic encephalopathies*, and *progressive myoclonic epilepsies*. Finally, some conditions may result in seizures but are not likely to result in epilepsy: chronic unprovoked seizures.

Based on these categories, the epilepsies are divided into eight groups (Table 1-2), within each of which are a number of specific epilepsy syndromes based on specific clustering of seizure type(s), specific etiology, genetics, age, and evidence of brain pathology

(Table 1-2). Each age group is vulnerable to a limited number of epilepsies and epilepsy syndromes, and age at epilepsy onset is a useful parameter in beginning to determine a patient's epilepsy and epilepsy syndrome. Knowing the age at epilepsy onset and seizure type(s) limits classification of a patient's epilepsy and epilepsy syndrome to just a few choices. This principle is used in presenting the epilepsies and epilepsy syndromes by age at onset in Chapters 3 to 8 to reduce the choices for a given patient to a manageable number.

IV. EPIDEMIOLOGY

Prevalence, cumulative incidence, and incidence are the measures used to describe the epidemiology of epilepsy. Prevalence is the proportion of a population affected with epilepsy at a given time. Various studies report the prevalence of epilepsy as 5 to 8 in 1,000, or approximately 1.25 to 2 million people in the United States. The prevalence of epilepsy by age is shown in Fig. 1-1.

Cumulative incidence is the proportion of a population in which epilepsy develops over a given time (Fig. 1-1). The risk of epilepsy from birth through age 20 years is approximately 1% and reaches 3% at age 75. Approximately 3% of persons can be expected to have epilepsy at some time during their lives.

Incidence is the occurrence of new cases of epilepsy per unit of person-time. Incidence of epilepsy is usually estimated at 30 to 50 per 100,000 person-years. Incidence can also be reported by clinical seizure type (Fig. 1-2) (Table 1-3).

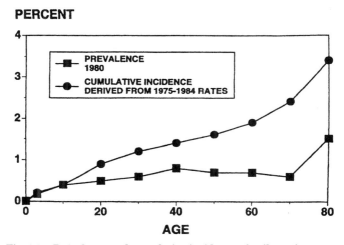

Fig. 1-1.   Prevalence and cumulative incidence of epilepsy in Rochester, Minnesota. (From Annegers JF. Epidemiology of epilepsy. In: Wyllie E, ed. *The treatment of epilepsy: principles and practice,* 3rd ed. Philadelphia: Lippincott Williams & Wilkins, 2001:131–138, with permission.)

INCIDENCE PER 100,000

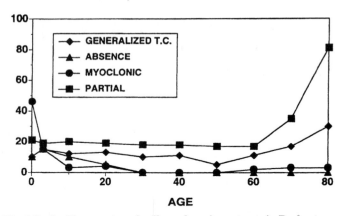

AGE

Fig. 1-2.   Incidence rates of epilepsy by seizure types in Rochester, Minnesota, 1935–1979. T.C., tonic–clonic. (From Annegers JF. Epidemiology of epilepsy. In: Wyllie E, ed. *The treatment of epilepsy: principles and practice*. 3rd ed. Philadelphia: Lippincott Williams & Wilkins, 2001:131–138, with permission.)

In Figs. 1-1 and 1-2, the prevalence and cumulative incidence of epilepsy and the incidence of partial seizures increase dramatically in the elderly; this phenomenon is discussed in more detail in Chapter 13.

V. GENETICS OF EPILEPSY

The genetic contribution to most epilepsy syndromes is unknown. However, considerable progress has been made in defining the genetics of certain epilepsy syndromes. Epilepsy

Table 1-3.   Incidence of epilepsy by seizure type

Seizure Type	Incidence
Simple partial	12.8
Complex partial	10.4
Multiple or unclassified partial	7.2
Tonic–clonic only	12.5
Incompletely generalized with or without associated tonic–clonic	6.1
Absence with or without associated tonic–clonic	3.4
Other	4.5

Note: Mean annual rate per 100,000 population. Calculated for Rochester, Minnesota, 1945–1964.
From Annegers JF. Epidemiology of epilepsy. In: Wyllie E, ed. *The treatment of epilepsy: principles and practice*, 3rd ed. Philadelphia: Lippincott Williams & Wilkins, 2001:131–138, modified with permission.

syndromes may be inherited in a simple mendelian fashion. Epilepsy syndromes also may be acquired through complex inheritance, in which more than one gene, with or without the influence of acquired factors, leads to the phenotype.

In a number of inherited syndromes, epilepsy may be the primary neurologic problem faced by the patient. For example, children with benign familial neonatal convulsions have seizures during the first few months of life but are otherwise normal. In the autosomal disorders identified thus far in which epilepsy is the primary condition, channelopathies appear to be the cause of the epilepsy. In a number of other genetic syndromes, epilepsy is part of a disorder with other neurologic problems. For example, children with Angelman syndrome and Rett syndrome have severe mental retardation and motor deficits in addition to the epilepsy. In a number of other genetic syndromes, epilepsy is part of a disorder with other neurologic problems.

The known genetic epilepsies are listed in Table 1-4.

VI. BASIC MECHANISMS OF EPILEPSY

Epilepsy is a paroxysmal disorder characterized by abnormal neuronal discharges. Although the causes of epilepsy are many, the fundamental disorder is secondary to abnormal synchronous discharges of a network of neurons. Epilepsy can be secondary to either abnormal neuronal membranes or an imbalance between excitatory and inhibitory influences.

In this section, we first review basic principles of generation and cessation of seizure activity: excitation and inhibition of neuronal membranes, excitation and inhibition of neurons by neurotransmitters, generation of EEG potentials, generation of interictal discharges, generation of seizure activity, and cessation of seizure activity. Specific seizure types are created by excitation and inhibition in specific neuronal networks, and this is reviewed for partial seizures and absence seizures in the second part of this section.

A. Principles of Generation and Cessation of Seizure Activity

1. Excitation and Inhibition of Neuronal Membranes

Neuronal membranes consist of lipid bilayers mixed with proteins that traverse the membrane and form ion channels. Each neuron has a resting potential that represents the voltage difference between the inside and outside of the cell. This potential difference exists because of the separation of positive and negative changes across the cell membrane. The extracellular space along the membrane is dominated by Na^+ and chloride (Cl^-) ions, whereas K^+, proteins, and organic acids are found in the intracellular space. Membranes are permeable to Na^+, Cl^-, and K^+ but impermeable to large organic ions and proteins. Because the lipid bilayers act as a barrier to the diffusion of ions, a net excess of positive charges outside and negative charges inside produces a resting membrane potential of approximately -50 to -80 mV.

Ion leaks across the membrane occur, moving from high concentration to low concentration: Na^+ leaks in and K^+ leaks out. With time, the inside and outside concentration (across the membrane)

Table 1-4. Mapped epilepsy syndromes

Type	Syndrome	Inheritance	Chromosome	Gene	Function
Idiopathic generalized	Benign familial neonatal convulsions (EBN1)	Autosomal dominant	20q	KCNQ2	Voltage-gated potassium channel
	Benign familial neonatal convulsions (EBN2)	Autosomal dominant	8q	KCNQ3	Voltage-gated potassium channel
	Childhood absence epilepsy with generalized tonic–clonic seizures	Complex	8q24		
	Childhood absence evolving to juvenile myoclonic epilepsy (JME)	Complex	1p		
	Juvenile absence epilepsy	Complex	21q22.1		
	JME	Complex	6p	GRIK1	GluR5 (kainate receptor)
	JME	Complex	15q14	CHRNA7	
	Familial adult myoclonic epilepsy	Autosomal dominant	8q24		
Situation-related seizures	Febrile (FEB1)	Autosomal dominant	8q13–21		
	Febrile (FEB2)	Autosomal dominant	19p13.3	SCN1B	Sodium channel β subunit
	Febrile (FEB3)	Autosomal dominant	2q24		
	Generalized epilepsy plus febrile seizures	Autosomal dominant	2q21–33		

	Syndrome	Inheritance	Locus	Gene
Localization-related (partial)	Generalized epilepsy with febrile seizures plus	Autosomal dominant	19q13.1	
	Benign infantile familial convulsions (BIFC)	Autosomal dominant	9q11–13	
	BIFC plus paroxysmal choreoathetosis	Autosomal dominant	16q	
	Autosomal-dominant nocturnal frontal lobe epilepsy (ADNFLE) (ENFL1)	Autosomal dominant	20q13.3	CHRNA4
	ADNFLE (ENFL2)	Autosomal dominant	15q24	
	Autosomal-dominant temporal lobe epilepsy	Autosomal dominant	10q22–24	
	Familial partial epilepsy with variable foci	Autosomal dominant	2?	
	Rolandic benign epilepsy of childhood with centrotemporal spikes (BECTS)	Complex	15q14	CHRNA7?
Progressive	Unverricht–Lundborg (EPM1)	Recessive	21q22.3	CSTB (Cystatin B (unstable minisatellite expansion))
	Lafora disease (EPM2)	Recessive	6q24	EPM2A (Tyrosine phosphatase)

From Treiman L, Treiman D. Genetic aspects of epilepsy. In: Wyllie E, ed. *The treatment of epilepsy: principles and practice.* Philadelphia: Lippincott Williams & Wilkins, 2001:115–130, with permission.

may change. The Na^+-K^+ pump extrudes Na^+ from the cell and brings in K^+, counterbalancing the leakage. The pump, which moves Na^+ and K^+ against their net electrochemical gradients, requires energy that is derived from hydrolysis of adenosine triphosphate. A reduction in the negativity of this polarized state is called depolarization; an increase in the negativity of the resting potential is known as hyperpolarization. Membrane permeability changes that allow Na^+ to enter the cell lead to depolarization, and membrane changes that allow K^+ to exit the cell or Cl^- to enter the cell result in hyperpolarization.

In addition to selectively permeable ion channels in the resting state, gated channels exist in several configurations. The term gating is used to describe the transition of a channel between these different states. Most gated changes are closed when the membrane is at rest. Each ion channel has at least one open state and two closed states. In voltage-gated channels, the voltage across the membrane determines whether a conformational change in the membrane occurs that may open the channel. In the case of the voltage-gated Na^+ channel (Fig. 1-3), the channel remains closed until the membrane begins to depolarize. The

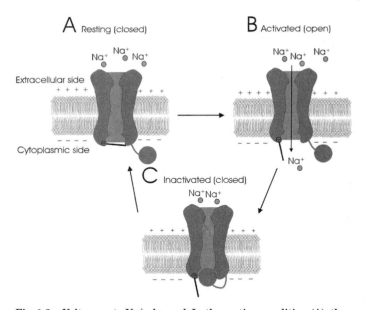

Fig. 1-3. Voltage-gate Na^+ channel. In the resting condition (A), the activation gate (*black bar*) is closed, and the inactivation gate (*ball and chain*) is open. No Na^+ flows because of the closed activation gate. With depolarization of the membrane, a conformational change of the channel occurs, and the activation gate opens (B). Na^+ flow then occurs. This is followed by inactivation by closure of the inactivation gate (C), prohibiting the further flow of Na^+ ions. With repolarization of the membrane, the inactivation gate opens, the activation gate closes, and the channel is ready for another cycle (A).

channel then opens and Na^+ enters, causing more depolarization resulting in an action potential (Fig. 1-4). Shortly after opening, the Na^+ channels becomes inactivated, and no further Na^+ currents occur. Only when the membrane is hyperpolarized does the channel become de-inactivated and return to its resting state.

2. Excitation and Inhibition of Neurons by Neurotransmitters

Protein segments extend out of the membrane and serve as receptor sites. Ionotropic receptors directly alter the conductance of the ion channel when bound to a neurotransmitter. Examples of ionotropic receptors include the γ-aminobutyric acid ($GABA_A$) receptors that increase Cl^- conductance and the N-methyl-D-aspartate (NMDA) receptors that increase the permeability to Na^+ and Ca^{2+}. Neurotransmitters (such as GABA) that cause hyperpolarization of the neuron give rise to inhibitory postsynaptic potentials (IPSPs), which result in a greater intracellular negativity than baseline. Neurotransmitters that lead to depolarization (such as excitatory amino acids) give rise to excitatory postsynaptic potentials (EPSPs), which result in an inward flow of positive charges through the synaptic membrane, leaving a relatively negative extracellular environment. Whether a neuron generates an action potential is determined by the relative balance of EPSPs and IPSPs. Figure 1-5 demonstrates current flow with EPSPs and IPSPs.

A second type of neurotransmitter receptor is the metabotropic receptor. When a transmitter binds to the metabotropic receptor, it activates a second-messenger system [guanyl nucleotide–binding protein (G protein)]. The activated G protein may then open an ion channel or activate an enzyme, such as a cyclase (cyclic adenosine monophosphate) or hydrolase, to affect the generation of additional messenger molecules within a cell. Examples of receptors that activate second-messenger systems include $GABA_B$ receptors, peptide and catecholaminergic receptors, and the metabotropic receptors activated by glutamate. Note that $GABA_A$ receptors are ionotropic receptors that enhance Cl^- conductance, and $GABA_B$ receptors are metabotropic receptors that are coupled through G proteins to calcium or K^+ ion channels.

3. Generation of Electroencephalogram Potentials

The EEG is based on volume conduction of ionic currents generated by nerve cells through the extracellular space. Recorded EEG potentials arise from extracellular current flow from summated EPSPs and IPSPs. The EEG does not record activity from single neurons but is dependent on the summation of thousands to millions of postsynaptic potentials (PSPs), and therefore represents activity from a large neuronal aggregation. Although nerve action potentials have higher voltage changes than EPSPs and IPSPs, the lack of summation and short duration of the action potentials usually adds little to EEG activity. During seizures, when synchronous firing of large ensembles of cells occurs, actions potentials may contribute to EEG discharges.

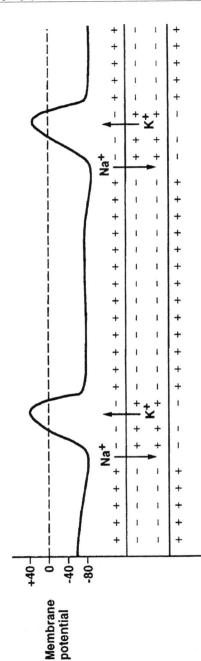

Fig. 1-4. Propagation of action potential along the axon as a result of changing membrane potentials. At rest, the inside of the neuron is negative compared with the extracellular space. An action potential is generated during transient breakdown in gradient between potassium (K^+) and sodium (Na^+) ions.

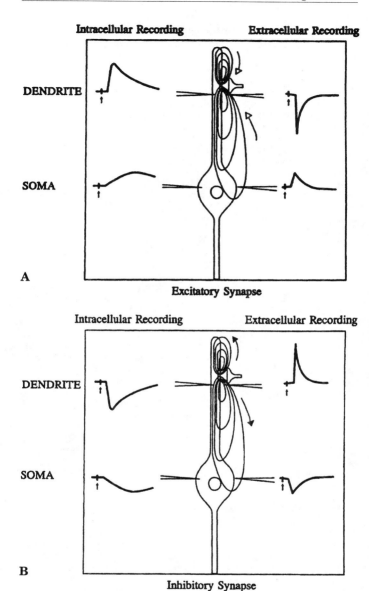

Fig. 1-5.   **Examples of current flow as a result of excitatory postsynaptic potential (A) and inhibitory postsynaptic potential (B) on the apical dendrites.**

4. Generation of Interictal Discharges

The hallmark of the epileptic neuron in experimental models of epilepsy is massive depolarization. During an interictal discharge, the cell membrane near the soma undergoes a relatively high-voltage (approximately 10 to 15 mV) and relatively long (100 to 200 microseconds) depolarization associated with bursts of spike activity (Fig. 1-6). This depolarization is much longer than the depolarization seen with EPSPs, which is in the range of 10 to 16 μsec. The long depolarization has the effect of generating a train of action potentials that are conducted away from the soma along the axon of the neuron. This large depolarization is called the paroxysmal depolarization shift (PDS). The general similarities in the neuronal events underlying interictal epileptogenesis in chronic epileptiform foci, studied both in experimental animals and in the human cortex, suggest that similar mechanisms give rise to such discharges.

Extensive intracellular studies of experimental epilepsy have been done in foci produced by the application of penicillin to cat neocortex and hippocampus. Within a few minutes after the focal application of penicillin to the cortex, high-voltage sharp waves appear in the EEG, associated with intracellularly recorded PDSs. The interictal PDS is followed by a large hyperpolarization, which serves to limit the duration of interictal paroxysms. It is important to remember that an epileptic area is made up of numerous abnormal neurons that discharge in an abnormal synchronous manner. The PDS may occur because of intrinsic membrane abnormalities in a group of neurons or because of excessive excitatory input (or reduced inhibitory input) to a group of neurons.

With time, a progressive loss of hyperpolarization after the PDS may occur in the epileptic focus. During seizures, the epileptic neurons undergo prolonged depolarization with waves of action potentials during the tonic phase of the seizure and oscillations of membrane potentials with bursts of action potentials, separated by quiet periods, during the clonic phase. An EEG recorded at the scalp at this time shows continuous spikes, which generally coincide with the tonic stage of a generalized tonic–clonic seizure. During the next stage, large inhibitory potentials occur (with slowing or flattening on surface EEG) and alternate with recurrent, rhythmic PDSs (with spikes on surface EEG). This pattern generally coincides with the clonic stage of the seizure.

5. Generation of Seizure Activity

Although the events that lead from the interictal to ictal state are not well understood, a number of possible mechanisms may be involved. These abnormalities may include disturbances of the neuronal membranes or excitatory or inhibitory neurotransmitter (Fig. 1-7). Decreases in synaptic inhibition, increases in synaptic excitation, alteration in K^+ or Ca^{2+} currents, or changes in the extracellular ion concentrations may trigger prolonged depolarizations. These changes may occur not only in the microenvironment at the epileptic focus, but also at distant sites through synaptic pathways. These "downstream" changes may be responsible for the generalization of the seizures. Different behavioral and EEG features of the seizure depend on spread of

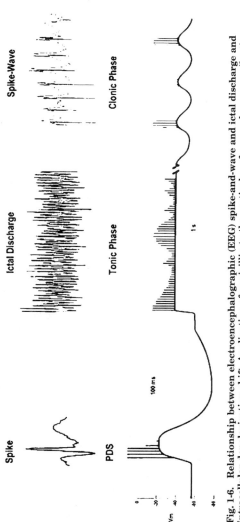

Fig. 1-6. Relationship between electroencephalographic (EEG) spike-and-wave and ictal discharge and intracellular depolarization shift. Application of penicillin to the cortical surface produces an epileptic focus. The paroxysmal depolarization shift (PDS) is similar to an excitatory postsynaptic potential and elicits a burst of action potentials. An EEG spike is elicited by the PDS. The EEG spike corresponds to the depolarization while the slow wave following the spike corresponds to the repolarization following the depolarization. If the PDS persists and is not followed by hyperpolarization, repetitive spikes and a clinical seizure occur. During the next stage, large inhibitory potentials occur and alternate with recurrent rhythmic paroxysmal depolarization shifts. This pattern generally coincides with the clonic state of the seizure.

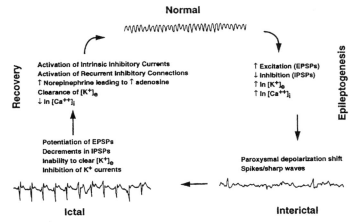

Fig. 1-7. Possible mechanisms of interictal and ictal events. [Ca^{2+}]$_i$, intracellular Ca^{2+}; EPSPs, excitatory postsynaptic potentials; IPSPs, inhibitory postsynaptic potentials; [K$^+$]$_e$, extracellular K$^+$.

the discharge and which specific cortical or subcortical nuclei developed synchronous discharges.

6. Cessation of Seizure Activity

The mechanisms that cause seizures to stop are poorly understood. Generalized convulsions are commonly assumed to terminate as a result of active inhibitory processes, and these mechanisms, as well as depolarization block, are assumed to be responsible for the end of the seizures and the marked voltage suppression on the EEG postictally. As shown in Fig. 1-7, seizures may end with activation of inhibitory circuits in the neuron or neuronal network; with changes in the extracellular environment, such as reduction of extracellular K$^+$; or with elimination of intracellular Ca^{2+}.

Some evidence also exists that endogenous agents, such as norepinephrine or adenosine, which have anticonvulsant action in experimental animal models, may be involved in stopping seizures. Seizures could result in activation of the locus ceruleus–cortical norepinephrine system, increasing extracellular adenosine and resulting in decreased excitation.

B. Neuronal Networks and Special Seizure Types

Although epilepsy clearly begins at the cellular level, it must be remembered that epilepsy is a disorder of a network of neurons. The importance of networks is particularly evident in the cases of partial seizures and absence seizures.

1. Partial Seizures and the Kindling Model

Much has been learned about the development of the epileptic focus by using the penicillin model discussed earlier, in section **VI.A.4**. However, the kindling model may provide better insights into how networks of neurons are altered during epileptogenesis, especially in partial seizures. Kindling consists of the repeated administration of an initially subconvulsive electrical stimulus to any of several brain structures, resulting in the development of EEG seizures (afterdischarges) and the progressive intensification of behavioral seizures, eventually culminating in a generalized seizure. Although electrical stimulations are most commonly used to induce kindling, the repeated administration of a variety of epileptogenic agents (such as pentylenetetrazol, flurothyl lidocaine, cocaine, and picrotoxin) or cholinergic agents may also lead to the gradual development of generalized seizures. Once the enhanced sensitivity has developed, the effect is long lasting, and the animal can be classified as kindled. Kindling is not limited to the original kindling agent but may result in increased seizure susceptibility to other kindling agents. Kindling is now widely accepted as an animal model of partial epilepsy.

In the kindling model, three mechanisms underlie the development of partial seizures. First, evidence indicates that enhanced NMDA receptor–mediated transmission takes place in dentate granule cells. This suggests that excitatory input into the hippocampus will be heightened in the dentate. A second mechanism is the loss of hilar neurons that normally activate inhibitory basket cells. Loss of these hilar neurons leads to loss of inhibition of dentate granule cells and increased hippocampal excitation. The third mechanism in kindling is the synaptic reorganization of granule cell–excitatory cell output. After kindling, an aberrant growth of granule cell axons (called *mossy fibers*) back into the inner molecular layer of the dentate has been noted. The sprouting of mossy-fiber axons is readily observed with the Timm method, a histochemical technique that selectively stains mossy-fiber axon terminals because of their high zinc content. Because the neurotransmitter of the mossy fibers is presumably glutamate, these aberrant synaptic conditions may contribute to the state of hyperexcitability that either provokes or facilitates abnormal discharges. The net effect of such synaptic reorganization has been shown to be excitatory in the kindling model.

2. Absence Seizures

The observation that 3-Hz spike-and-wave discharges in absence seizures appear simultaneously and synchronously in all electrode locations led early investigators to speculate that the pathophysiologic mechanisms of absence seizures must involve "deep" structures with widespread connections between the two hemispheres (see Chapter 2, Fig. 2-1). A number of more recent studies have suggested that the basic underlying mechanism in absence seizures involves thalamocortical circuitry and the generation of abnormal oscillatory rhythms in the neuronal network. The neuronal circuit is responsible for the generation of the oscillatory thalamocortical burst-firing observed during absence seizures. The circuit involved in thalamocortical burst-firing includes cortical pyramidal neurons, thalamic relay neurons, and the nucleus reticularis thalami (NRT). The principal synaptic connections of the thalamocortical circuit include glutamatergic fibers between neocortical pyramidal cells and the NR;

GABAergic connections between cells of the NRT that activate $GABA_A$ receptors; and GABAergic fibers from NRT neurons that activate $GABA_A$ and $GABA_B$ receptors on thalamic relay neurons (Fig. 1-8). The NRT is in a position to greatly influence the flow of information between the thalamus and cerebral cortex. The NRT cells have rhythmic burst firing (oscillatory firing) during periods of sleep and continuous single spike firing (tonic firing) during wakefulness.

The cellular events that underlie the ability of NRT neurons to shift between an oscillatory and a tonic firing mode are the low-threshold (T) Ca^{2+} spikes that are present in thalamocortical and NRT neurons. These T Ca^{2+} channels are a key mem-

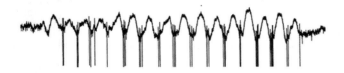

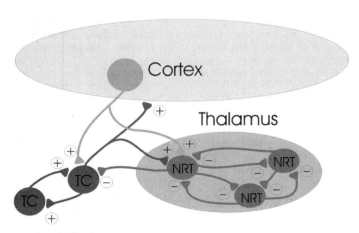

Fig. 1-8.   **Principal neuronal populations and connections of thalamocortical circuitry responsible for absence seizures. Pyramidal cells in the cortex are reciprocally connected by excitatory synapses with the thalamic relay neurons (TC). γ-Aminobutyric acid (GABA)-ergic neurons in the nucleus reticularod thalami reticular (NRT) are excited by pyramidal cells in the cortex and by TC neurons. The NRT inhibit the TC relay neurons. Inhibition of the TC relay neurons is mediated by both GABAA and GABAB receptors and voltage- and Ca^{++}-dependent K^+ conductances. The resulting hyperpolarization deactivates the low threshold calcium current, which results in depolarization and action potentials. These bursts are capable of reexciting the reticular thalamic nucleus, thus continuing the cycle of oscillations, resulting in spike-and-wave complexes.**

brane property involved in burst-firing excitation and are associated with the change from oscillatory to burst-firing in thalamocortical cells. Mild depolarization of these neurons is sufficient to activate these channels and to allow the influx of extracellular Ca^{2+}. Further depolarization produced by Ca^{2+} inflow will exceed the threshold for firing a burst of action potentials. After T-channels are activated, they become inactivated rather quickly; hence the name *transient*. De-inactivation of T-channels requires a relatively lengthy hyperpolarization. $GABA_B$ receptor–mediated hyperpolarization is a primary factor in the de-inactivation of T-channels.

The abnormal oscillatory rhythms in absence seizures could be caused by abnormalities of the T-type Ca^{2+} channels or enhanced $GABA_B$ function. In some animal models of absence seizures, T-channel Ca^{2+} activation in the NRT differs significantly from that in control animals. These aberrant T-channels likely are the basis for absence seizures. In other models, an increase in $GABA_B$ receptors in thalamic and neocortical neuronal populations has been noted compared with those in controls. As would be predicted from the thalamocortical circuits involved in absence seizures, in animal models of absences, $GABA_B$ agonists produce an increase in seizure frequency, whereas $GABA_B$ antagonists reduce seizure frequency. Other neurotransmitter systems (i.e., serotonergic, noradrenergic, and cholinergic) can influence the thalamocortical circuits and therefore influence absence seizure frequency. However, the GABA system appears to be the critical system in the pathogenesis of absence seizures.

Recurrent collateral GABAergic fibers from the NRT neurons activate $GABA_A$ receptors on adjacent NRT neurons. Activating $GABA_A$ receptors in the NRT therefore results in an inhibition of inhibitory output to the thalamic relay neurons. Because of the decreased $GABA_B$ activation, a reduced likelihood would exist that Ca^{2+} de-inactivation would occur. This would result in decreased oscillatory firing. However, direct $GABA_A$ and $GABA_B$ activation of thalamic relay neurons would be expected to have detrimental effects, increasing hyperpolarization and therefore increasing the likelihood of de-inactivation of the T-channels.

As would be expected from these animal findings, clinical observations indicate that three drugs efficacious in the treatment of absence seizures, such as valproate, ethosuximide, and trimethadione, suppress T-currents. In addition, some clinical evidence suggests that vigabatrin, which increases endogenous GABA levels and thereby increases the activation of $GABA_B$ receptors in the thalamic relay neurons, worsens absence seizures in patients. However, clonazepam, which preferentially activates GABA levels in the NRT, can be a highly effective antiabsence drug.

C. Effects of Development
Children are at high risk for seizures during the first months and years of life. The propensity for seizures in the immature brain has been demonstrated in a number of experimental models. The underlying mechanisms responsible for this increased excitability during this period of life are not completely under-

stood but are clearly age dependent. During the early postnatal period, at a time when the immature brain is highly susceptible to seizures, GABA exerts paradoxic excitatory action, raising a hypothesis that enhanced excitability is due to the excitatory rather than inhibitory actions of GABA. The lack of an efficient time-locked inhibition, the delayed maturation of postsynaptic $GABA_B$-mediated currents, and the high input resistance of small compact neurons will facilitate the generation of action potentials and synchronized activities. At more developed stages, in rodents during the second postnatal week, enhanced excitation may play an additional role in the propensity of the immature brain for seizures. With maturation, axonal collaterals and attendant synapses regress.

REFERENCES

1. Annegers JF. Epidemiology of epilepsy. In: Wyllie E, ed. *The treatment of epilepsy: principles and practice.* 3rd ed. Philadelphia: Lippincott Williams & Wilkins, 2001:131–138.
2. Ayala GF, Dichter M, Gummit RJ, et al. Genesis of epileptic interictal spikes: new knowledge of cortical feedback systems suggests a neurophysiologic explanation of brief paroxysms. *Brain Res* 1973;52:1–17.
3. Ben-Ari Y, Holmes GL. Effects of seizures on developmental processes in the immature brain. *Lancet Neurol* 2006;5:1055–1063.
4. Browne TR, Holmes GL. Primary care: epilepsy. *N Engl J Med* 2001;344:590–595.
5. Commission on Classification and Terminology of the International League Against Epilepsy. Proposal for revised clinical and electroencephalographic classification of epileptic seizures. *Epilepsia* 1981;22:489–501.
6. Commission on Classification and Terminology of the International League Against Epilepsy. Proposal for revised classification of epilepsies and epileptic syndromes. *Epilepsia* 1989;30:389–390.
7. Crunelli V, Leresche N. A role for $GABA_B$ receptors in excitation and inhibition of thalamocortical cells. *TINS* 1991;14:16–21.
8. Engel J Jr. A proposed diagnostic scheme for people with epileptic seizures and with epilepsy: report of the ILAE Task Force on Classification and Terminology. *Epilepsia* 2001;42:796–803.
9. Hauser WA. The prevalence and incidence of convulsive disorders in children. *Epilepsia* 1994;35(suppl 2):S1–S6.
10. Holmes GL. Models for generalized seizures. *Suppl Clin Neurophysiol* 2004;57:415–424.
11. Holmes GL, Ben-Ari Y. The neurobiology and consequences of epilepsy in the developing brain. *Pediatr Res* 2001;49:320–325.
12. Holmes GL, Khazipov R, Ben-Ari Y. Basic neurophysiology and the cortical basis of EEG. In: Blume AS, Rutkove SB, eds. *The clinical neurophysiology primer.* Totowa, NJ: Humana Press, 2000:719–733.
13. Hosford DA, Clark S, Cao Z, et al. The role of $GABA_B$ receptor activation in absence seizures of lethargic (lh/lh) mice. *Science* 1992;257:398–401.

14. Huguenard JR, Prince DA. Clonazepam suppresses $GABA_B$-mediated inhibition in thalamic relay neurons through effects in nucleus reticularis. *J Neurophysiol* 1994;71:2576–2581.

15. Jackson JH. Lectures of the diagnosis of epilepsy. In: Taylor J, ed. *Selected writings of John H. Jackson*, Vol 1. New York: Basic Books, 1951:276–307.

16. Jones SW, Swanson TH. Basic cellular neurophysiology. In Wyllie E, ed. *The treatment of epilepsy: principles and practice*. Philadelphia: Lippincott Williams & Wilkins, 2001:3–24.

17. Kohling R. Voltage-gated sodium channels in epilepsy. *Epilepsia* 2002;43:1278–1295.

18. Lehmann-Horn F, Jurkat-Rott K. Voltage-gated ion channels and hereditary disease. *Physiol Rev* 1999;79:1317–1372.

19. Lin FH, Cao Z, Hosford DA. Increased number of $GABA_B$ receptors in the lethargic (lh/lh) mouse model of absence epilepsy. *Brain Res* 1993;608:101–106.

20. Panayiotopoulos CP. *A clinical guide to epileptic syndromes and their treatment*. Oxfordshire: Blandon Medical Publishing, 2002.

21. Privetera M. Complications of epilepsy. *Epilepsia* 2000; 41(suppl 2):1–68.

22. Snead OC III. Basic mechanisms of generalized absence seizures. *Ann Neurol* 1995;37:146–157.

23. So NK. Epileptic auras. In: Wyllie E, ed. *The treatment of epilepsy: principles and practice*. Philadelphia: Lippincott Williams & Wilkins, 2001:299–308.

24. Song I, Kim D, Choi S, et al. Role of the alpha1G T-type calcium channel in spontaneous absence seizures in mutant mice. *J Neurosci* 2004;24:5249–5257.

25. Strauss DJ, Day SM, Shavelle RM, et al. Remote symptomatic epilepsy: does seizure severity increase mortality? *Neurology* 2003;60:395–399.

26. Treiman L, Treiman D. Genetic aspects of epilepsy. In: Wyllie E, ed. *The treatment of epilepsy: principles and practice*. Philadelphia: Lippincott Williams & Wilkins, 2001:115–130.

27. Wyllie E, ed. *The treatment of epilepsy: principles and practice*. 3rd ed. Philadelphia: Williams & Wilkins, 2001.

28. Kandel ER, Schwartz JH, Jessell TM. *Principles of neural science*. 4th ed. New York: McGraw-Hill, 2000.

Types of Seizures

An epileptic seizure is classified as a single event based on clinical and electroencephalographic (EEG) information. The classification of epileptic seizures used throughout this book is the 1981 revision of the Clinical and Electroencephalographic Classification of Epileptic Seizures of the International League Against Epilepsy (henceforth, International Classification of Epileptic Seizures). In 2001, the International League Against Epilepsy proposed a new classification of epileptic seizure types. This classification has not been accepted yet and is cumbersome in its present form for general use. We have elected to continue the use of the 1981 classification in this volume.

The International Classification of Epileptic Seizures is presented in Table 2-1. Seizures are first classified into two broad categories: (a) partial seizures (seizures beginning in a relatively small location in the brain), and (b) generalized seizures (seizures that are bilaterally symmetric and without local onset). Seizures are then further classified by the exact clinical and EEG manifestations of the seizure. The clinical and EEG manifestations of the principal types of epileptic seizures recognized by the International Classification of Epileptic Seizures are presented in this chapter.

I. PARTIAL (FOCAL, LOCAL) SEIZURES

A. Simple Partial (Focal) Seizures

1. Definitions

Simple partial seizures are caused by a focal cortical discharge that results in seizure symptoms appropriate to the function of the discharging area of brain, without impairment of consciousness. Simple partial seizures may consist of motor, sensory, autonomic, or psychic symptoms and signs. The same symptoms and signs may occur in both simple partial seizures and complex partial seizures (CPSs). The crucial distinction is that impairment of consciousness occurs in the latter but not in the former. *Impaired consciousness* is defined as the inability to respond normally to exogenous stimuli by virtue of altered awareness or responsiveness. *Responsiveness* refers to the ability of the patient to carry out simple commands or willed movements, and *awareness* refers to the patient's contact with and recall of events during the period in question.

2. Seizure Phenomena

Seizure manifestations are dependent on the region of the cortex in which they originate and its functions. Following the International Classification of Epileptic Seizures, the manifestations of simple partial seizures can be divided into four groups: (a) with motor signs, (b) with somatosensory or special sensory symptoms, (c) with autonomic symptoms or signs, and (d) with psychic symptoms.

**Table 2-1.   International classification
of epileptic seizures**

I. Partial (focal, local) seizures
   A. Simple partial seizures (consciousness not impaired)
      1. With motor signs
      2. With sensory symptoms
      3. With autonomic symptoms or signs
      4. With psychic symptoms
   B. Complex partial seizures (temporal lobe or psychomotor
      seizures; consciousness impaired)
      1. Simple partial onset, followed by impairment of
         consciousness
         a. With simple partial features (A.1–A.4), followed by
            impaired consciousness
         b. With automatisms
      2. With impairment of consciousness at onset
         a. With impairment of consciousness only
         b. With automatisms
   C. Partial seizures evolving to secondarily generalized
      seizures (tonic–clonic, tonic, or clonic)
      1. Simple partial seizures (A) evolving to generalized
         seizures
      2. Complex partial seizures (B) evolving to generalized
         seizures
      3. Simple partial seizures evolving to complex partial
         seizures, evolving to generalized seizures
II. Generalized seizures (convulsive or nonconvulsive)
   A. Absence (petit mal) seizures
   B. Myoclonic seizures
   C. Tonic seizures
   D. Atonic seizures
   E. Clonic seizures
   F. Tonic–clonic (grand mal) seizures
III. Unclassified epileptic seizures (caused by incomplete data)

From Commission on Classification and Terminology of the International
League Against Epilepsy. Proposal for revised clinical and electroencephalographic classification of epileptic seizures. *Epilepsia* 1981;22:489–501, modified with permission.

A. SIMPLE PARTIAL SEIZURES WITH MOTOR SIGNS.   These are
among the most frequently encountered varieties of simple partial seizure. The symptoms are, at least initially, always strictly
contralateral to the hemispheric focus and may represent the
expression of excitatory (positive–irritative) phenomena,
inhibitory (negative–suppressive or paralytic) phenomena, or a
combination of the two.

   The simplest form of simple partial seizure with motor signs
is clonus, which consists of rhythmic alternating contraction
and relaxation of muscle groups controlled by the precentral
gyrus. The episodes may be self-limited (clonic focal seizure),
recurrent (focal motor status epilepticus), or continuous

(epilepsia partialis continua). Spread of the discharge along contiguous areas of the precentral gyrus gives rise to the characteristic march of spreading involvement of muscle groups in jacksonian seizures. Transient paralytic phenomena (Todd paralysis) are a common postictal manifestation of an excitatory clonic seizure, especially if it is severe or repeated. With somatic inhibitory seizures, sensory loss or dysesthesia and weakness occur.

Versive seizures consist of conjugate eye movements and turning of the head to the same side. Parietal and temporal lobe seizures may produce homolateral or contralateral versive movements, and occipital seizures usually produce contralateral versive movements.

Postural seizures consist of asymmetric dystonic posturing of the limbs, which may be associated with vocalization or speech arrest.

Aphasic seizures consist primarily of speech arrest or inability to verbalize while consciousness is fully retained, or both. Aphemia (speech arrest), as well as vocalization (phonatory seizures), also may occur.

B. SIMPLE PARTIAL SEIZURES WITH SOMATOSENSORY OR SPECIAL SENSORY SYMPTOMS. Somatosensory seizures are usually described as "numbness," "tingling," "pins and needles," or "like a weak electric shock" and may arise from the postcentral (most often) or precentral areas. Less frequently, a sense of movement, desire to move, or inability to move is present. The initial somatosensory sensation may be the only manifestation of a seizure. The focal discharge may spread to the adjacent sensory cortex, producing a jacksonian march of sensory phenomena. The focal discharge also may spread to the adjacent motor cortex, producing motor symptoms.

Visual seizures beginning with simple visual symptoms are indicative of a focus in the occipital lobe. Visual simple partial seizures consisting of crude positive symptoms, such as flashes of lights or colors in the contralateral hemifield, are more frequently described than are negative symptoms, such as scotomas or hemianopia. Visual illusions (distortions of visual input) and hallucinations (perception of a stimulus not actually present) usually represent seizure phenomena arising from the posterior temporal area.

Auditory seizures arising near the cortex of Heschl region of the first temporal gyrus may produce simple auditory phenomena usually described as a "humming," "buzzing," or "hissing." More complex auditory illusions or hallucinations result from discharges arising in the auditory association areas of the temporal lobe.

Olfactory and gustatory seizures consist of olfactory and gustatory illusions or hallucinations, usually in the form of unpleasant odors and tastes.

Vertiginous seizures may consist only of a vague feeling of dizziness or light-headedness. Vertiginous sensations without alteration of consciousness are extremely frequent expressions of vestibular irritative phenomena (peripheral or central), although they have been described also as true epileptic manifestations of seizure foci in the middle or posterior portion of the first temporal gyrus (tornado epilepsy).

C. **SIMPLE PARTIAL SEIZURES WITH AUTONOMIC SYMPTOMS OR SIGNS.** Autonomic symptoms accompanying simple partial seizures may consist of epigastric sensations, flushing or pallor, sweating, pupil dilation, diaphoresis, piloerection, nausea, vomiting, borborygmi, or incontinence.

D. **SIMPLE PARTIAL SEIZURES WITH PSYCHIC SYMPTOMS.** Psychic symptoms of simple partial seizures may include dysphasia, dysmnesia, cognitive symptoms, affective symptoms, illusions, or structured hallucinations.

Dysphasic symptoms may take the form of speech arrest, vocalization, or palilalia (involuntary repetition of a syllable or phrase).

Dysmnesic symptoms, distortions of memory, may take the form of a temporal disorientation, a dreamy state, a flashback, the sensation that an experience has occurred before (*déja vu*, if visual; *déja entendu*, if auditory), or the sensation that a familiar sensation is new (*jamais vu*, if visual; *jamais entendu*, if auditory). Occasionally, a patient may experience a rapid recollection of episodes from the past (panoramic vision).

Cognitive symptoms may include dreamy states, distortions of time sense, and sensations of unreality, detachment, or depersonalization.

Affective symptoms may include fear, pleasure, displeasure, depression, rage, anger, irritability, elation, and eroticism. Some individuals may have inappropriate affective reactions to environmental stimuli, possibly because of misinterpretation of cues during the clouded consciousness of a seizure. Fear is the most frequent affective symptom and may be accompanied by objective signs of autonomic activity such as pupil dilation, pallor, flushing, piloerection, palpitation, and hypertension.

Unlike the affective symptoms of psychiatric disease, the symptoms of partial seizures occur in attacks lasting a few minutes, tend to be unprovoked by environmental stimuli, and usually abate rapidly. Less commonly, patients describe exhilaration, elation, serenity, satisfaction, and pleasure (ecstatic seizures, Dostoyevsky epilepsy). The enjoyable sensations may be similar to or different from sexual pleasure. Sexual pleasure during an aura may consist of either sexual arousal or orgasm. Violent affect and behavior during partial seizures are discussed later, in section **I.B.4.c**. Illusions are distorted perceptions in which objects are perceived as deformed. Polyopic illusions, such as monocular diplopia, macropsia, micropsia, and distortions of distance, may occur. Distortions of sound, including microacusia and macroacusia, may be experienced. Depersonalization, a feeling that the person is outside the body, may occur. The patient may experience altered perception of the size or weight of a limb.

Structural hallucinations are perceptions without corresponding external stimuli and may affect somatosensory, visual, auditory, olfactory, or gustatory senses. Seizures arising from primary receptive areas tend to give rather primitive hallucinations, whereas seizures arising from association areas tend to give more elaborate symptoms.

E. COMPLEX PARTIAL SEIZURES WITH SIMPLE PARTIAL ONSET. If a simple partial seizure arising in a circumscribed portion of one lobe spreads to involve larger portions of the brain, and if consciousness becomes impaired, the seizure is classified as a CPS with simple partial onset.

F. SIMPLE PARTIAL SEIZURES EVOLVING TO SECONDARILY GENERALIZED SEIZURES. Simple partial onset seizures may spread further and become secondarily generalized (tonic–clonic, tonic, or clonic).

3. Electroencephalographic Phenomena

A. INTERICTAL ELECTROENCEPHALOGRAM. Abnormal interictal EEGs are found in as many as 80% to 90% of patients with simple partial seizures when multiple EEGs (including long-term monitoring) are performed and all types of abnormalities are considered. Only 50% or fewer of individual routine interictal EEGs show an abnormality. Focal spike or sharp discharges, slowing, or suppression of normal background are the usual abnormalities. Focal EEG findings are absent in many patients for several reasons: (a) spikes are an intermittent phenomenon, (b) spikes or slow waves originating from small areas of cortex may be markedly attenuated at the scalp, and (c) spikes or slow waves may originate from cortical areas distant from the convexity and be unrecorded at the scalp. Additional routine recordings, sleep deprivation, and long-term EEG recording increase the yield of abnormal EEG findings in a patient with a normal initial EEG.

B. ICTAL ELECTROENCEPHALOGRAM. At the time of onset of clinical seizures, a majority of patients with focal seizures show a transformation in the scalp EEG from an interictal pattern to a sustained rhythmic pattern. The initial frequency of rhythmic ictal transformation (RIT) is most often in the range of 13 to 30 Hz but may be slower. The RIT shows a progressive increase in amplitude and a decrease in frequency as clinical seizures develop. Spread to adjacent areas of the brain is indicated by the development of RIT in those areas. Termination of rhythmic ictal activity may be associated with the gradual development of slow-wave and spike–slow-wave activity that gradually decreases in frequency and then gives way to postictal slowing, depression of voltage, or both. Rhythmic ictal activity can also subside abruptly. In the minority of cases that show no RIT, the interictal pattern of mixed sharp and slow activity (or normal background) persists without observable change during the clinical seizure.

4. Basic Mechanisms
See Chapter 1, section **VI**.

5. Differential Diagnosis
Simple partial seizures in adults must be differentiated from migraine, syncope, transient ischemic attacks, Ménière disease, and psychogenic seizures. In children, tics, chorea, and tremor sometimes cause diagnostic confusion. The differential diagnosis for epileptic seizures is discussed in Chapter 9.

6. Epilepsy Syndromes

The epilepsy syndromes are listed in Chapter 1, Table 1-2. Partial seizures usually occur as part of the following groups of syndromes: symptomatic and probably symptomatic focal epilepsies (see Chapter 3), idiopathic focal epilepsies of infancy and childhood (see Chapters 4, 5, and 6), familial (autosomal dominant) focal epilepsies (see Chapters 3, 4, and 5).

7. Etiology, Management, and Prognosis

Etiology, management, and prognosis are reviewed in Chapter 3.

B. Complex Partial Seizures (Psychomotor or Temporal Lobe Seizures)

1. Definitions

The central feature of CPSs is *impairment of consciousness*, which is defined as the inability to respond normally to exogenous stimuli by virtue of altered awareness or responsiveness. *Responsiveness* refers to the ability of the patient to carry out simple commands or willed movement, and *awareness* refers to the patient's contact with events during the period in question and its recall.

The period of impairment of consciousness may or may not be preceded by symptoms or signs of a simple partial seizure. No other manifestations may appear during the period of impaired consciousness, or automatisms (i.e., nonreflex actions performed "automatically," without conscious volition, and for which the patient has no recollection) may be present.

2. Seizure Phenomena

A. CLASSIFICATION.   The International Classification of Epileptic Seizures divides CPSs into four groups (Table 2-1): (a) CPSs with simple partial onset followed by impairment of consciousness only, (b) CPSs with simple partial onset followed by impaired consciousness and automatisms, (c) CPSs with impairment of consciousness at onset with impairment of consciousness only, and (d) CPSs with impairment of consciousness at onset with automatisms. Three major areas describe seizure phenomena during CPSs: (a) impairment of consciousness, (b) types of simple partial onset, and (c) automatisms.

B. IMPAIRMENT OF CONSCIOUSNESS.   During the period of impaired consciousness, a patient may look vacant or frightened. Although sometimes able to recount vague sensations, these patients do not realize that anything more has occurred.

C. TYPES OF SIMPLE PARTIAL ONSET.   Simple partial onset with motor signs, with somatosensory or special sensory symptoms, with autonomic symptoms or signs, and with psychic symptoms are discussed earlier, in sections **I.A.2.a–d**. Psychic symptoms can occur without impairment of consciousness as part of a simple partial seizure. More commonly, psychic symptoms occur in association with impaired consciousness as part of a CPS. The frequent association of psychic symptoms and motor automatisms with CPSs is responsible for the formerly used term *psychomotor seizure*.

D. AUTOMATISMS. An automatism is a more- or less-coordinated, involuntary motor activity occurring during the state of clouding of consciousness, either in the course of or after an epileptic seizure, usually followed by amnesia of the event. The automatism may be simply a continuation of an activity that was going on when the seizure occurred, or it may be a new activity developed in association with the ictal impairment of consciousness. Usually, the activity is commonplace, often provoked by the subject's environment or by sensations during the seizure; fragmentary, primitive, infantile, or antisocial behavior is occasionally seen. Automatisms can be detected in more than 90% of CPSs recorded on videotape.

Five types of phenomena may occur during an automatism: alimentary, mimetic, gestural, ambulatory, and verbal. Alimentary phenomena include automatic chewing movements, increased salivation, and borborygmus. Mimetic phenomena include movements of the face resulting in expressions of fear, bewilderment, discomfort, or vacant tranquility; laughing (gelastic seizures); and crying (lacrimonic seizures). Gestural phenomena include repetitive movements of the hands and fingers and sexual gestures. Ambulatory phenomena include wandering or running (cursive seizures), and the patient may unknowingly run out into traffic or into obstacles. Verbal phenomena include short phrases, expletives, or swearing, commonly repeated in an automatic fashion. The spontaneously vocalized words may reflect a previous experience.

E. DROP ATTACKS. Sudden loss of consciousness, accompanied by loss of postural tone and falls, may occur during a CPS. Such patients usually have had seizures for several years before the falls begin, suggesting an increasing rate of spread over time.

F. COMPOUND FORMS OF COMPLEX PARTIAL SEIZURES. Most CPSs exhibit a combination of the symptoms listed earlier. Delgado-Escueta et al. (2) found that most CPSs were compound forms of two types.

During the early phase of a type I attack, the patient was essentially motionless and initially unresponsive to superficial and deep pain. After approximately 10 seconds, a second phase of 10- to 60-second duration was observed. During this time, the patient remained unresponsive and showed automatisms such as repeated chewing, blinking, and swallowing. During the third and longest phase of a type I seizure (0.5 to 12.0 minutes), impairment of consciousness of a less profound nature was observed. Automatisms could be interrupted, and the patient sometimes reacted to environmental cues. This phase is best described as a *cloudy state*.

Type II attacks consisted of reactive automatisms during impaired consciousness. A motionless, staring state was not observed, although stereotyped movements occurred. Automatisms occurring during the cloudy states of type II attacks and during the third phase of type I attacks were considered reactive, because the behavior appeared purposeful. Amnesia for the entire attack ensued. Motor responses were coordinated and were sufficient to carry out the patient's intended actions; appropriate and inappropriate responses were both seen.

G. COMPLEX PARTIAL SEIZURES EVOLVING TO GENERALIZED SEIZURES.
The seizure discharges of a CPS may become secondarily generalized, producing a generalized seizure (tonic–clonic, tonic, or clonic; see section **I.C**, later).

H. COMPLEX PARTIAL SEIZURES STATUS EPILEPTICUS. See Chapter 12.

3. Electroencephalographic Phenomena

A. INTERICTAL. Interictal manifestations of CPSs include focal spikes, sharp waves, and slowing. These abnormalities most often are found in the anterior temporal region, but many occur in other areas. Abnormalities may be localized or bilateral (synchronous or asynchronous). Discharges arising from the mesial surface of the frontal lobe may appear as generalized discharges on surface EEG.

B. ICTAL ELECTROENCEPHALOGRAM. During a clinical CPS, any of the following can be recorded from scalp EEG electrodes: (a) sustained rhythm of spikes or sharp waves and rhythmic slowing, (b) attenuation of amplitude (suppression), (c) rhythmic slow waves; (d) 10- to 30-Hz fast activity, (e) spike–wave complexes, (f) other changes or variants of these five, or (g) no change (10% to 30% of patients). These patterns may be focal, lateralized, bilateral, or diffuse.

C. POSTICTAL ELECTROENCEPHALOGRAM. The postictal EEG usually consists of generalized or localized slow activity. Localized postictal slowing provides information about lateralization or localization of the site of origin of the CPS in approximately 40% of recordings.

D. SPECIAL ELECTROENCEPHALOGRAPHIC TECHNIQUES. Approximately 50% of routine EEGs performed on patients with CPSs are abnormal. This yield can be increased to 90% by using repeated studies, sleep deprivation (allowing 4 hours or less sleep the night before study), additional temporal electrodes (usually T1 and T2; alternatively, sphenoidal electrodes), and long-term EEG monitoring. When CPSs are suspected clinically and a routine EEG is normal, a sleep-deprived EEG with temporal leads should be ordered. If this is normal, long-term EEG monitoring should be considered.

4. Neurobehavioral Aspects of Complex Partial Seizures

Patients with CPSs often have (a) damage to limbic structures (with resulting cognitive and behavioral problems), (b) seizures involving limbic structures, and (c) psychosocial difficulties caused by (a) and (b). Thus, a number of complex neurobehavioral issues are associated with CPSs.

A. EMOTIONAL ACTIVATION OF COMPLEX PARTIAL SEIZURES.
Patients with CPSs are vulnerable to emotional activation of seizure activity because the anatomic structures involved during CPSs are those that subserve normal emotional responses. Conversely, reducing emotional stress (which may happen during hospitalization) may decrease the occurrence of CPSs.

B. INTERICTAL PERSONALITY. Several authors have described "an interictal personality" of patients with CPSs, characterized by such features as "stickiness," humorlessness, dependence, obsessionalism, circumstantiality, philosophic interests, religiosity, hypermoralism, anger, personalized significance attached to trivial events, hypergraphia, altered sexual interest (hyposexuality or hypersexuality), and emotionality.

Although some patients with CPSs do exhibit these traits, it is important to remember that many individuals without CPS have similar personalities. More studies are needed, however, to determine the prevalence of these traits in nonselected patients, their specificity for CPSs, and the pathophysiology and psychodynamics of the traits. Pharmacologic or surgical control of seizures does not alter these personality traits.

C. VIOLENT BEHAVIOR.   Attempts to restrain a patient who has clouded sensorium during or after a tonic–clonic seizure or CPSs may result in defensive and aggressive behavior. Well-organized, unprovoked, directed acts of violence are rarely a manifestation of epilepsy, however. Episodic dyscontrol syndrome (rage attacks) is not a form of CPS (see Chapter 9).

D. MEMORY LOSS.   Poor memory and memory loss are frequent complaints of the patient with CPSs. Short-term memory loss and subjective difficulty with memory have been attributed to hippocampal dysfunction in temporal lobe epilepsy. A major abnormality found on formal psychometric testing is poor performance on confrontation-naming tests in patients with CPSs and a left-temporal EEG focus. This anomia, in turn, may result in impairment on many verbal subtests of intelligence and memory.

E. PSYCHOSIS.   A psychosis resembling paranoid schizophrenia has been noted in some patients with CPSs. Some have reported, and some have denied, that the psychosis of CPSs can be differentiated from schizophrenia because patients with CPSs retain more affect and are less socially isolated than are patients with schizophrenia.

F. EPISODES OF AIMLESS WANDERING (PORIOMANIA).   Patients with CPSs may experience prolonged episodes of aimless wandering followed by retrograde amnesia for this behavior. This may represent a prolonged postictal automatism and has been reported to respond to antiepileptic medication.

5. Basic Mechanisms
See Chapter 1, section **VI**.

6. Differential Diagnosis
In adults, CPSs must be differentiated from absence seizures, syncope, transient ischemic attacks, episodic dyscontrol syndrome, psychosis, Ménière disease, and psychogenic seizures. In children, night terrors and sleepwalking must also be considered. These elements of the differential diagnosis are discussed in Chapter 9.

7. Epilepsy Syndromes
The epilepsy syndromes are listed in Chapter 1, Table 1-2. Partial seizures usually occur as part of the following groups of syndromes: symptomatic and probably symptomatic focal epilepsies (see Chapter 3); idiopathic focal epilepsies of infancy and childhood (see Chapters 4, 5, and 6); and familial (autosomal dominant) focal epilepsies (see Chapters 3, 4, and 5).

C. Partial Seizures Evolving to Secondarily Generalized (Tonic–Clonic, Grand Mal) Seizures

1. Definitions

Tonic–clonic seizures consist of an initial increase in tone of certain muscles (tonic phase) followed by bilateral symmetric jerking of the extremities (clonic phase).

Secondarily generalized tonic–clonic seizures begin with focal seizure activity and may be accompanied by clinical or EEG evidence of simple complex seizures, CPSs, or both.

Tonic–clonic seizures most often occur as part of symptomatic focal epilepsies. However, tonic–clonic seizures may occur as part of many other adult epilepsy syndromes. Regardless of epilepsy syndrome, tonic–clonic seizures share a number of common features, reviewed in this section. Special features of tonic–clonic seizures associated with symptomatic focal epilepsies are reviewed in this section. Special features of tonic–clonic seizures associated with other specific epilepsy syndromes are reviewed with the specific epilepsy syndrome in Chapters 3 through 8.

2. Seizure Phenomena

A. AURA.   Secondarily generalized tonic–clonic seizures may begin with signs or symptoms of focal seizure phenomena appropriate to the focus of origin (simple partial seizure phenomena, CPS phenomena, or both). However, most patients cannot recall an aura.

B. TONIC PHASE.   The tonic phase usually consists of a brief phase in flexion, followed by a longer phase in extension. Consciousness is lost during the tonic phase. The flexion phase usually begins in the face (eyes open, ocular globes rotated upward, mouth held rigidly open); neck (held rigid in semiflexion); and trunk (chest bent forward on pelvis). The flexion phase then spreads to the extremities, involving the arms more than the legs and the proximal muscles more than the distal muscles. The arms are elevated, adducted, and externally rotated, and the legs and thighs are flexed, adducted, and externally rotated.

The extension phase begins in the axial musculature with extension of the back and neck. The mouth snaps shut (the tongue may be bitten). The thoracic and abdominal muscles then contract, sometimes producing a "tonic cry" as air is forced over the vocal cords. The arms are lowered and adducted. The forearm may remain flexed or may be extended and pronated. Fingers may be clenched on the extended wrists or extended on flexed wrists. The legs are extended, adducted, and externally rotated.

During the period of transition from the tonic to the clonic phase (vibratory tonic period), tetanus becomes less complete. Tonic rigidity is replaced by a fine tremor, which increases in amplitude and decreases in frequency from 8 to 4 Hz. The tremor is caused by intermittent decreases in tone. It begins in the extremities and spreads proximally.

C. CLONIC PHASE.   During the clonic phase, muscle relaxation completely interrupts tonic contraction. The rhythmic return of muscle tone causes the appearance of rhythmic jerks, which become further and further apart until the seizure ends. The tongue may be bitten during clonic masseter movements. Each jerk may be accompanied by a cry.

D. AUTONOMIC PHENOMENA. Autonomic phenomena begin in the preictal phase, are maximal at the end of the tonic phase, and decrease abruptly at the onset of the clonic phase. Autonomic phenomena that may be observed during a tonic–clonic seizure include increased blood pressure, increased heart rate, increased bladder pressure, increased sphincter tone, flushing, cyanosis, piloerection, perspiration, increased salivation, and increased bronchial secretion.

Apnea begins with violent expiration at the onset of the tonic phase and persists during the tonic and clonic phases (except for violent, forced expirations with clonic jerks), and often into the early postictal period. Apnea cannot be explained entirely on the basis of muscular contractions; a central mechanism is probably involved in maintaining it.

E. IMMEDIATE POSTICTAL PHASE. Complete muscular relaxation does not occur immediately in the postictal phase. About 5 seconds after the last clonic jerk, a new period of tonic contraction begins, lasting from several seconds to 4 minutes. Muscle tone is most increased in the cephalic muscles, and the tongue may be bitten. The trunk and arms may be extended but not as violently as during the tonic phase.

Between the last clonic jerk and the immediate postictal tonic phase, the bladder sphincter muscles relax; at this point, incontinence may occur.

Respirations return during the immediate postictal phase. The combination of a clenched jaw and increased secretions results in partial obstruction of respiration. Respirations are stertorous, and accessory muscles of respiration are activated. Blood pressure and skin resistance return to normal, but tachycardia persists. Cyanosis changes to pallor. Loss of consciousness remains complete, and pupillary and cutaneous reflexes are absent. Deep tendon reflexes are variably modified.

F. LATER POSTICTAL PHASE. In the later postictal phase, flaccidity is more or less complete. The cardiac rate returns to normal. Deep tendon reflexes are usually diminished, and the plantar response is sometimes extensor. The patient may awaken by passing through successive stages of coma, confusional state, and drowsiness or may pass directly into sleep without awakening.

G. DURATION OF PHASES. The average durations of the various phases of a tonic–clonic seizure are as follows: tonic phase, 10 to 30 seconds; clonic phase, 30 to 50 seconds; immediate postictal phase, 1 to 5 minutes; later postictal phase, 2 to 10 minutes; total, 5 to 15 minutes. Individual phase duration and clinical expression are highly variable in partial seizures secondarily generalized, suggesting multiple routes of spread.

H. TONIC–CLONIC STATUS EPILEPTICUS. See Chapter 12.

3. Complications

The possible complications of tonic–clonic seizures are summarized here in order of likelihood. Tonic–clonic status epilepticus increases the risk of all these complications.

A. ORAL TRAUMA. The tongue, lip, or cheek may be macerated.

B. HEAD TRAUMA. Skull fractures, contusions, and epidural or subdural hematomas may result from head injury caused by falls or clonic activity.

C. STRESS FRACTURES. Compression fractures of thoracic or lumbar vertebrae may occur; they are often asymptomatic and more common in the elderly.

D. ASPIRATION PNEUMONIA. Aspiration of secretions or regurgitated stomach contents may occur when the airway's normal protective reflexes are inhibited postictally; they may be life-threatening.

E. POSTICTAL PULMONARY EDEMA. Postictal pulmonary edema is a rare complication (immediate or delayed) manifested by dyspnea, cough, bloodstained sputum, and abnormal chest radiograph. This complication usually requires only oxygen therapy and must be differentiated from aspiration pneumonia.

4. Electroencephalographic Phenomena

A. INTERICTAL PHASE. Focal spikes, sharp waves, or slowing may be present during the interictal phase (see simple partial seizures and CPSs, sections **I.A.3** and **I.B.3** earlier).

B. INITIAL PHASE. During the initial ictal phase of a secondarily generalized tonic–clonic seizure, the EEG may show focal attenuation, sharp waves, or slow activity.

C. TONIC PHASE. The tonic phase begins with a 1- to 3-second period of EEG flattening (desynchronization) or with low-voltage fast activity. Then surface negative waves at about 10 Hz appear and increase rapidly in amplitude (epileptic recruiting rhythm). After approximately 10 seconds, the recruiting rhythm is combined with an apparently separate rhythm of slow waves, increasing in amplitude and decreasing in frequency from 3 to 1 Hz. The slow rhythm becomes progressively more prominent, and the recruiting rhythm becomes progressively less prominent, until the recruiting rhythm appears only as brief bursts of rapid activity between surface-negative slow waves.

D. CLONIC PHASE. During the clonic phase, bursts of 10-Hz recruiting rhythm alternate with slow waves. Bursts of recruiting rhythm are associated with generalized jerks, and slow waves are associated with relaxation. The slow waves become slower, and the bursts of recruiting rhythm become farther apart.

E. POSTICTAL PHASE. Typically, the EEG is isoelectric for a few seconds to 1 minute after the last clonic jerk (cortical exhaustion). Then low-voltage, very slow activity appears. The EEG progressively picks up in voltage and frequency.

5. Basic Mechanisms
See Chapter 1, section **VI**.

6. Differential Diagnosis
Partial seizures evolving to secondarily generalized seizures occurring as part of symptomatic focal epilepsies must be differentiated from primarily generalized tonic–clonic seizures occurring as part of generalized/idiopathic epilepsies. Secondarily

generalized seizures are suggested by (a) evidence of structural brain damage (neurologic examination, imaging studies); (b) onset with symptoms or signs suggesting simple partial seizure, CPS, or both; and (c) focal sharp or slow activity on interictal EEG. Primarily generalized seizures are suggested by (a) absence of evidence of structural brain damage, (b) family history of seizures, (c) coexisting myoclonic or absence seizures, (d) occurrence shortly after awakening, (e) bilateral myoclonic jerks at seizure onset, and (f) generalized spike–wave or polyspike wave on interictal EEG.

Tonic–clonic seizures must also be distinguished from syncope and psychogenic seizures in patients of all ages. In children, tonic–clonic seizures must be distinguished from breath-holding spells and prolonged QT syndrome. The differential diagnosis for tonic–clonic seizures in children is discussed in Chapter 9.

7. Epilepsy Syndromes

The epilepsy syndromes are listed in Chapter 1, Table 1-2. Partial seizures usually occur as part of the following groups of syndromes: symptomatic and probably symptomatic focal epilepsies (see Chapter 3); idiopathic focal epilepsies of infancy and childhood (see Chapters 4, 5, and 6); and familial (autosomal dominant) focal epilepsies (see Chapters 3, 4, and 5).

8. Etiology, Management, and Prognosis

These topics are reviewed in Chapter 3, sections I.E–G.

II. GENERALIZED SEIZURES (CONVULSIVE OR NONCONVULSIVE)

A. Absence (Petit Mal) Seizures

1. Definitions

Absence seizures are generalized seizures, indicating bihemispheric, initial involvement clinically and on EEG. They have a rapid onset and offset and most frequently are characterized by a change in facial expression, motionless blank staring, and automatisms. Absence seizures are divided into typical and atypical (Table 2-2). Many children with absence seizures can be further categorized as having a characteristic epileptic syndrome.

Table 2-2. Classification of absence seizures

  I. Typical absence seizures
    A. Simple: impairment of consciousness only
    B. Complex
       1. With mild clonic components
       2. With changes in tone
       3. With automatisms
       4. With autonomic components
 II. Atypical absence seizures
III. Absence status epilepticus

2. Seizure Phenomena

A. TYPICAL ABSENCE SEIZURES. Although typical absence seizures may occur at any age, they rarely start before the age of 2 years or after the teenage years. The hallmark of the typical absence seizure is the suppression of mental function, usually to the point of complete abolition of awareness, responsiveness, and memory. The seizures start abruptly, without an aura, and typically last from a few seconds to half a minute, although, at times, they last more than 1 minute. Ongoing activity is suddenly interrupted; the child changes facial expression and becomes transfixed (like a statue). In a simple typical absence seizure, the child stares with a motionless, distant appearance. At the end of the seizure, the child usually returns to the gesture, sentence, or other activity that the seizure interrupted. Postictal fatigue never occurs, although the child may be momentarily confused by the "time loss." This "time loss" may serve as a clue to the child that a seizure occurred, even though complete amnesia for events during the seizure may be experienced.

Maximal impairment of responsiveness usually occurs during the first few seconds of an absence seizure, regardless of whether the total duration of the seizure is brief or long. At times, the suspension of mental function is less complete, especially at the end of certain longer attacks. At this time, mild confusion without complete loss of awareness may occur. When this happens, the child may be able to continue simple and automatic behavior. At times, the impairment of consciousness is so slight that it passes unnoticed by observers and may be detected only during EEG monitoring.

Simple absence seizures are relatively rare. The majority of typical absence seizures are complex, consisting of clonic or myoclonic activity, automatisms, and changes in postural tone. Automatisms occur frequently in absence seizures. Automatic behavior may consist of licking the lips, chewing, grimacing, scratching, or fumbling with the clothes. The longer the seizure, the more likely that automatisms will occur. More-complex activity, such as dealing cards or moving chess pieces, may occur if the activity is ongoing at the onset of the seizure. Although speech may continue to occur during an absence seizure, the speed usually slows.

B. ATYPICAL ABSENCE SEIZURES. Atypical absences are those seizures in which the onset, the cessation, or both are not as abrupt as in typical absences, and in which changes in tone are more pronounced than in typical absences. Atypical absences, like typical absences, may be associated with automatisms, clonic components, and autonomic components, as well as changes in tone. However, automatisms are not as frequently seen in atypical absences as in typical absences. Atypical absence seizures frequently have a longer duration than typical absences, sometimes lasting several minutes.

C. ABSENCE STATUS EPILEPTICUS. This topic is reviewed in Chapter 12.

3. Electroencephalographic Phenomena

A hallmark of absence seizures is the sudden onset of either generalized symmetric spike–wave or multiple spike-and-slow-wave complexes. In typical absence seizures, the spike-and-wave complexes usually occur at a frequency of 3 Hz (range, 2.5 to 3.5 Hz; Fig. 2-1. At times, the discharge may begin with frontal spikes, occurring either unilaterally or bilaterally. Only when the spikes are persistently focal and precede the generalized discharge by several seconds should the diagnosis of a partial seizure with secondary generalization be considered. Likewise, after a generalized discharge, 1 or 2 seconds of rhythmic frontal delta activity without spikes may occur.

Hyperventilation is a potent activator of typical absence seizures. Failure to induce an absence seizure with several trials of hyperventilation of 3 to 5 minutes' duration in an untreated patient makes the diagnosis of absence seizures unlikely. Photic stimulation may also induce absence seizures, although the frequency for activation is not as high as with hyperventilation.

Focal spikes, particularly in the frontal region, or bilateral frontal spike-and-wave discharges are commonly seen in children with absence seizures. It has been suggested that these represent remnants of generalized discharges that did not fully propagate to the surface of the brain.

Unlike the usual 3-Hz spike-and-wave discharges that occur in typical absence seizures, slow spike-and-wave discharges occurring at 1.5 to 2.5 Hz are more characteristic of atypical absence seizures (Fig. 2-2). The interictal EEG is usually abnormal in patients with atypical absences.

4. Basic Mechanisms

The pathophysiology of absence seizures is discussed in Chapter 1, section **VI**.

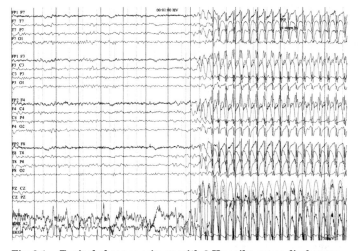

Fig. 2-1. Typical absence seizure with 3-Hz spike–wave discharges. Seizure occurred during hyperventilation. During the seizure, the child stops hyperventilating.

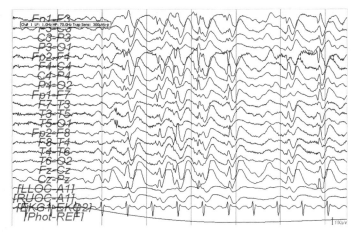

Fig. 2-2. Slow spike–wave discharges in a child with Lennox–Gastaut syndrome.

5. Differential Diagnosis

Absence seizures must be differentiated from CPSs and daydreaming. The differential diagnosis of absence seizures from CPSs is discussed in Chapter 9.

Daydreaming is associated with boredom, can be "broken" with stimulation, and is not associated with motor activity. Children with autistic spectrum disorder often have episodes in which they withdraw from ongoing activities and stare vacantly. However, automatisms typically do not occur during these seizure-like behaviors. Absence seizures, however, can sometimes be terminated with stimulation and tend to increase during periods of relaxation and tiredness. A normal EEG that includes several trials of 3 to 5 minutes of hyperventilation, however, virtually rules out absence seizures.

6. Epilepsy Types and Epilepsy Syndrome

The epilepsy syndromes are listed in Chapter 1, Table 1-2. Typical absence seizures usually occur as part of the following syndromes: childhood absence epilepsy, juvenile absence epilepsy, juvenile myoclonic epilepsy syndrome, and epilepsy with myoclonic absences (see Chapters 6 and 7). Atypical absence seizures occur as part of the Lennox–Gastaut syndrome (see Chapter 6).

7. Etiology

The lack of structural pathology and the age-specific window observed in most patients with typical absence seizures implicate a hereditary etiology. Patients with atypical absence seizures have a higher likelihood of acquired disease. Often, patients with atypical absence seizures will have the Lennox–Gastaut syndrome, which is discussed in Chapter 6.

8. Management and Prognosis

See Chapters 6 and 7.

B. Myoclonic Seizures

1. Definition

Myoclonic seizures are characterized by sudden, brief (less than 350 μsec), shocklike contractions that may be generalized or confined to the face and trunk, or to one or more extremities, or even to individual muscles or groups of muscles. Myoclonic seizures result in short bursts of synchronized electromyographic (EMG) activity, which often involves simultaneous activation of agonist and antagonist muscles. The contractions of muscles are quicker than the contractions of clonic seizures.

2. Seizure Phenomena

Any group of muscles can be involved in a myoclonic seizure. Myoclonic seizures may be dramatic, causing the patient to fall to the ground, or quite subtle, resembling tremors. Because of the brevity of the seizures, determining whether consciousness is impaired is impossible.

Although myoclonic seizures can sometimes be the only seizure type present, they often occur in combination with other seizure types.

3. Electroencephalographic Phenomena

Myoclonic seizures are typically associated with generalized spike-and-wave or multiple spike-and-wave discharges on the EEG. In early myoclonic epileptic encephalopathy, the EEG demonstrates a burst-suppression pattern.

Myoclonic jerks may be correlated with bursts of generalized epileptiform discharges. However, the link between the EEG discharges and myoclonic jerks recorded by using EMG techniques, the so-called EEG–EMG dissociation, may be obvious. However, back-averaging of EEG at the time of the EMG discharge may demonstrate a time link between the two events. Myoclonic seizures are frequently associated with enhanced photosensitivity.

4. Differential Diagnosis

Myoclonic jerks are so brief that they may be missed by parents and physicians. Once they are seen, diagnosis is usually not difficult. Like simple partial seizures, myoclonic seizures may occasionally be confused with tics. Tics are repetitive, patterned motor activity, often involving multiple groups. Unlike seizures, tics can be voluntarily suppressed. Shuddering attacks are common in toddlers and consist of pronounced shivering. Typically, the child keeps his arms flexed and his shoulders adducted. The episodes last from seconds to minutes, and typically occur when the child is excited. Usually, both tics and shuddering attacks can be differentiated from simple partial seizures by clinical criteria. However, in cases in which the diagnosis is in doubt, an EEG can be useful. In both tics and shuddering attacks, the EEG is normal.

5. Etiology

Myoclonic seizures can be seen in both acquired and familial disorders. Virtually any etiologic agent that leads to brain damage can be associated with myoclonic seizures. Therefore, myoclonic seizures are a part of many epilepsy types and many epilepsy syndromes.

6. Epilepsy Syndromes

The epilepsy syndromes are listed in Chapter 1, Table 1-2. Myoclonic seizures occur at all ages, from neonates to the elderly. Myoclonic seizures may be part of the following syndrome groups: idiopathic generalized, epileptic encephalopathies, and progressive myoclonus epilepsies. See Chapters 4 to 7, Tables 4-1, 5-1, 6-1, and 7-1.

7. Management and Prognosis

See Chapters 3 through 7.

C. Tonic and Atonic Seizures

1. Definitions

Tonic seizures are brief seizures consisting of the sudden onset of increased tone in the extensor muscles. If standing, the patient typically falls to the ground. The duration of these seizures is longer than myoclonic seizures. The EMG activity is dramatically increased in tonic seizures. Conversely, atonic seizures consist of the sudden loss of muscle tone. The loss of muscle tone may be confined to a group of muscles, such as the neck, resulting in a head drop, or it may involve all trunk muscles, leading to a fall to the ground.

2. Seizure Phenomena

Tonic seizures frequently begin with a tonic contraction of the neck muscles, leading to fixation of the head in an erect position, widely opened eyes, and jaw clenching or mouth opening. Contraction of the respiratory and abdominal muscles often follows and may lead to a high-pitched cry and brief periods of apnea. The tonic contractions may extend to the proximal musculature of the upper limbs, elevating the shoulders and abducting the arms. Asymmetric tonic seizures vary, from a slight rotation of the head to a tonic contraction of all the musculature of one side of the body. Occasionally, tonic seizures terminate with a clonic phase. Eyelid retraction, staring, mydriasis, and apnea are commonly associated with the motor activity and may be the most prominent features. The seizures may cause falls and injury.

Tonic seizures are typically activated by sleep and may occur repetitively throughout the night. They are much more frequent during non–rapid-eye-movement sleep than during wakefulness and usually do not occur during rapid-eye-movement sleep. During tonic seizures, the patient is unconscious, although arousal from light sleep may occur. Because these seizures are often very brief, they frequently go undetected. Tonic seizures are usually brief, lasting from a few seconds to 1 minute, with an average duration of about 10 seconds. In seizures lasting longer than a few seconds, impairment of consciousness is usually apparent. Postictal impairment with confusion, tiredness, and headache is common. The degree of postictal impairment is usually related to the duration of the seizure.

Atonic seizures begin suddenly and without warning and cause the patient, if standing, to fall quickly to the floor. Because total lack of tone may occur, the patient has no means of self-protection, and injuries often occur. The attack may be fragmentary and lead to dropping of the head with slackening of the jaw, or dropping of a limb. In atonic seizures, a brief loss of EMG activity should occur. Consciousness is impaired during the fall, although the patient may regain alertness immediately on hitting the floor.

Tonic and atonic seizures can occur in patients of all ages. However, they most often begin during childhood, as part of one of several epilepsy syndromes listed in section **II.C.6**.

3. Electroencephalographic Phenomena

The interictal EEG of patients with tonic seizures is usually quite abnormal, consisting of slowing of the background, with multifocal spikes, sharp waves, and bursts of irregular spike-and-wave activity. The EEG ictal manifestations of tonic seizures usually consist of bilateral synchronous spikes of 10 to 25 Hz of medium to high voltage, with a frontal accentuation (Fig. 2-3). Simple flattening or desynchronization may also occur. Occasionally, multiple spike-and-wave or diffuse, slow activity may occur during a tonic seizure.

Atonic seizures are usually associated with rhythmic spike-and-wave complexes varying from slow (1 to 2 Hz) to more

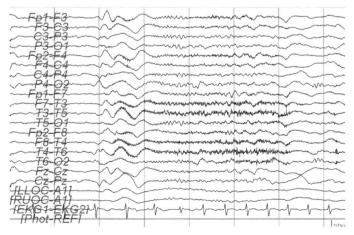

Fig. 2-3.   Generalized burst of rapid spikes in a patient with tonic seizures.

rapid, irregular spike-and-wave or multiple spike-and-wave activity.

4. Differential Diagnosis

Tonic seizures are usually not difficult to diagnose. Sometimes children with very severe encephalopathies have episodes of opisthotonic posturing that may resemble tonic seizures. Recording an episode usually helps distinguish the two events; tonic seizures are associated with spike–wave discharges or a discharge of rapid spikes, whereas no epileptiform discharges should be seen during opisthotonic posturing.

Spasmodic torticollis consists of episodes of head tilting that last from hours to days. During the episodes, the child is irritable but retains consciousness. Often a history of torticollis or migraine is found in the family. The EEG is normal in spasmodic torticollis.

Paroxysmal choreoathetosis is a rare, usually familial, disorder characterized by episodic attacks of severe dystonia, choreoathetosis, or both. Two types have been described: paroxysmal dystonic choreoathetosis of Mount and Reback, and paroxysmal kinesigenic choreoathetosis. In paroxysmal dystonic choreoathetosis, the patient has a sudden onset of severe, often painful, dystonia that may affect the arms, legs, or trunk and speech. Consciousness is not impaired during the attacks, which last from minutes to hours and are often precipitated by alcohol, caffeine, excitement, stress, or fatigue. The disorder is inherited through an autosomal-dominant pattern. Paroxysmal kinesigenic choreoathetosis is characterized by the sudden assumption of dystonic posturing or choreoathetosis. The kinesigenic attacks are usually shorter in duration than the dystonic form and are frequently induced by sudden movements or a startle. These attacks can occur hundreds of times daily.

Spasmus nutans is a disorder occurring in toddlers that is characterized by head tilt, head nodding, and nystagmus, which is often asymmetric. The head nodding may be confused with atonic seizures. Spasmus nutans is usually a self-limiting condition, disappearing after a period of 4 months to several years.

5. Etiology

Virtually any disorder that can lead to brain damage may result in tonic and atonic seizures. Common etiologies include hypoxic–ischemic encephalopathy, head injuries, encephalitis, strokes, congenital brain anomalies, and metabolic disturbances.

6. Epilepsy Syndromes

The epilepsy syndromes are listed Chapter 1, Table 1-2. Tonic and atonic seizures most often occur as part of the Lennox–Gastaut syndrome (see Chapter 6). Tonic seizures also may occur as part of neonatal seizures (see Chapter 4) or febrile convulsions (see Chapter 8). Atonic seizures also may occur as part of myoclonic–akinetic epilepsy syndrome (see Chapter 6). Finally, a form of partial seizure exists in which loss of tone plays a prominent role.

7. Management and Prognosis

See Chapters 4, 6, and 8.

D. Clonic Seizures

Clonic seizures occur almost exclusively in neonates and young children. The attack begins with loss or impairment of consciousness, associated with sudden hypotonia or a brief, generalized tonic spasm. This is followed by 1 minute to several minutes of bilateral jerks, which are often asymmetric and may predominate in one limb. During the attack, great variability may be seen in the amplitude, frequency, and spatial distribution of these jerks from moment to moment. In other children, particularly those aged 1 to 3 years, the jerks remain bilateral and synchronous throughout the attack. Postictally, recovery may be rapid, or a prolonged period of confusion or coma may occur.

E. Tonic–Clonic (Grand Mal) Seizures

1. Definitions, Seizure Phenomena, Electroencephalographic Phenomena, and Differential Diagnosis

The tonic–clonic seizures associated with generalized seizures are similar in most clinical and EEG respects to tonic–clonic seizures associated with partial seizures. The differences in these two seizure types are reviewed earlier, in section **I.C.6**.

2. Epilepsy Types and Epilepsy Syndromes

The epilepsy groups and epilepsy syndromes are listed in Chapter 1, Table 1-2. Generalized-onset tonic–clonic seizures may occur as part of the following epilepsy groups: generalized/idiopathic, reflex, and seizures not necessarily requiring a diagnosis of epilepsy.

3. Management and Prognosis

General management of tonic–clonic seizures is reviewed in Chapter 3. Prognosis of specific syndromes containing tonic–clonic seizures is reviewed in Chapters 3, 5, 6, and 7.

REFERENCES

1. Commission on Classification and Terminology of the International League Against Epilepsy. Proposal for revised clinical and electroencephalographic classification of epileptic seizures. *Epilepsia* 1981;22:489–501.
2. Delgado-Escueta AV, Bascal FE, Treiman D. Complex partial seizures on closed-circuit television and EEG: a study of 691 attacks on 79 patients. *Ann Neurol* 1982;11:292–300.
3. Engel J. A proposed diagnostic scheme for people with epileptic seizures and with epilepsy: report of the International League Against Epilepsy Task Force on Classification and Terminology. *Epilepsia* 2001;42:1212–1218.
4. Gambardella A, Reutens DC, Anderman F, et al. Late-onset drop attacks in temporal lobe epilepsy: a reevaluation of the concept of temporal lobe syncope. *Neurology* 1994;44:1074–1078.
5. Gastaut H. Generalized convulsive seizures without local onset. In: Vinken PJ, Bruyn GW, eds. *Handbook of clinical neurology*. Vol 15: *The epilepsies*. Amsterdam: Elsevier, 1974:107–129.
6. Gastaut H. Generalized nonconvulsive seizures without local onset. In: Vinken PJ, Bruyn GW, eds. *Handbook of clinical neu-*

rology. Vol 15: *The epilepsies*. Amsterdam: Elsevier, 1974: 130–144.

7. Holmes GL. Myoclonic, tonic, and atonic seizures in children. *J Epilepsy* 1988;1:173–195.

8. Paolicchi JM. The spectrum of nonepileptic events in children. *Epilepsia* 2002;43(suppl 3):60–64.

9. Penry JK, Porter RJ, Dreifuss FE. Simultaneous recording of absence seizures with videotape and electroencephalography: a study of 374 seizures in 48 patients. *Brain* 1975;98:427–447.

10. Theodore WH, Porter RJ, Albert P, et al. The secondarily generalized tonic-clonic seizure: a videotape analysis. *Neurology* 1994;44:1403–1407.

11. Wyllie E, ed. *The treatment of epilepsy: principles and practice*. Philadelphia: Lippincott Williams & Wilkins, 2001. (Contains reviews of each seizure type.)

Epilepsies with Onset at All Ages: Symptomatic and Probably Symptomatic Focal Epilepsies

One group of epilepsies has onset in patients of all ages: symptomatic and probably symptomatic focal epilepsies. These epilepsies are listed in Table 3-1.

Based on seizure and electroencephalographic (EEG) characteristics, age, and evidence of brain pathology, a patient with symptomatic focal epilepsies often can be classified into one of several epilepsy syndromes, according to the presumed site in which seizures originate: mesial temporal lobe, lateral temporal lobe, frontal lobe, parietal lobe, or occipital lobe. Rasmussen syndrome and hemiconvulsion–hemiplegia syndrome also are included in this epilepsy group.

I. TEMPORAL LOBE EPILEPSIES

A. General Characteristics

Simple partial, complex partial, or secondarily generalized seizures (reviewed in Chapter 2) may occur, with onset frequently in childhood or young adulthood. Seizures may occur randomly, at intervals, or in clusters. Simple partial seizures are characterized by autonomic or psychic symptoms, or both, and by certain sensory phenomena, such as olfactory and auditory illusions or hallucinations. The most common sensation is a rising epigastric discomfort.

B. Routine Electroencephalogram Characteristics

Routine EEGs may show (a) no abnormality; (b) slight or marked asymmetry of the background activity; or (c) temporal spikes, sharp waves, or slow waves (unilateral or bilateral, synchronous or asynchronous; may not be confined to temporal areas).

C. Subtypes

1. Mesial Temporal Seizures

Mesial temporal seizures are the most common form of temporal lobe epilepsy and generally conform to the following general description. Seizures are characterized by rising epigastric discomfort, nausea, marked autonomic signs, and other symptoms including borborygmi, belching, pallor, fullness of the face, flushing, arrest of respiration, pupil dilation, fear, panic, and olfactory–gustatory hallucinations. Scalp EEG often shows unilateral or bilateral spikes most prominent in the anterior temporal leads.

One variant of amygdala–hippocampal seizures is called the *mesial temporal lobe epilepsy syndrome*. Such patients demon-

Table 3-1.   Groups of epilepsy syndromes and specific epilepsy syndromes with onset at all ages and accompanying seizure types

Symptomatic and probably symptomatic focal epilepsy syndromes
Mesial temporal lobe epilepsy syndromes (SPS, CPS, TCS)
Lateral temporal lobe epilepsy syndromes (SPS, CPS, TCS)
Frontal lobe epilepsy syndromes (SPS, CPS, TCS)
Parietal lobe epilepsy syndromes (SPS, CPS, TCS)
Occipital lobe epilepsy syndromes (SPS, CPS, TCS)

CPS, complex partial (psychomotor, temporal lobe) seizure; SPS, simple partial (focal) seizure; TCS, tonic–clonic (grand mal) seizures.

strate mesial temporal sclerosis (Fig. 3-1). They typically have a strong family history of epilepsy showing an autosomal-dominant inheritance with incomplete penetrance. The patient has seizures (often complicated) during infancy or childhood. After a silent period lasting 2 to 15 years, unprovoked partial seizures begin in late childhood or early adolescence. The seizures are refractory to medical treatment in 20% to 30% of patients.

2. Lateral Temporal Seizures

Lateral temporal seizures begin as simple partial seizures characterized by auditory hallucinations or illusions, dreamy state, visual misperceptions, or language disorders (dominant-hemisphere focus). These may progress to complex partial seizures if propagation to mesial temporal or extratemporal structures occurs. Lateral temporal seizures usually lack several of the features typical of mesial temporal seizures, including automatisms, contralateral dystonia, swerving head movements, body shifting, hyperventilation, and postictal cough or sigh. The scalp EEG often shows unilateral or bilateral spikes most prominent in the middle or posterior temporal leads.

A special subtype is termed *autosomal-dominant partial epilepsy with auditory features (ADPEAF)*. Onset is in typically in the second decade of life. The syndrome is characterized by auditory symptoms. The auditory phenomenon may consist of unformed sounds such as monotonous buzzing or fringing, distortions of sound such as a change in volume or pitch, or formed sounds such as voices from the past or specific singers. Other sensory or psychic symptoms, motor activity, and autonomic dysfunction may develop. Paroxysmal activity may be seen in the EEG interictally in the temporal or occipital leads. The condition responds to antiepileptic drugs, but may require prolonged administration. Genetic analysis has found linkage to chromosome 10q24 with mutations in the *LGI1* gene (leucine-rich gene, glioma inactivated). The gene is involved in ligand binding and protein–protein interactions and likely is involved in development of the nervous system. *LGI1* is the only gene yet identified in temporal lobe epilepsy and is the only non–ion-channel gene identified in idiopathic epilepsy.

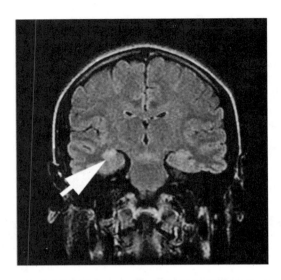

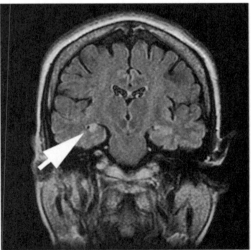

Fig. 3-1.   MRI of patient with mesial temporal sclerosis. FLAIR images showing signal changes in the right mesial temporal region (*arrows*).

3. Lateralizing Features

Useful lateralizing features for the temporal lobe seizures include unilateral clonic activity (seizure focus contralateral in all patients); unilateral dystonic or tonic posturing (seizure focus contralateral in 90% or 86%, respectively); unilateral automatisms (seizure focus ipsilateral in 80%); and ictal speech preservation (seizure focus contralateral to the language-dominant hemisphere in 80%). Versive head rotation occurring less than 10 seconds before seizures secondarily generalize predicts a contralateral focus. Ictal speech arrest or postictal speech impairment is associated with a seizure focus ipsilateral to the language-dominant hemisphere in two thirds of patients. Postictal speech preservation is associated with a seizure focus contralateral to the language-dominant hemisphere in two thirds of patients. Seizure manifestations not providing reliable lateralizing information include eye deviation, type of aura, and versive head movements occurring at times other than immediately before seizures secondarily generalize.

4. Cysticercosis

As mentioned in the opening paragraph of this chapter, the manifestations of partial seizures depend on the region of the cortex in which they originate. This is true for cysticercosis, a common cause of partial seizures in developing countries and certain regions of the United States in which it is endemic. The diagnosis is best established with imaging studies.

II. FRONTAL LOBE EPILEPSIES

A. Clinical Characteristics

Frontal lobe epilepsies are characterized by simple partial, complex partial, or secondarily generalized seizures (reviewed in Chapter 2), or combinations of these. Features suggesting frontal lobe epilepsies are (a) frequent seizures, often in stage 2 sleep; (b) short seizure duration; (c) minimal or no postictal confusion after a complex partial seizure; (d) rapid secondary generalization; (e) prominent motor manifestations that are tonic or postural; (f) complex gestural automatisms (may be sexual) at onset; (g) frequent falling during the seizure; and (h) frequent episodes of status epilepticus.

B. Electroencephalogram Characteristics

The interictal EEG of frontal lobe epilepsy patients may show (a) no abnormality; (b) background asymmetry; and (c) spikes, sharp waves, or paroxysmal fast activity that can be unilateral or bilateral, unilobular, or multilobular. Patients whose seizures originate from the dorsolateral convexity tend to have interictal epileptiform abnormalities that localize to the region of seizure onset. Patients whose seizures begin in the medial frontal region tend to have either no epileptiform activity or multifocal epileptiform discharges. Vertex or midline epileptiform discharges also can be seen with medial frontal foci. Frontal foci not infrequently exhibit spikes or sharp waves in the temporal leads.

C. Subtypes

1. Supplementary Motor Seizures

Supplementary motor seizures are typically brief, lasting only 10 to 40 seconds. The patient demonstrates abrupt tonic posturing of one or more extremities; the arms are affected more often than the legs. Characteristically, arms and legs are tonically adducted. During the tonic phase, the patient may cry or moan loudly. Consciousness is usually preserved, but the patient may be unable to speak. A versive movement, usually away from the side of ictal onset, may precede secondary generalization. The tonic posturing may be preceded by sensory symptoms in an extremity. Supplementary motor seizures occur frequently, and for a patient to experience five to ten episodes per day is not rare. Many seizures occur during sleep. Commonly, these seizures are medically intractable.

2. Cingulate

Cingulate seizure patterns are complex partial with complex motor gestural automatisms at onset. Autonomic signs are common, as are changes in mood and affect.

3. Anterior Frontopolar Region

Anterior frontopolar seizure patterns include forced thinking or initial loss of contact and adversive movements of head and eyes, with possible evolution, including contraversive movements and axial clonic jerks, and falls and autonomic signs.

4. Orbitofrontal

The orbitofrontal seizure pattern is one of complex partial seizures with initial motor and gestural automatisms, olfactory hallucinations and illusions, and autonomic signs. Automatisms may include unformed or formed speech (including expletives) and walking around the room.

5. Combined Mesial Frontal

Seizures originating in any of the four mesial frontal structures described earlier sometimes show phenomena described for other mesial frontal structures. Functional spread of discharges likely occurs among the areas.

6. Dorsolateral

Dorsolateral seizure patterns may be tonic or, less commonly, clonic, with versive eye and head movements and speech arrest.

7. Opercular

Opercular seizure characteristics include mastication, salivation, swallowing, laryngeal symptoms, speech arrest, epigastric aura, fear, and autonomic phenomena. Simple partial seizures, particularly partial clonic facial seizures, are common and may be ipsilateral. If secondary sensory changes occur, numbness may be a symptom, particularly in the hands. Gustatory hallucinations are particularly common with seizures in this area.

8. Motor Cortex

Motor cortex epilepsies are characterized mainly by simple partial seizures, and their localization depends on the side and topography of the area affected. In cases of the lower prerolandic area, speech arrest, vocalization or dysphasia, tonic–clonic movements of the face on the contralateral side, or swallowing may occur. Generalization of the seizure frequently occurs. In the rolandic area, partial motor seizures with march, or jacksonian, seizures occur, particularly beginning in the contralateral upper extremities. In the case of seizures involving the paracentral lobule, tonic movements of the ipsilateral foot may occur, as well as contralateral leg movements. Postictal paralysis is frequent.

9. Kojewnikow Syndrome

Kojewnikow syndrome represents a particular form of rolandic partial epilepsy both in adults and in children and is related to a variety of lesions in the motor cortex. Its principal features are (a) motor partial seizures, always well localized; (b) often late appearance of myoclonus in the same site at which somatomotor seizures occur; (c) an EEG with normal background activity and a focal paroxysmal abnormality (spikes and slow waves); (d) occurrence at any age in childhood and adulthood; (e) frequently demonstrable etiology (tumor, vascular); and (f) no progressive evolution of the syndrome (clinical, EEG, or psychological, except in relation to the evolution of the causal lesion).

10. Rasmussen Encephalitis

In Rasmussen encephalitis, in a previously normal child, usually approximately 6 to 10 years old, therapy-resistant focal seizures rapidly develop, usually motor or sensorimotor, with a slowly progressive motor deficit implicating the same cerebral hemisphere. A mild or moderate mental deficit appears later. The EEG shows prominent and persistent arrhythmic delta waves, loss of background features, and abundant spikes. Later, seizures may implicate widely separate portions of the same hemisphere. Pathologic specimens may show gliosis, inflammation, or spongiform changes. The disease may progress to death, stabilize, or improve over time. High-dose intravenous human immunoglobulin may be beneficial for this condition.

11. Autosomal-Dominant Frontal Lobe Nocturnal Epilepsy

Autosomal-dominant frontal lobe nocturnal epilepsy is a syndrome in which nocturnal seizures develop within the first two decades of life, although the seizures often persist throughout adulthood. The seizures usually occur during sleep, but in severe cases, seizures may occur while awake. The clinical features are similar to other frontal epilepsies. A nonspecific aura that may include somatosensory, special sensory, psychic, or autonomic phenomena is commonly present. After the aura, gasping, groaning, other vocalization, prominent motor phenomena (thrashing, hyperkinetic movements, tonic stiffening, clonic jerking), or reflex agitation with rapid changes in position may occur. The condition usually responds well to carbamazepine.

The gene defect has been mapped to chromosome 20q13 *(CHRNA4)* and 1q21 *(CHRNB2)* with mutations in the genes coding for the α_4 and β_2 subunits of the neuronal nicotinic acetylcholine receptors. Analysis of the functional properties of these mutant acetylcholine receptors associated with autosomal-dominant nocturnal frontal lobe epilepsy indicates that a gain of function with increased sensitivity to acetylcholine may be the origin of the neuronal network dysfunction causing the seizures.

III. PARIETAL LOBE SEIZURES

A. General Characteristics

Parietal lobe epilepsy syndromes usually are characterized by simple partial and secondarily generalized seizures (reviewed in Chapter 2). Most seizures remain simple and exhibit sensory phenomena. Most frequently, seizures are of the anterior parietal subtype.

B. Electroencephalogram Characteristics

Interictal EEGs may show (a) normal results; (b) focal slowing; or (c) focal spikes and sharp waves that are unilateral or bilateral, synchronous or asynchronous. Slow and sharp activity spreading beyond parietal leads is not uncommon. Vertex or midline epileptiform abnormalities can be seen with somatosensory seizures arising from the mesial surface of the parietal lobe.

C. Subtypes

1. Anterior Parietal Seizures

Anterior parietal seizures involve the posterior central gyrus and are predominantly sensory with positive or negative phenomena. Positive phenomena may include tingling; a feeling of electricity; desire to move a body part; the sensation that a body part is being moved; tongue or facial sensations, or both; and pain. Negative phenomena include loss of muscle tone, numbness, the feeling that a body part is absent, or loss of awareness of a part of or half of the body (asomatognosia).

The parts most frequently involved are those with the largest cortical representation (hand, arm, face), and seizures may spread along the posterior central gyrus, producing a jacksonian march of symptoms as adjacent structures are progressively affected.

2. Posterior Parietal Seizures

Posterior parietal seizures are frequently accompanied by prominent staring and relative immobility. Visual phenomena may occur, including formed hallucinations and metamorphopsia (visual distortions) and confusion.

3. Inferior Parietal Seizures

Inferior parietal seizures may demonstrate severe vertigo and disorientation in space, and abdominal sensations.

4. Paracentral Seizures

Paracentral seizures may demonstrate contralateral genital sensations or rotary or postural motor activity, and have a tendency to become secondarily generalized.

5. Dominant Hemisphere Parietal Seizures

Seizures arising from the dominant parietal lobe may demonstrate receptive or conductive language disturbances.

6. Nondominant Hemisphere Parietal Seizures

Metamorphopsia (distortion of body parts) and asomatognosia (inability to recognize body parts) often indicate involvement of the nondominant parietal lobe.

IV. OCCIPITAL LOBE SEIZURES

A. General Characteristics

Occipital lobe seizures are characterized by positive and negative visual phenomena. Positive phenomena include elementary visual hallucinations often described as bright lights or colored lights. Negative phenomena include amaurosis, scotomas, and hemianopsia. The visual phenomena usually are contralateral to the side of the seizure and may remain stationary or move across the field. Persistent (hours) amaurosis can be a postictal phenomenon.

Other occipital seizure manifestations include tonic and clonic eye deviation, head deviation, blinking, a sensation of eye movement, and nystagmoid eye movements. Eye and head movements usually are contralateral to the side of the seizure focus in occipital seizures. (This may not be the case for seizures arising in other areas.)

B. Electroencephalogram Characteristics

Surface EEGs most often demonstrate extensive posterior temporal–occipital paroxysmal activity. This pattern may be difficult to distinguish from temporal lobe epilepsy of posterior temporal origin.

C. Subtypes

Seizure discharges within the occipital lobe produce a limited number of signs and symptoms. However, such discharges may spread to the temporal, frontal, supplementary motor, or parietal areas and produce seizures typical of these areas. The most common mode of spread is infrasylvian to the ipsilateral temporal lobe, producing automatisms typical of temporal lobe seizures (psychoparetic, psychomotor). Visual signs or symptoms at onset of a seizure suggest occipital origin.

D. Evaluation

The approach to benign occipital epilepsy of children is discussed in Chapter 6. Symptomatic (due to a structural lesion) occipital epilepsy is suggested by the presence of neurologic deficits, limbic spread of seizures, and short and frequent seizures. Structural lesions causing occipital seizures include developmental malformations, perinatal lesions, posttraumatic lesions, strokes, tumors, Sturge–Weber syndrome, epilepsy with bilateral occipital calcification, mitochondrial disorders [mitochondrial encephalomyelopathy with ragged-red fibers and strokelike episodes (MELAS), myoclonic epilepsy and ragged-red fibers (MERRF)], and Lafora disease (neural ceroid lipofuscinosis). If a structural lesion is suspected, magnetic resonance imaging is the preferable scan because developmental anomalies (a common finding) do not show well on computed tomography.

V. ETIOLOGY OF PARTIAL SEIZURES AND SYMPTOMATIC FOCAL EPILEPSIES

A. Overall

By definition, partial seizures and symptomatic focal epilepsies are symptomatic of a cerebral lesion. The usual etiologies are developmental defects, trauma, cerebrovascular disease, tumors, and infection. Figure 3-2 is an MRI showing focal cortical dysplasia in a child with frontal lobe epilepsy. The incidence of these etiologies varies with age (Fig. 3-3).

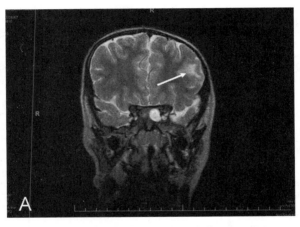

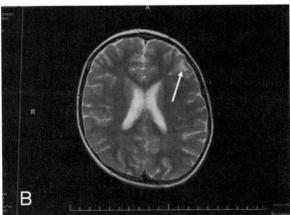

Fig. 3-2.   MRI of a child with complex partial seizures of frontal lobe origin. MRI shows frontal lobe dysplasia (*arrows*) on the coronal (A) and axial (B) views.

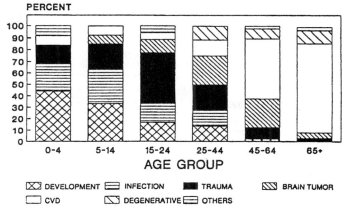

PERCENT

Fig. 3-3. Etiologies of symptomatic epilepsy in various age groups. CVD, cerebrovascular disease. (From Annegers JF. The epidemiology of epilepsy. In: Wyllie E, ed. *The treatment of epilepsy: principles and practice*. Philadelphia: Lippincott Williams & Wilkins, 2001:131–138, with permission.)

B. Neuropathologic Examination of Surgical Excision Specimens

Surgical excision of epileptogenic foci has been a recognized therapy for refractory epilepsy for several decades (see Chapter 10). Neuropathologic examinations of surgical specimens provide an insight into the etiologies of such epilepsies.

Mesial temporal sclerosis is the most common finding, being present in approximately one half of patients. *Mesial temporal sclerosis* refers to the pathologic entity of hippocampal sclerosis and atrophy (often visible on imaging studies) with loss of neurons in the CA1 region and end-folium (CA3/CA4), but with relative sparing of the CA2 region. Loss of dentate hilar neurons (end-folium sclerosis) is a common feature, and, in some patients, may be the only apparent hippocampal lesion. The etiology of mesial temporal sclerosis is controversial. Evidence suggests that prolonged seizures, including prolonged febrile seizures, may cause mesial temporal sclerosis.

Congenital lesions (principally hamartomas, heterotopias, and focal cortical dysplasia) account for 15% to 20% of recognized lesions and are particularly common in children. Neoplasms (principally glial) account for 10% to 15% of recognized lesions. Trauma accounts for only 5% to 10% of pathologic findings.

VI. MANAGEMENT OF PARTIAL SEIZURES AND SYMPTOMATIC FOCAL EPILEPSIES

A. Seizure First Aid and Prevention of Complications

1. General

The first responsibilities of a person who is present when a patient is seizing are to prevent physical injury, to ensure safety, and to observe accurately. Never leave the patient alone. Call for help if it is needed.

2. Complex Partial Seizures

During complex partial seizures, medical personnel should prevent falls caused by loss of tone or incoordination. Patients exhibiting automatisms (walking, standing, smoking) should be monitored. Physical restraint should be used only as a last resort because patients demonstrating automatisms may become violent if restrained.

3. Tonic–Clonic Seizures

Placing a soft oral airway in the patient's mouth prevents oral trauma and promotes drainage of secretions during tonic–clonic seizures. This should be done only if the airway can be placed without force (usually impossible, because the mouth closes tightly early in the tonic phase). Forcing an airway between teeth results in oral trauma. Falling patients should be caught before they hit the floor. Hands or other soft objects can be used to prevent trauma to the head or other parts caused by clonic movements. Patients should be placed in the lateral decubitus or prone position as soon as possible to promote drainage of secretions and to prevent aspiration. Complications of tonic–clonic seizures (oral trauma, head trauma, stress fractures, aspiration pneumonia, pulmonary edema—see Chapter 2) should be looked for as soon as possible.

B. Pharmacologic Management

1. Basic Approach and Pharmacologic Principles

See Chapter 10.

2. Drugs of Choice

The drugs of first choice for adults are carbamazepine, oxcarbazepine, lamotrigine, levetiracetam, and topiramate, based on comparative trials. Because of the side-effect profiles, antiepileptic drugs such as primidone, phenytoin, and valproate are considered second-tier drugs. In children, comparative studies have demonstrated that carbamazepine, phenytoin, and valproic acid are equally efficacious. Phenobarbital and primidone are also efficacious, but side effects such as irritability, hyperactivity, and lethargy limit these drugs to second-line therapy. For further details, see Chapter 10; a review of adult therapy by Mattson (26).

3. Drug Administration

For further details on these drugs, see Chapter 11.

C. Medically Refractory Epilepsy

1. Definition

Patients with localization-related/symptomatic epilepsy who continue to have seizures after trials of three or more marketed antiepileptic drugs by following the principles outlined in Chapter 10 are considered *medically refractory*. Approximately

15% of patients with localization-related/symptomatic epilepsy (partial seizures) fall into this category. The probability that a fourth drug will completely control seizures is less than 10%. Therefore, such patients require reevaluation of their diagnosis and management.

2. Diagnostic Reevaluation

Many cases of medically refractory epilepsy are caused by improper diagnosis. The patient should be reevaluated by the treating physician or a neurologic consultant to reexamine the differential diagnostic alternative diagnoses discussed in Chapter 9. Psychogenic seizures and absence seizures are the most common causes of improper diagnosis.

3. Alternative Therapies

A. SURGICAL MANAGEMENT. Surgical management should be considered first because the probability that a fourth drug will completely control seizures is less than 10%. The probability that a resection procedure will completely control seizures is greater than 50% in patients meeting the criteria for such procedures. See Chapter 10 for a full discussion.

B. OTHER THERAPIES. The ketogenic diet (see Chapter 10), experimental antiepileptic drugs, behavior therapy, and hormone therapy are other alternatives for patients who are not surgical candidates. Surgery and other alternative treatments generally are available only at specialized epilepsy centers.

VII. PROGNOSIS OF PARTIAL SEIZURES AND SYMPTOMATIC FOCAL EPILEPSIES

A. First Unprovoked Seizure

The risk of seizure recurrence by 36 months is 25% in persons with no risk factors after having a first unprovoked seizure. In persons with risk factors, the risk of seizure recurrence usually is much greater. Risk factors include evidence of prior neurologic insult (determined by history, neurologic examination, imaging studies); abnormal EEG; and multiple seizures or status epilepticus as the initial event. Treatment after first partial seizures remains controversial because of the uncertainty regarding the risk of another seizure and the side effects of antiepileptic medication. However, randomized clinical trials do indicate that antiepileptic drugs reduce risk of seizure recurrence. See Chapter 10 for further details.

B. After Two or More Unprovoked Seizures

Persons with two or more unprovoked seizures almost always are treated. The two Veterans Administration Cooperative Studies (25) indicate that 35% to 60% of adult patients with partial seizures will have complete seizure control after 1 year, with carbamazepine or phenytoin monotherapy as the initial and only treatment.

Satisfactory results (an acceptable number of seizures or none, acceptable side effects) are obtained in approximately 70% of patients with a single drug, either the initial choice or an alternative. Patients in whom the first drug is not effective have only a 14% chance of becoming seizure free with the second or third drug. With a third drug is added, another 5% are satisfactorily controlled. Overall, approximately 30% of patients have inadequate control despite trials of several drugs used alone. Such patients are considered to be medically refractory or to have pharmacoresistant epilepsy.

Risk factors for poor control of partial seizures include abnormal EEG, evidence of a structural brain lesion, number and duration of seizures before diagnosis and before control with medication, neurologic deficit from birth, failure of treatment with first drug, and secondarily generalized tonic–clonic seizures.

C. Successful Medication Withdrawal after Remission
See Chapter 10.

D. Mortality

1. General
Available studies are not optimal but generally report increased mortality in patients with symptomatic epilepsies. This mortality is caused, at least in part, by the underlying symptomatic disease (congenital malformations, tumors, cerebrovascular disease) and its complications. Studies regarding increased rate of suicide are conflicting.

2. Sudden Unexplained Death
The risk of sudden unexplained death is between 1 in 500 and 1 in 1,100 person-years for all persons with epilepsy, and 1 in 200 person-years for patients with refractory seizures. Although sudden unexplained death can occur at all ages, the risk is greater for persons between the ages of 15 and 45 years with poorly controlled tonic–clonic seizures (usually secondarily generalized). Structural lesions and severe or frequent seizures appear to be risk factors. Available evidence suggests that most sudden deaths are temporally related to seizures and often occur in sleep. Postulated mechanisms include cardiac arrhythmias, pulmonary edema, and suffocation. Cardiac abnormalities recorded during partial seizures include asystole, atrial fibrillation, sinus arrhythmia, supraventricular tachycardia, atrial premature depolarizations, ventricular premature depolarizations, and bundle branch block.

E. Neuropsychological Function
Animal studies suggest that repeated partial seizures may result in neuronal damage. Human studies are difficult to evaluate because of the confounding effects of the original structural lesion, antiepileptic drug effects, and impaired social adjustment. The effects of repeated partial seizures on neuropsychological function remain unknown.

VIII. HEMICONVULSION–HEMIPLEGIA SYNDROME
This syndrome is reviewed in Chapter 6.

REFERENCES

1. Acharya JN, Wyllie E, Luders H, et al. Seizure symptomatology in infants with localization-related epilepsy. *Neurology* 1997; 48:189–196.
2. Annegers JF. The epidemiology of epilepsy. In: Wyllie E, ed. *The treatment of epilepsy: principles and practice*. Philadelphia: Lippincott Williams & Wilkins, 2001:131–138.
3. Bautista RE, Spencer DD, Spencer SS. EEG findings in frontal lobe epilepsies. *Neurology* 1998;50:1765–1771.
4. Bertrand D, Picard F, Le Hellard S, et al. How mutations in the nAChRs can cause ADNFLE epilepsy. *Epilepsia* 2002;43(suppl 5):112–122.
5. Bien CG, Widman G, Urbach H, et al. The natural history of Rasmussen's encephalitis. *Brain* 2002;125(pt 8):1751–1759.
6. Brodtkorb E, Gu W, Nakken KO, et al. Familial temporal lobe epilepsy with aphasic seizures and linkage to chromosome 10q22–q24. *Epilepsia* 2002;43:228–235.
7. Carpio A, Escobar A, Hauser WA. Cysticercosis: a critical report. *Epilepsia* 1998;39:1025–1040.
8. Cendes F, Lopes-Cendes L, Andermann E, et al. Familial temporal lobe epilepsy: a clinically heterogenous syndrome. *Neurology* 1998;50:554–557.
9. Cockerall OC, Johnson AL, Sander WAS, et al. Prognosis of epilepsy: a review and further analysis of the first nine years of the British National Practice Study of Epilepsy, a prospective population-based study. *Epilepsia* 1997;38:31–46.
10. Commission on Classification and Terminology of the International League Against Epilepsy. Proposal for revised clinical and EEG classification of epileptic seizures. *Epilepsia* 1981; 22:489–501.
11. Commission on Classification and Terminology of the International League Against Epilepsy. Proposal for revised classification of epilepsies and epileptic syndromes. *Epilepsia* 1989;30:389–399.
12. Donner EJ, Smith CR, Snead OC III. Sudden unexplained death in children with epilepsy. *Neurology* 2001;57(3):430–434.
13. Dulac O. Use of antiepileptic drugs in children. In: Levy RH, Mattson RH, Meldrum BS, Perruca E, eds. *Antiepileptic drugs*, 5th ed. Philadelphia: Lippincott Williams & Wilkins, 2002: 119–131.
14. Foldvary N, Lee N, Thwaites G, et al. Clinical and electrographic manifestations of lesional neocortical temporal lobe epilepsy. *Neurology* 1997;49:757–763.
15. French JA, Williamson PD, Thadani VM, et al. Characteristics of mesial temporal lobe epilepsy, I: results of history and physical examination. *Ann Neurol* 1993;34:774–780.
16. Hauser WA, Hesdorffer DC. Remission, intractability, mortality, and comorbidity of epilepsy. In: Wyllie E, ed. *The treatment of epilepsy: principles and practice*. Philadelphia: Lippincott Williams & Wilkins, 2001:139–145. (Contains a review of sudden unexplained death.)
17. Hayman M, Scheffer IE, Chinvarum Y, et al. Autosomal dominant nocturnal frontal lobe epilepsy: demonstration of focal frontal onset and intrafamilial variation. *Neurology* 1997;49:969–975.

18. Ho SS, Berkovic SF, Newton MR, et al. Parietal lobe epilepsy: clinical features and localization by ictal SPECT. *Neurology* 1994;44:2277–2284.

19. Kobayashi E, Lopes-Cendes I, Gurrierro CAM, et al. Seizure outcome and hippocampal atrophy in familial temporal lobe epilepsy. *Neurology* 2001;56:166–172.

20. Kuzniecky R. Symptomatic occipital lobe epilepsy. *Epilepsia* 1998;39(suppl 4):24–31.

21. Kuzniecky RI, Barkovich AJ. Pathogenesis and pathology of focal malformations of cortical development and epilepsy. *J Clin Neurophysiol* 1996;13:468–480.

22. Kwan P, Brodie MJ. Early identification of refractory epilepsy. *N Engl J Med* 2000;342:314–319.

23. Laskowitz DT, Sperling MR, French JA, et al. The syndrome of frontal lobe epilepsy: characteristics and surgical management. *Neurology* 1995;45:780–787.

24. Marks WJ, Laxner KO. Semiology of temporal lobe seizures: value in lateralizing the seizure focus. *Epilepsia* 1998;39: 721–726.

25. Mattson RH, V.A. Epilepsy Cooperative Studies No. 118 and 264 Group. Prognosis for total control of complex partial and secondarily generalized tonic-clonic seizures. *Neurology* 1996; 47:68–76.

26. Mattson RH. Antiepileptic drug monotherapy in adults: selection and use in new-onset epilepsy. In: Levy RH, Mattson RH, Meldrum BS, et al., eds. *Antiepileptic drugs*, 5th ed. Philadelphia: Lippincott Williams & Wilkins, 2002:72–95.

27. Nei M, Ho RT, Sperling MR. EKG abnormalities during partial seizures in refractory partial epilepsy. *Epilepsia* 2000;41: 542–548.

28. Poza JJ, Saenz A, Martinez-Gil A, et al. Autosomal dominant lateral temporal epilepsy: clinical and genetic study of a large Basque pedigree linked to chromosome 10q. *Ann Neurol* 1999; 45:182–188.

29. Salanova V, Morris HH, Van Ness P, et al. Frontal lobe seizures: electroclinical syndromes. *Epilepsia* 1995;36:16–24.

30. So NK. Mesial frontal epilepsy. *Epilepsia* 1998;39(suppl 4): 44–61.

31. Spencer S. Temporal lobectomy: selection of candidates. In: Wyllie E, ed. *The treatment of epilepsy: principles and practice*. Philadelphia: Lippincott Williams & Wilkins, 2001:1077–1094.

32. Sveinbjornsdottir S, Duncan JS. Parietal and occipital lobe epilepsy: a review. *Epilepsia* 1993;34:493–521.

33. Theodore WH, Porter RJ, Albert P, et al. The secondarily generalized tonic-clonic seizure: a videotape analysis. *Neurology* 1994; 44:1403–1407.

34. Walczak TS, Leppik IE, D'Amelio M, et al. Incidence and risk factors in sudden unexplained death in epilepsy: a prospective cohort study. *Neurology* 2001;56:519–525.

35. Westmoreland BF. The EEG findings in extratemporal seizures. *Epilepsia* 1998;39(suppl 4):1–8.

36. Winawer MR, Ottman R, Hauser WA, et al. Autosomal dominant epilepsy with auditory features: defining the syndrome. *Neurology* 2000;54:2173–2176.

37. Wolf P. Behavioral therapy. In: Engel J, Pedley TA, eds. *Epilepsy: a comprehensive textbook*. Philadelphia: Lippincott-Raven, 1997: 1359–1364.

38. Wyllie E, ed. *The treatment of epilepsy: principles and practice*. Philadelphia: Lippincott Williams & Wilkins, 2001. (Contains reviews of seizure types and the epilepsies.)

Epilepsies with Neonatal Onset (Birth to 2 Months): Focal and Generalized Epilepsies

Both focal and generalized seizures (see Chapter 1) are described in this chapter. Five syndromes have onset in the neonatal period; they are listed in Table 4-1.

I. NEONATAL SEIZURES

Children are at high risk for seizures during the first months and years of life. Because of the birthing process, the infant is at risk for a number of insults such as trauma, hypoxic–ischemic insults, intracranial hemorrhages, and infection. In addition, a large number of pathologic processes occurring in neonates may be seen initially with seizures. For example, congenital brain anomalies, inborn errors of metabolism, and genetic conditions may lead to recurrent seizures during the neonatal period. Because neonatal seizures are often associated with serious neurologic disorders, they are the most ominous neurologic signs in newborns. Because seizures may be the first and only sign of a central nervous system disorder, their recognition is extremely important. Despite advances made in the areas of obstetrics and perinatal care, seizures continue to be a significant predictor of poor neurologic outcome.

A multitude of changes occur in neuronal and glial growth and differentiation, myelination, and neurochemical composition of the brain during the third trimester of pregnancy and postnatal months. Because of immaturities in anatomic, chemical, and bio-electric connections in and between cortical and subcortical structures, it is not surprising that neonatal seizures differ markedly from those occurring in older subjects. They differ mainly in their clinical manifestations, in their etiologies, and in their short- and long-term prognosis.

A. Definition

Neonatal seizures refer to seizures that occur between birth and 2 months of age.

B. Seizure Phenomena

A considerable difference is apparent in the behavior observed during seizures in neonates and the behaviors seen in older children and adults. Infants are unable to sustain organized generalized epileptiform discharges, and generalized tonic–clonic and absence seizures do not occur. The age-dependent clinical and electroencephalographic (EEG) features of seizures in neonates are a result of the immaturity of cortical organization and myelination.

Table 4-1.   Groups of epilepsy syndromes and specific epilepsy syndromes with neonatal onset (birth to 2 months) and accompanying seizure types

Neonatal seizures syndrome (CLON, MYO, TON)
Benign familial neonatal convulsions syndrome (CLON)
Benign neonatal seizures (nonfamilial) syndrome (CLON)
Benign partial epilepsy of infancy (CPS, TCS)
Early myoclonic encephalopathy syndrome (MYO)
Otahara syndrome (CLON)

CLON, clonic seizure; CPS, complex partial seizure; TCS, tonic–clonic seizure; MYO, myoclonic seizure; TON, tonic seizure.

Neonatal seizures are classified as clonic, tonic, and myoclonic. Clonic seizures consist of rhythmic jerking of groups of muscles and occur in either a focal or a multifocal pattern. In multifocal clonic seizures, movements may migrate from one part of the body to another. Although focal seizures may be seen with localized brain insults, such as neonatal strokes, they may also be seen in disorders that diffusely affect the brain, such as asphyxia, subarachnoid hemorrhage, hypoglycemia, and infection. In tonic seizures, asymmetric posturing of the trunk or deviation of the eyes to one side develop in infants. Myoclonic seizures are similar to those seen in older children, consisting of rapid jerks of muscles. The myoclonic seizures can consist of bilateral jerks, although occasionally unilateral or focal myoclonus can occur.

Sick neonates often display repetitive, stereotyped behavior that may be confused with seizures. These behaviors include repetitive sucking and other oral–buccal–lingual movements, assumption of an abnormal posture, pedaling movements of the legs or paddling movements of the arms, blinking, momentary fixation of gaze with or without eye deviation, nystagmus, and apnea. However, when these behaviors are observed during EEG recordings, epileptiform activity is usually not recorded. Likewise, when tonic posturing involves all four extremities and the trunk, an associated EEG-epileptiform discharge rarely appears. Myoclonus not associated with epileptiform discharges also can be seen in sick neonates.

C. Electroencephalographic Phenomena

Whereas the diagnosis of seizures relies primarily on clinical observation, the EEG may be extremely valuable in confirming the presence of epileptic seizures. In addition, the EEG is very useful in the detection of electrographic seizures in paralyzed infants or in assessing response to antiepileptic medications.

1. Interictal Abnormalities

Background EEG patterns are very helpful in determining prognosis after neonatal seizures. Electroencephalograms demonstrating isoelectric, low-voltage burst suppression and excessive discontinuity are associated with poor prognoses, whereas records with normal backgrounds are associated with excellent outcomes.

The prognostic value of the EEG improves when similar findings are found on serial studies.

As with older children and adults, interictal spikes are seen more frequently in infants with seizures than in those without seizures. However, differentiating "normal" spikes and sharp waves from those with pathologic significance may be difficult. Strict criteria for differentiating normal sharp waves and spikes from those that are pathologic have yet to be established. For example, frontal sharp waves that shift from hemisphere to hemisphere (often termed "frontal sharp transients") and multifocal spikes and sharp waves that occur only during the burst phase of quiet sleep (tracé alternant or tracéé discontinue) are considered normal by most electroencephalographers. In addition, normal infants, both term and preterm, may have infrequent, sporadic spikes and sharp waves.

Criteria used to classify spikes and sharp waves as abnormal include spikes and sharp waves that are focal and persist through all sleep states, rolandic-positive sharp waves, and focal or multifocal spikes during the low-amplitude phase of discontinuous sleep. Pathologic spikes often occur in bursts. As with older children, spikes and sharp waves can be seen in neonates who never have detected seizures.

Positive spikes occurring over the rolandic area are often associated with underlying white matter disease, such as periventricular leukomalacia or intraventricular hemorrhages. Positive rolandic spikes typically are not associated with seizures.

2. Ictal Discharges

Epileptiform activity that is rhythmic and has a distinct beginning and ending is considered an ictal event. In addition, most ictal discharges have some degree of evolution in frequency or morphology of the waveforms. Although no consensus yet exists on the minimal length of time required for the discharge to be considered ictal, we define an EEG ictus as 10 seconds of rhythmic epileptiform activity.

Ictal epileptiform activity can be divided into four basic types: focal spike or sharp-wave discharges, focal low-frequency discharges, focal rhythmic discharges, and multifocal discharges. Although the type of ictal discharge has not been shown to be specific to etiology, this classification system is useful for the purposes of description. Focal spike or sharp-wave discharges consist of rhythmic spikes or sharp waves that originate focally. The frequency of the discharge usually exceeds 2 Hz, and spread of the focal discharge to other regions occasionally occurs. The spread of ictal discharges in the immature brain is usually much slower than in older children and adults. Focal low-frequency discharges consist of focal spikes or sharp waves that occur at a low frequency (approximately 1 Hz). Differentiation of this ictal discharge from periodic lateralized epileptiform discharges is based primarily on evolution and duration. Periodic lateralized epileptiform discharges demonstrate no evolution, typically last longer than 10 minutes, and are considered nonepileptic activity.

Focal low-frequency ictal discharges usually demonstrate an evolution during the discharge in frequency, amplitude, or wave-

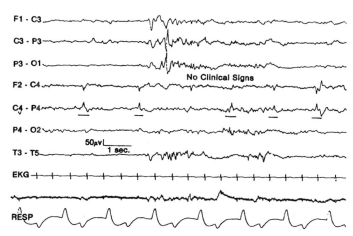

No Clinical Signs

50μV
1 sec.

EKG

RESP

Fig. 4-1.   Focal low-frequency discharge arising from right central region. EKG, electrocardiogram; RESP, respiration.

form morphology (Fig. 4-1). Focal rhythmic patterns consist of rhythmic, monomorphic waves varying from 0.5 to 15.0 Hz. The ictal patterns often vary in frequency during the course of the discharge. In some patients, the ictal discharges "migrate" from one area of the cortex to another. The discharge may have a resemblance to "normal" activity and has been referred to as focal *pseudo-beta-alpha-theta-delta discharges*. However, unlike the normal background activity seen on the neonatal EEG, ictal beta-alpha-theta-delta discharges are paroxysmal, rhythmic, and usually monomorphic in character (Fig. 4-2). Multifocal patterns consist of EEG discharges originating independently or, rarely, simultaneously from two or more foci.

Focal epileptiform activity does not necessarily imply focal pathology. Infants may have focal epileptiform discharges in the face of systemic disorders such as hypoglycemia or hypoxic–ischemic injuries. Cerebral infarctions are frequently associated with focal seizures and lateralized epileptiform discharges in term infants.

Electroencephalographic seizures often occur without any clear clinical accompaniment. In general, EEG seizures without clinical accompaniment have a poorer prognosis than electrical seizures with behavioral changes.

D. Differential Diagnosis

A challenge to the clinician in evaluating the neonate with seizures is differentiating seizures from other stereotyped repetitive behavior in the neonate. Many infants with central nervous system disorders have episodes of chewing, repetitive sucking, and other oral–buccal–lingual movements; assumption of an abnormal posture; pedaling movements of the legs or paddling movements of the arms; blinking; momentary fixation of gaze with or without eye deviation; or nystagmus that is not seizure

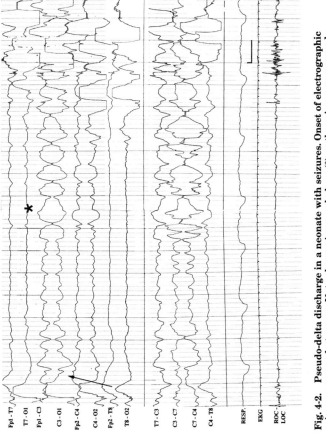

Fig. 4-2. Pseudo-delta discharge in a neonate with seizures. Onset of electrographic seizure occurred at *arrow*. Note change in morphology (*) as the seizure progressed.

activity. The EEG is enormously helpful in distinguishing seizure from nonseizure activity.

Jitteriness may be seen in newborns after mild hypoxic–ischemic events or during drug withdrawal. Jitteriness usually involves all four extremities and can be suppressed by holding the extremity. If doubt exists about the diagnosis, an EEG can be useful.

Benign neonatal sleep myoclonus refers to a condition in which, during the first few months of life, myoclonic jerks develop in infants only during sleep. The EEG is very useful in differentiating benign neonatal sleep myoclonus from seizure-related myoclonus. In the former, the myoclonic jerks during sleep are not associated with any epileptiform discharges.

Hyperexplexia or startle disease is a rare neurologic condition mapped to chromosome 5q33–55. It is characterized by pathologic startle responses to unexpected stimuli and generalized stiffness. Symptoms are usually present from birth. Symptoms can range from mild to severe.

E. Etiology

Many seizures are the result of insults occurring before, during, or after birth. The seizures may be the response to a transient metabolic or systemic disorder. Etiologic factors are usually readily identifiable at this age, and fewer than one third of neonatal seizures are cryptogenic or idiopathic in origin. Outcome correlates best with etiologic factors, rather than the frequency, severity, and duration of the seizures, in contrast with what occurs in older subjects.

Neonatal seizures require a prompt evaluation for etiology. Although neonatal seizures are rarely life threatening, the underlying condition can lead to serious neurologic impairment if it is not treated. For example, the neonate with meningitis benefits more from treatment of the meningitis than from treatment of the seizures.

Table 4-2 lists common etiologies of neonatal seizures.

F. Management

The first step in the evaluation should be a careful history and physical examination. A family history of neonatal seizures is suggestive of benign familial neonatal seizures (see section **I.B**), whereas a history of maternal drug ingestion may implicate drug discontinuation as a cause of seizures. Maternal infections or a difficult delivery may be helpful in determining etiology. Chorioretinitis or a skin rash may suggest a congenital infection such as toxoplasmosis, and needle marks in the scalp raise the possibility of inadvertent injection of a local anesthetic, such as lidocaine, during delivery.

Infants with inherited metabolic diseases may also be seen at (or shortly after) birth with seizures or severe hypotonia. Most affected babies, however, appear normal at birth and subsequently deteriorate, with hypoglycemia, acidosis, neurologic or cardiac problems, or liver disease. In the newborn period, inborn errors of metabolism can therefore easily be misdiagnosed as sepsis or birth asphyxia. Table 4-3 lists hereditary metabolic diseases in which seizures are common.

Table 4-2. **Etiologic agents associated with neonatal seizures**

Etiology	Comments
Asphyxia	Hypoxic–ischemic encephalopathy is the most common cause of neonatal seizures.
Hypocalcemia	Hypocalcemia has two major peaks of incidence in the newborn. The first occurs during the first 3 days of life and is associated with prenatal morbidity or perinatal insults. Late-onset hypocalcemia (5–14 days) occurs primarily in term infants consuming a nonhuman milk preparation with a suboptimal ratio of phosphorus to magnesium. Hypomagnesemia may accompany or occur independent of hypocalcemia
Hypoglycemia	Most authors cite glucose levels less than 20 mg/dL in preterm infants and 30 mg/dL in term babies as indicating hypoglycemia. Like hypocalcemia, hypoglycemia is often associated with other neonatal disorders
Hyponatremia/hypernatremia	Hyponatremia, like hypocalcemia, usually occurs in association with other disorders. Hypernatremia is usually iatrogenic, most frequently secondary to improper mixing of formula
Intracranial hemorrhages	Although many subarachnoid hemorrhages are mild and inconsequential except for causing transient seizures, some result in a difficult course with hydrocephalus and brain parenchymal damage. Intraventricular hemorrhage is the most common type of intracranial hemorrhage and accounts for a large percentage of morbidity and mortality primarily, but not exclusively, in preterm infants

continued

Table 4-2. *Continued*

Etiology	Comments
Congenital infection	Intrauterine or postnatal central nervous system infections may lead to seizures. Intrauterine causes include rubella, toxoplasmosis, cytomegalovirus, herpes simplex, human immunodeficiency virus, and coxsackievirus B. Intrauterine infections are usually associated with other systemic signs: microcephaly, jaundice, rash, hepatomegaly, and chorioretinitis
Postnatal infection	Common postnatal infections include *Escherichia coli* and group B β-hemolytic *Streptococcus*. Any infant without a clear etiology of seizures requires prompt lumbar puncture. Sepsis without meningitis may also lead to seizures
Congenital malformation	Virtually all disorders of neuronal migration and organization (e.g., polymicrogyria, neuronal heterotopias, lissencephaly, holoprosencephaly, and hydranencephaly) may lead to severe neonatal seizures
Metabolic disorders	Although the differential diagnosis of neonatal seizures includes inherited metabolic disorders, these are rare and usually produce other significant symptoms, such as peculiar odors, protein intolerance, acidosis, alkalosis, lethargy, or stupor. In most cases of metabolic disease, pregnancy, labor, and delivery are normal. Whereas food intolerance may be the earliest indication of a systemic abnormality, seizures are commonly the first specific clue to central nervous system involvement. If untreated, metabolic disorders commonly lead to lethargy, coma, and death. In surviving infants, weight loss, poor growth, and failure to thrive are common

continued

Table 4-2. *Continued*

Etiology	Comments
Drug withdrawal	A significant cause of neonatal seizures in urban hospitals is withdrawal from narcotic-analgesics, sedative-hypnotics, and alcohol. Infants born to heroin- or methadone-addicted mothers have an increased risk of seizures, although the most common neurologic findings are jitteriness and irritability. Infants of methadone-addicted mothers may have late withdrawal symptoms, with seizures occurring as long as 4 weeks after birth. Maternal use of cocaine has been associated with neonatal seizures
Inadvertent injections	Although rare, seizures may be a prominent feature in infants poisoned with local anesthetics. Inadvertent fetal anesthetic injection usually occurs in deliveries at the time of local anesthesia administered for episiotomy. The infant at birth has bradycardia, apnea, and hypotonia. Seizures usually occur within the first 6 hours and are generally tonic. The infants may have mydriasis and loss of lateral eye movements and pupillary light reflexes

Table 4-3. Hereditary metabolic and degenerative diseases associated with epilepsy

Aminoacidopathies
Organoacidopathies
Biotinidase deficiency
Pyridoxine dependency
Alper syndrome
Menke disease
Peroxisomal diseases
Mitochondrial diseases
Glucose transporter deficiency
Sulfite oxidase deficiency
3-Phosphogycerate dehydrogenase deficiency

After the history and physical examination, the appropriate diagnostic studies should be performed, and treatment for the seizures begun. Although the history and clinical examination will dictate which studies are most appropriate, in most cases, venous blood should be obtained for a complete blood cell count, glucose, electrolytes, ammonia, liver-function tests, bilirubin, and culture. If metabolic disease is suspected, arterial blood gases, serum amino acids, and urine organic acids should be obtained. A spinal-fluid examination is almost always indicated if the etiology of the seizures is not known. Neuroimaging, preferably with magnetic resonance imaging (MRI), can be very useful in evaluating the child for malformations of cortical development, intracranial hemorrhages, and cerebrovascular disorders such as neonatal stroke (Fig. 4-3).

All infants with suspected seizures should have an EEG, especially the paralyzed infant who cannot demonstrate abnormal movements. The EEG may confirm that stereotyped behavior is associated with electrical discharges. Conversely, if the behavior in question is not associated with EEG changes, the need for antiepileptic drugs may be eliminated.

Pyridoxine, 100 mg, should be given to all infants with neonatal seizures of unknown etiology. Pyridoxine-dependent epilepsy, characterized by a combination of various seizure types, usually occurs in the first hours of life and is unresponsive to standard anticonvulsants, responding only to immediate administration of pyridoxine hydrochloride. The dependence is permanent, and the

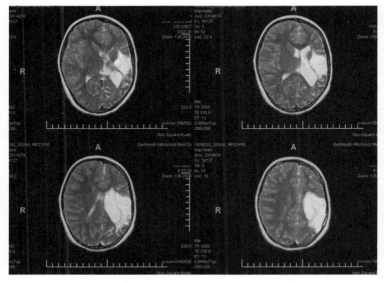

Fig. 4-3.   Example of a left middle cerebral infarction that occurred prenatally. Infant was initially seen with clonic seizures of the right hand.

interruption of daily pyridoxine supplementation leads to the recurrence of seizures. Some patients show developmental delay. Pipecolic acid (PA) and α-amino adipic semialdehyde (AASA) are markedly elevated in urine, plasma, and cerebrospinal fluid, and thus can be used as biomarkers of the disorder.

Pyridoxine-dependent seizures (PDSs) have mutations in the atiquitin (*ALDH7A1*) gene. Mutations abolish the activity of antiquitin as a Δ1–piperideine-6-carboxylate (P6C)-α-aminoadipic semialdehyde (α-AASA) dehydrogenase. The accumulating P6C inactivates pyridoxal-5′-phosphate (PLP), an essential cofactor in neurotransmitter metabolism.

G. Treatment

The decision to treat or not to treat is usually based on a number of factors, including duration and frequency of seizures; associated autonomic dysfunction, such as hypertension or apnea; etiology; and EEG abnormalities. Whether the treatment of neonatal seizures alters prognosis is not yet known; however, because outcome is related to etiology, the cause of the seizure must be identified and treated, if possible.

If seizures are brief and not associated with autonomic dysfunction, the clinician may decide not to treat or to treat with a short-acting benzodiazepine. Conversely, infants with frequent seizures, especially if the seizures interfere with ventilation, require prompt and vigorous treatment.

Despite significant advances in the treatment of epilepsy in older children and adults, treatment of neonatal seizures remains unsatisfactory. Phenobarbital and phenytoin are the primary drugs used in neonates, although neither is highly efficacious. Loading with 20 mg/kg of phenobarbital results in a serum level of approximately 20 mg/mL. It is recommended that phenobarbital be given in two 10-mg/kg boluses, with each bolus administered over a 5–minute period (2 to 3 mg/kg/min). If seizures persist, giving additional phenobarbital may be helpful. Phenytoin is typically used if phenobarbital is not effective and, like phenobarbital, is administered in two boluses of 10 mg/kg. Although hypotension and cardiac arrhythmias rarely occur with phenytoin administration in neonates, it is recommended that each bolus of phenytoin be given at a rate no faster than 2 mg/kg/min. This loading dose of 20 mg/kg results in blood levels of 15 to 20 mg/mL.

Infants requiring oral maintenance with antiepileptic drugs are given phenobarbital, 5 mg/kg/d. Because of increasing clearance of phenobarbital with age, trough-serum levels of the drug should be checked monthly, or more frequently if seizures continue. The combination of slow and incomplete absorption with rapid clearance of the drug makes it extremely difficult to administer phenytoin orally.

Other drugs, including diazepam, levetiracetam, lorazepam, primidone, topiramate, carbamazepine, lidocaine, and paraldehyde, have been tried in the treatment of neonatal seizures. However, little information is available regarding the efficacy of additional drugs after metabolic abnormalities are corrected, ventilation and perfusion are satisfactory, and loading with phenobarbital and phenytoin is complete.

H. Prognosis

By far the most significant factor in determining prognosis is the etiology of the seizures. For example, infants with seizures secondary to congenital brain malformations, hypoxia–ischemia, or postnatal meningitis do far worse than infants with seizures secondary to small subarachnoid hemorrhages or transient hypocalcemia.

The EEG is a powerful prognostic tool in neonates with seizures. For prognostic purposes, the background EEG patterns are more significant than the patterns of EEG epileptiform discharges. Infants with frequent or prolonged seizures generally have a poorer outcome than do infants with infrequent seizures. However, exceptions do occur; infants with benign familial neonatal seizures and benign neonatal convulsions often have very frequent seizures but have an excellent prognosis. Finally, infants with normal neurologic examinations at the time of discharge from the newborn unit do better than do infants with abnormal examinations.

II. BENIGN FAMILIAL NEONATAL CONVULSIONS

Unlike in older children, few epileptic syndromes have been described in neonates. This is because most neonatal seizures are not epilepsy but rather reactions to acute insults. However, five epileptic syndromes have been described in neonates and infants, three with favorable prognoses and two with poor outcomes: benign familial neonatal convulsions (also called *benign familial neonatal seizures*), benign neonatal convulsions, benign partial epilepsy of infancy, early infantile epileptic encephalopathy (EIEE), and early myoclonic epileptic encephalopathy (EMEE).

The diagnosis of benign familial neonatal convulsions in a neonate with seizures is based on five criteria: (a) normal neurologic examination, (b) negative evaluation for another etiology of the seizures, (c) normal developmental and intellectual outcome, (d) family history of newborn or infantile seizures with benign outcome, and (e) onset of seizures during the neonatal or early infantile period. Although most infants with seizures have them during the first week of life, a small percentage of patients have a later onset. This disorder represents one of the few legitimate epileptic syndromes of the neonate. Linkage analysis in large families of patients with benign neonatal convulsions has demonstrated two loci for the disorder, located on chromosomes 20q13.3 and 8q24. The genes encode voltage-gated K^+ channels expressed in the brain (*KCNQ2* and *KCNQ3*). The seizures are usually frequent for a few days and then stop. The infant is usually alert and vigorous between the seizures. Clonic seizures, focal or multifocal, are the most frequent seizure type, although generalized seizures have been reported. The seizures are generally brief, lasting for approximately 1 to 2 minutes, but they may occur as often as 20 to 30 times a day.

The interictal EEG is of little assistance in making the diagnosis of benign familial neonatal convulsions because it may or may not be abnormal. No specific diagnostic features have been reported. When abnormal, the findings are frequently transient. Ictal records are characterized by an initial flattening on the

EEG followed by bilateral discharges of spikes and sharp waves. This condition may represent a generalized seizure disorder.

III. BENIGN NEONATAL SEIZURES (NONFAMILIAL)

Benign neonatal *seizures (nonfamilial)*, are characterized by seizures occurring in term, otherwise healthy infants. The seizures are usually partial clonic in type, and they may be confined to one body part or migrate from one region to another. Apnea may occur with the clonic activity or be the sole manifestation of the seizure. The seizures often escalate into a crescendo of activity. Initially, the patient is normal between the seizures. The seizures then increase in frequency until the child goes into status epilepticus. The flurry of seizures usually lasts less than 24 hours, although less frequent seizures may continue for a few days.

A search for etiology is not revealing. Although the seizures may be very frequent, they usually resolve after a few days. Because the seizures often begin on the fifth day of life, some authors have described these seizures as "fifth-day fits."

Like benign familial neonatal convulsions, EEG findings in benign, idiopathic neonatal seizures have been variable. An EEG pattern thought to be associated with this syndrome has been described. The "theta pointu alternant" pattern consists of dominant theta activity that is discontinuous, unreactive, often asynchronous, and has intermixed sharp waves. However, the theta pointu alternant pattern is not specific for benign seizures and can be seen after a variety of neonatal encephalopathies.

Benign familial neonatal seizures and benign neonatal seizures (nonfamilial) are both diagnoses of exclusion. Even with a family history of benign neonatal seizures, other, more ominous, disorders should be ruled out.

IV. BENIGN PARTIAL EPILEPSY OF INFANCY

Benign partial epilepsy of infancy may begin during the first months of life, although median age at onset is 5 months. Seizures typically disappear within 3 months. The seizure type is complex partial seizures, which may or may not secondarily generalize. Decreased responsiveness, lateral eye deviation, and cyanosis are characteristic of the seizures. The interictal EEG is typically normal.

V. EARLY MYOCLONIC EPILEPTIC ENCEPHALOPATHY

Early myoclonic epileptic encephalopathy is a devastating condition characterized by frequent myoclonic seizures and a burst-suppression pattern on the EEG. Like EIEE, the syndrome can be caused by a number of etiologies. Nonketotic hyperglycinemia should be considered in patients with either EMEE or EIEE. The prognosis is quite poor, with most children either dying or evolving into infantile spasms or Lennox–Gastaut syndrome.

VI. EARLY INFANTILE EPILEPTIC ENCEPHALOPATHY OR OTAHARA SYNDROME

Otahara syndrome is a rare and devastating form of severe epileptic encephalopathy of early childhood. Tonic seizures occur 10 to 300 times per day. A burst-suppression EEG pattern is consistently present, awake and asleep. MRI scans reveal serious developmental anomalies. Progressive mental and neurologic deterioration occurs. Half of patients die within a few months. Survivors are severely impaired. No known therapies exist. Antiepileptic drugs and steroids do not have beneficial effects in these patients.

REFERENCES

1. Hirsch E, Velez A, Sellal F, et al. Electroclinical signs of benign neonatal familial convulsions. *Ann Neurol* 1993;34:835–841.
2. Holmes GL, Lombroso CT. Prognostic value of background patterns in the neonatal EEG. *J Clin Neurophysiol* 1993;10:323–352.
3. Holmes GL. Neonatal seizures. *Semin Pediatr Neurol* 1994;1: 72–82.
4. Leonard JV, Morris AA. Diagnosis and early management of inborn errors of metabolism presenting around the time of birth. *Acta Paediatr* 2006;95:6–14.
5. Lombroso CT, Holmes GL. Value of EEG in neonatal seizures. *J Epilepsy* 1993;6:39–70.
6. Miles DK, Holmes GL. Benign neonatal seizures. *J Clin Neurophysiol* 1990;7:369–379.
7. Mills PB, Struys E, Jakobs C, et al. Mutations in antiquitin in individuals with pyridoxine-dependent seizures. *Nat Med* 2006; 12:307–309.
8. Mizrahi EM, Kellaway P. Characterization and classification of neonatal seizures. *Neurology* 1987;37:1837–1844.
9. Okumura A, Watanabe K, Negoro T, Hayakawa F, Kato T, Natsume J. The clinical characterizations of benign partial epilepsy in infancy. *Neuropediatrics* 2006;37:359–363.
10. Painter J, Pippenger C, Wasterlain C, et al. Phenobarbital and phenytoin in neonatal seizures: metabolism and tissue distribution. *Neurology* 1981;31:1107–1112.
11. Plecko B, Paul K, Paschke E, et al. Biochemical and molecular characterization of 18 patients with pyridoxine-dependent epilepsy and mutations of the antiquitin (ALDH7A1) gene. *Hum Mutat* 2007;28:19–26.
12. Ryan SG. Ion channels and the genetic contribution to epilepsy. *J Child Neurol* 1999;14:59–66.
13. Scher MS. Neonatal seizures. In Wyllie E, ed. *The treatment of epilepsy: principles and practice*. Philadelphia: Lippincott Williams & Wilkins, 2001:577–600.

Epilepsies with Onset during Infancy (2 to 12 Months)

The epilepsies and epilepsy syndromes with onset during infancy (2 to 12 months) and accompanying seizure types are listed in Table 5-1.

I. SYMPTOMATIC AND PROBABLY SYMPTOMATIC FOCAL EPILEPSIES

Focal/symptomatic epilepsies can occur at any age. Three seizure types occur with these epilepsies: simple partial (focal); complex partial (psychomotor, temporal lobe); and tonic–clonic (grand mal). The clinical and electroencephalographic (EEG) features of these three seizure types are reviewed in Chapter 2. Differential diagnostic entities to consider in children and adults when diagnosing these seizure types are listed in Chapter 2 and reviewed in Chapter 9.

Depending on locus of onset, five symptomatic and probably symptomatic epilepsy syndromes have been recognized (Table 5-1). Clinical and EEG features, management, and prognosis of these syndromes are reviewed in Chapter 3.

One special symptomatic focal epilepsy deserves special consideration. The *hemiconvulsion–hemiplegia syndrome* (HHS) is a rare form of symptomatic epilepsy that usually begins during the first 2 years of life. A sudden and prolonged unilateral clonic seizure is followed by unilateral hemiparesis. The event occurs suddenly in an otherwise healthy child. In 80% of patients, unilateral seizures later develop to complete the *hemiconvulsion-hemiplegia epilepsy syndrome* (HHES). Perhaps because of better treatment of status epilepticus, the condition is now rare.

II. GENERALIZED/SYMPTOMATIC EPILEPSIES

Four generalized/symptomatic epilepsies (West syndrome, tonic seizures, atonic seizures, and Lennox–Gastaut syndrome) are true age-dependent epileptic conditions. West syndrome and Lennox–Gastaut syndrome always begin during early childhood, and the vast majority of patients with tonic and atonic seizures have seizure onset during the first year of life.

These conditions are classified as generalized seizures because the clinical and EEG features typically suggest widespread involvement of the cortex. However, in many of these patients, the seizures have a partial onset with rapid secondary generalization.

A. West Syndrome (Infantile Spasms)

Clinical and EEG features of seizures in children vary as a function of age. A good example of these age-related phenomena is infantile spasms, a unique seizure disorder confined to early childhood; infantile spasms are an age-specific disorder occurring in children only during the first 2 years of life. The peak age at onset is between 4 and 6 months, and approximately 90% of

Table 5-1.   Groups of specific epilepsy syndromes and specific epilepsy syndromes with onset during infancy (2–12 months) and accompanying seizure types

I. Symptomatic and probably symptomatic focal epilepsies
   A. Mesial temporal lobe epilepsy syndromes (SPS, CPS, TCS)
   B. Lateral temporal lobe epilepsy syndromes (SPS, CPS, TCS)
   C. Frontal lobe epilepsy syndromes (SPS, CPS, TCS)
   D. Parietal lobe epilepsy syndromes (SPS, CPS, TCS)
   E. Occipital lobe epilepsy syndromes (SPS, CPS, TCS)
II. Generalized/symptomatic epilepsies
   A. West syndrome (infantile spasms) (spasm)
   B. Tonic seizures (TON)
   C. Atonic seizures (ATO)
   D. Lennox–Gastaut syndrome (TON, TCS, MYO, ABS, ATO)
III. Generalized, either idiopathic or symptomatic
   A. Benign myoclonic epilepsy of infancy (MYO)
   B. Severe myoclonic epilepsy of infancy (MYO, SPS, TCS, ABS)
   C. Myoclonic–astatic epilepsy syndrome (MYO, ATO)
IV. Seizures not necessarily requiring a diagnosis of epilepsy: febrile convulsions (TCS, TON)

ABS, absence seizure; ATO, atonic seizure; CPS, complex partial (psychomotor, temporal lobe) seizures; MYO, myoclonic seizure; SPS, simple partial (focal) seizure; TCS, tonic–clonic (grand mal) seizure; TON, tonic seizure.

infantile spasms begin before 12 months of age. The incidence of infantile spasms is estimated at 0.4 in 1,000 live births.

1. Definition

The characteristic features of this syndrome are myoclonic seizures, hypsarrhythmic EEG, and mental retardation. This triad is sometimes referred to as *West syndrome.* As will be seen, however, not all cases conform strictly to this definition. The disorder is also referred to in the literature as *massive spasms, salaam seizures, flexion spasms, jackknife seizures, massive myoclonic jerks,* and *infantile myoclonic seizures.*

2. Seizure Phenomena

Infantile spasms may vary considerably in their clinical manifestations. Some seizures are characterized by brief head nods; other seizures consist of violent flexion of the trunk, arms, and legs. The diagnosis may often be delayed because the parents and even the family physician may not recognize spasms as seizures. What usually does not vary is that in each child, the spasms are stereotyped. In addition, spasms characteristically occur in flurries.

Although it resembles a myoclonic or tonic seizure, the spasm is a distinct type of seizure. A myoclonic jerk is a rapid, shocklike contraction of limited duration, whereas the tonic seizure is a prolonged muscle contraction of growing intensity. The true spasm consists of a characteristic muscular contraction that lasts from 1 to 2 seconds and reaches a peak more slowly than a myoclonic jerk, but more rapidly than a tonic seizure.

The seizures in infantile spasms are of three types: flexor, extensor, and mixed flexor–extensor. Flexor spasms consist of brief contractions of flexor musculature of the neck, trunk, arms, and legs. Spasms of the muscles of the upper limbs result either in adduction of the arms in a self-hugging motion or in abduction of the arms to either side of the head with the arms flexed at the elbow. Extensor spasms consist predominantly of extensor muscle contractions, producing abrupt extension of the neck and trunk with extensor abduction or adduction of the arms, legs, or both. Mixed flexor–extensor spasms include flexion of the neck, trunk, and arms and extension of the legs, or flexion of the legs and extension of the arms with varying degrees of flexion of the neck and trunk. Asymmetric spasms occasionally occur and resemble a fencing posture. Infantile spasms are frequently associated with eye deviation or nystagmus.

Asymmetric spasms can be seen when the muscular contractions do not occur simultaneously on the two sides of the body. This type of spasm is usually observed in symptomatic infants with severe brain lesions, agenesis of the corpus callosum, or both. Focal signs, such as eye or head deviation, may accompany symmetric and asymmetric spasms. Asymmetric spasms generally are isolated, but they can also follow or precede a partial seizure, or sometimes appear simultaneously with a partial or generalized seizure.

Infantile spasms frequently occur in clusters, and the intensity and frequency of the spasms in each cluster may increase to a peak before progressively decreasing. The number of spasms per cluster varies considerably, with some clusters having more than 30 spasms. The number of clusters per day also varies, with some patients having more than 20 clusters per day. Clusters can occur at night, although they rarely occur during sleep. Crying or irritability during or after a flurry of spasms is commonly observed.

3. Electroencephalographic Phenomena

Infantile spasms are associated with markedly abnormal EEGs. The most commonly seen interictal pattern is hypsarrhythmia, which consists of very high-voltage, random, slow waves and multifocal spikes and sharp waves (Fig. 5-1). The chaotic appearance of the EEG abnormality gives the impression of total disorganization of cortical voltage and rhythms. During sleep, bursts of polyspike and slow waves occur. Somewhat surprising, in view of the marked background abnormalities, is the persistence of sleep spindles in some patients. During rapid eye movement (REM) sleep, a marked diminution or complete disappearance of the hypsarrhythmic pattern may diminish markedly or disappear. Infantile spasms are associated with a decrease of the total sleep time, as well as a decrease in REM sleep. Variations in hypsarrhythmia have been described, including patterns with interhemispheric synchrony, a consistent focus of abnormal discharge, episodes of attenuation, and high-voltage slow activity with few sharp waves or spikes. The variant patterns of hypsarrhythmia are frequent and do not correlate with prognosis.

Although a hypsarrhythmic or modified hypsarrhythmic pattern is the most common type of interictal abnormality seen in

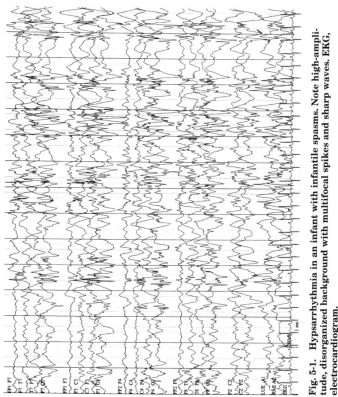

Fig. 5-1. Hypsarrhythmia in an infant with infantile spasms. Note high-amplitude, disorganized background with multifocal spikes and sharp waves. EKG, electrocardiogram.

infantile spasms, this EEG pattern may not be present in some patients with infantile spasms. Some patients with infantile spasms do not have hypsarrhythmia early in the course of the disorder, but the pattern develops later. Although hypsarrhythmia is primarily associated with infantile spasms, it occurs in other disorders as well.

Like the interictal pattern, the ictal EEG changes during infantile spasms are variable. The most characteristic ictal EEG pattern of the spasms consists of a positive wave over the vertex-central region; low-amplitude fast (14 to 16 Hz) activity, or a diffuse flattening, called *decremental activity*, may also be seen.

The presence of focal features is one of the variations of the basic hypsarrhythmic patterns and may be associated with partial seizures. Partial seizures may precede, accompany, or follow the cluster of spasms. This observation suggests that cortical "pacemakers" may be important in the development of infantile spasms.

EEGs are not static in this disorder and may evolve over time. Some patients with spasms may not have hypsarrhythmia at the onset of their disorder. Other patients may have slow EEG recordings with rare epileptiform activity that then develops into hypsarrhythmic patterns. Follow-up EEG recordings may be necessary to demonstrate hypsarrhythmia.

4. Basic Mechanisms

The clinical and ictal EEG features of infantile spasms are suggestive of a generalized seizure disorder, yet some children with infantile spasms respond to surgical removal of a cortical lesion. For that reason, the brainstem, which has widespread projections throughout the central nervous system, has been implicated as playing an important role in the genesis of infantile spasms. An underlying disruption of neuronal function within specific nuclei of the pontine reticular formation could result in interference with descending pathways that exert control over spinal reflexes and result in infantile spasms. In addition, the hypsarrhythmic EEG pattern could be the result of abnormal input to the thalamic and cortical neurons through ascending projections.

5. Differential Diagnosis

Because infantile spasms differ significantly from the clinical features of other seizures in young children, it is not surprising that parents and primary caregivers may miss the diagnosis. Yet the pediatrician or family physician rarely has the opportunity actually to see the spasms and must depend on the description by the parents. With increasing use of home videotaping and greater awareness of the problem, the delay in diagnosis is being reduced. Occasionally, the clinical course is atypical, and the spasms do not occur in clusters, or involve only slight movements or episodes of akinesia. In these patients, the EEG is helpful, because it is invariably abnormal.

A few other conditions may be confused with infantile spasms. *Early myoclonic epileptic encephalopathy* (EMEE) and *early infantile epileptic encephalopathy* (EIEE) have a clinical similarity to infantile spasms. EMEE is characterized clinically by the occurrence of sporadic and erratic fragmentary myoclonus, usually in association with other seizure types. The seizures usually begin in the neonatal period. The EEG demonstrates burst-suppression. A variety of etiologic agents have been associated with the disorder, including metabolic diseases, cerebral dysgenesis, and hypoxic–ischemic insults. The prognosis in the disorder is severe; most infants die within 1 year or have severe neurologic sequelae.

EIEE, also termed *Ohtahara syndrome*, is reviewed in Chapter 4.

Benign nonepileptic infantile spasms is a syndrome that begins in infancy with flexion spasms. However, the syndrome differs from West syndrome by the absence of mental retardation or regression and the presence of normal EEGs during both wakefulness and sleep.

Benign neonatal sleep myoclonus, which was discussed with neonatal seizures, in Chapter 4, section **I.D**, may be confused with infantile spasms. The EEG is very helpful in distinguishing the two conditions.

6. Etiology

On the basis of history, physical examination, and laboratory studies, cases of infantile spasms have been conventionally classified into those in which no preceding neurologic disorder or identified etiologic factor (idiopathic) is apparent, and those in which a preexisting, presumptively responsible pathologic event or disorder is demonstrated (symptomatic cases). Some authors use another category, cryptogenic, to refer to children who have developmental delay or an abnormal neurologic examination before the onset of spasms, but in whom an etiology cannot be sufficiently identified.

As can be seen in Table 5-2, infantile spasms have been associated with a wide variety of etiologies. Virtually any disorder that can cause brain damage can be associated with infantile spasms. Infantile spasms are particularly prevalent among children with tuberous sclerosis complex, and tuberous sclerosis complex (TSC) accounts for up to 25% of infantile spasms cases. TSC is a congenital syndrome characterized by the widespread development of benign tumors in multiple organs, somewhat different that those seen in classic West syndrome. In TSC, focal seizures can precede, coexist with, or evolve into infantile spasms. EEG features of focal or multifocal spikes are most common when seizures are first identified, with hypsarrhythmia (often with focal features) evolving later.

TSC is difficult to diagnose during the first year of life because the characteristic skin lesion, adenoma sebaceum, never occurs before the age of 3 years. However, infants may have hypopigmented areas on the skin, which may be detectable only by using a Wood's lamp. If the diagnosis is suspected, further evidence for the disorder can come from a computed tomography (CT) scan, which may demonstrate intracranial calcifications; abdominal ultrasound, which may detect polycystic kidneys; or echocardiogram, which may demonstrate cardiac tumors. Magnetic

Table 5-2. Etiologic factors associated with infantile spasms

Prenatal
  Congenital cerebral anomalies
    Hydrocephalus
    Microcephaly
    Hydranencephaly
    Schizencephaly
    Polymicrogyria
    Sturge–Weber
    Incontinentia pigmenti
    Tuberous sclerosis
    Down syndrome
    Aicardi syndrome
    Hypoxic–ischemic encephalopathies
    Congenital infections
    Trauma
Perinatal
  Hypoxic–ischemic encephalopathies
  Meningitis
  Encephalitis
  Trauma
  Intracranial hemorrhages
Postnatal
  Neurometabolic disturbances
    Nonketotic hyperglycinemia
    Maple syrup urine disease
    Phenylketonuria
    Mitochondrial disorders
  Meningitis
  Encephalitis
  Degenerative disorders

resonance imaging (MRI) may show cortical tubers, although calcium is not well visualized by using this technique (Fig. 5-2). TSC is caused by mutations in one of the tumor-suppressor genes, *TSC1* or *TSC2*. About 80% of affected patients have a new mutation, and the remaining 20% have inherited a *TSC* gene mutation from a parent.

Aicardi syndrome should be considered in girls with infantile spasms. In addition to infantile spasms, girls have absence or partial absence of the corpus callosum, dorsal vertebral anomalies, and chorioretinal lacunar defects. The ocular lesions are frequently associated with colobomas of the optic nerve and microphthalmia. The syndrome appears to be X-linked, occurring primarily in girls. Another form of X-linked infantile spasms occurring in boys has been reported.

A controversy exists as to whether pertussis immunization can lead to infantile spasms. The vaccine is given at the time of peak incidence of infantile spasms, and therefore, a temporal coincidence would be expected in a large number of cases. In addition, determining the exact time of onset of the spasms is

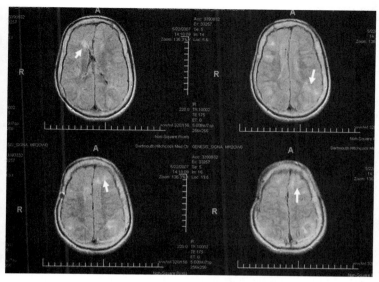

Fig. 5-2.   MRI of a child with tuberous sclerosis who was first seen with infantile spasms. *Arrows* **point to cortical tubers.**

often difficult. However, when closely documented cases are reviewed, the link between the pertussis vaccine and infantile spasms is quite weak. It remains possible that in a small number of children, especially if a striking neurologic reaction has occurred within 24 hours after the immunization, a causal relation exists. It is also possible that in some cases, the vaccine acts in conjunction with other, unidentified factors to precipitate the clinical onset of symptoms in children already predisposed to the disease. An acellular pertussis vaccine appears to reduce significantly the risk of adverse events associated with the vaccine.

The finding that some infants with neurologic disorders have infantile spasms, whereas others with similar brain disturbances do not, suggests that genetic susceptibility may be important.

7. Management

The infant with infantile spasms requires a thorough evaluation, including a developmental assessment, neurologic examination, and laboratory studies to try to determine etiology. In addition, the neurologic and developmental examinations at the time of diagnosis are important indicators of prognosis.

The skin should be closely inspected for hypopigmented lesions, which can occur in tuberous sclerosis. These lesions often cannot be seen unless the infant is examined with a Wood's lamp in a darkened room.

The laboratory studies needed are determined largely by the history and physical examination. Every child with a possible diagnosis of infantile spasms should have an EEG and neuroimaging. A normal EEG raises questions about the diagnosis and suggests that the child has benign myoclonus of early infancy.

An MRI is recommended in every patient with infantile spasms, because these studies may provide valuable information regarding the etiology. For example, cranial calcifications may indicate tuberous sclerosis or a congenital infection. In addition, brain anomalies such as agenesis of the corpus callosum, porencephaly, and hydranencephaly will be apparent on MRI. Abnormal neuroimaging occurs in 70% to 80% of patients with infantile spasms. The most common abnormality seen in large series is diffuse cerebral atrophy. Because ACTH can result in transient atrophy in the brain, it is recommended that the MRI be obtained before ACTH treatment.

Because pyridoxine dependency has rarely been associated with infantile spasms in children in whom an etiology cannot be definitely established, an infusion of 100 to 200 mg of pyridoxine intravenously during EEG monitoring may be useful. Infants with pyridoxine dependency should have an improvement in the seizures and EEG within minutes. Testing for pyridoxine dependency is discussed in Chapter 4.

Infants with seizures for which no adequate explanation can be found should undergo a metabolic evaluation. This includes urine and serum amino acid screening, serum ammonia, organic acid, lactate, pyruvate, and liver-function tests. A spinal-fluid examination should include glucose (which should be compared with a serum glucose level), protein, and cell count. Cerebrospinal fluid, amino acids, pyruvate, and lactate should be tested in children when metabolic disease is suspected. Because most children are given corticotropin (adrenocorticotropic hormone, ACTH), electrolytes, calcium, phosphorus, glucose, and urinalysis should be done.

8. *Treatment*

A. CORTICOTROPIN AND CORTICOSTEROIDS. Corticotropin (ACTH) and corticosteroids are the primary drugs used in the treatment of infantile spasms. Vigabatrin is an appropriate choice in children with infantile spasms secondary to tuberous sclerosis. Studies exist that indicate felbamate, lamotrigine, levetiracetam, tiagabine, topiramate, zonisamide, and vigabatrin may be effective for infantile spasms. However, none of these drugs has been proven effective in blinded, controlled studies.

The effects of ACTH and other therapies on long-term outcome remain controversial. For example, several authors have found no developmental differences between patients who did receive treatment and those who did not. For the large number of infants who exhibit preexisting brain damage, it is unlikely that any form of therapy will greatly influence the long-range outcome in terms of mental and motor development. The important question is whether the type of treatment for infantile spasms in children who were normal before the onset of the spasms, or who have a cryptogenic cause for the spasms, alters outcome. The majority of evidence suggests that treatment with

ACTH results in a lower incidence of seizures and better psychomotor development than does treatment with oral steroids, such as prednisone, or other antiepileptic drugs.

The dosage for treatment with corticosteroids or ACTH and the length of time treatment should continue have not been established. In view of the lack of consensus regarding dosage and treatment duration, the following approach is necessarily empiric. The recommended starting dose of ACTH is 40 IU per day given intramuscularly. A nonsynthetic form of ACTH gel should be used. If the seizures do not completely resolve by 2 weeks, the dose should be increased by 10-IU increments every week until the seizures cease or a daily dosage of 80 IU is reached. The ACTH is given for a minimum of 1 month after the cessation of seizures. At that time, a taper can begin, decreasing by 10 IU per week. Other clinicians start with a higher dose (150 IU/m^2/24 h, divided twice daily, followed by a gradual taper over a 2- to 4-week period). If the seizures persist despite administration of the maximum dose of ACTH, a trial of valproic acid or nitrazepam is recommended. If relapse occurs during the taper or after discontinuation of ACTH, the ACTH should be restarted at the dose that originally stopped the spasms. After the seizures have been controlled, the ACTH should be continued for a minimum of 1 month before tapering is attempted again. The response to ACTH is sometimes very dramatic, with cessation of seizures and marked improvement of the EEG within a few days.

Although treatment with ACTH and corticosteroids can be very effective in stopping spasms, it can result in many side effects, some of which can be very serious. Steroid therapy is invariably associated with cushingoid obesity. In addition, growth retardation, acne, and irritability may ensue. In short-term use of ACTH, these side effects are of no major concern. More serious side effects include infection, arterial hypertension, intracerebral hemorrhages, osteoporosis, gastrointestinal bleeding, hypokalemic alkalosis, and other electrolyte disturbances.

Children treated with ACTH or adrenal corticosteroids should be closely monitored. Twice-weekly blood pressure measurements and checks on stool guaiac, as well as periodic checks of electrolyte levels, should be performed. If hypertension or hypokalemic alkalosis develops, a reduction in dose is recommended. However, patients who have a relapse once the dose is decreased may be restarted on the effective dose and managed with antihypertensives, salt restriction, or both. If this is not effective, changing to synthetic glucocorticoids (methylprednisolone) that have a smaller sodium-retaining effect is prudent. Fever should be investigated promptly.

B. LAMOTRIGINE, LEVETIRACETAM, FELBAMATE, TIAGABINE, VALPROIC ACID, AND TOPIRAMATE. These medications have all been reported to be effective for infantile spasms and are available in the United States.

C. VIGABATRIN. Vigabatrin appears to be effective in children with tuberous sclerosis complex who have infantile spasms. It can also be used in children with infantile spasms caused by other etiologies. However, a serious risk exists for vigabatrin-associated retinal toxicity likely from intracellular accumulation of γ-aminobutyric acid (GABA) in amacrine cells of the retina. This toxicity results in visual field defects that may be irreversible. Because of this serious side effect, vigabatrin is used cautiously and for as short a period as possible in children with infantile spasms. The drug is not currently marketed in the United States.

D. SURGERY. Infants with intractable infantile spasms who have evidence of focal lesions may benefit from surgery. However, case reports exist of infants with focal lesions associated with infantile spasms and hypsarrhythmia who responded to medication or resolved spontaneously. Therefore, surgery should be contemplated only if antiepileptic drugs, including ACTH, are not effective. The early success of focal resections in cases of infantile spasms is a promising approach. However, further studies evaluating the long-term outcome of infants undergoing surgery are necessary.

9. Prognosis

Infantile spasms are among the most devastating seizure disorders to affect infants. The poor prognosis has been confirmed in virtually all follow-up studies. A significant number of infants demonstrate psychomotor retardation and continue to have seizures. In addition, a large number of patients have neurologic abnormalities on examination. Because a substantial majority of patients have brain injury before the onset of the spasms, it is not surprising that the prognosis is so poor. In all likelihood, these children would have had similar neurologic outcomes without the infantile spasms.

Prognosis is directly related to etiology. Authors who have coded their cases as symptomatic and idiopathic have found that idiopathic cases have a significantly better prognosis. Cryptogenic cases have a significantly better prognosis than do symptomatic cases. However, patients with Down syndrome typically respond well to therapy. Patients who are classified as doubtful usually have outcomes similar to the symptomatic cases. Neurologic status before the onset of infantile spasms is an important prognostic factor. Children with normal neurologic examinations and development have a much better prognosis than infants with developmental delay and abnormal neurologic examinations. A poor prognostic sign reported by some authors is early onset (before 6 months). However, age at onset appears to be related to etiology; the onset of the spasms is at a younger age in children with symptomatic etiologies than in those with cryptogenic etiologies. The occurrence of other types of seizures, in addition to the spasms and focal interictal EEG abnormalities, has been associated with a poor prognosis. In addition, reappearance of hypsarrhythmia between consecutive spasms in a cluster has been considered a favorable feature. Finally, some evidence exists that early cessation of the spasms is of prognostic significance. Therefore, early diagnosis and treatment are important.

In some children, the seizures evolve into other seizure types such as Lennox–Gastaut syndrome. Often, the tonic seizures in this syndrome are virtually identical to the tonic seizures seen with infantile spasms. The similarities of clinical and EEG features in the two syndromes strengthen the hypothesis that the two syndromes represent age-related manifestations of similar epileptogenic processes.

B. Tonic and Atonic Seizures

1. Definitions

Tonic seizures are brief seizures consisting of the sudden onset of increased tone in the extensor muscles. If standing, the patient typically falls to the ground. The duration of the seizures is longer than that of myoclonic seizures. Electromyographic activity is dramatically increased in tonic seizures. Conversely, atonic seizures consist of the sudden loss of muscle tone. The loss of muscle tone may be confined to a group of muscles, such as the neck, resulting in a head drop, or it may involve all trunk muscles, leading to a fall to the ground.

Although occasionally tonic and atonic seizures can be the only types of seizures experienced by the child, the majority of children with these seizure types have the Lennox–Gastaut syndrome, which is discussed briefly in section **II.C** and in detail in Chapter 6.

2. Seizure Phenomena

Tonic seizures frequently begin with a tonic contraction of the neck muscles, leading to fixation of the head in an erect position, widely opened eyes, and jaw clenching or mouth opening. Contraction of the respiratory and abdominal muscles often follows and may lead to a high-pitched cry and brief periods of apnea. The tonic contractions may extend to the proximal musculature of the upper limbs, elevating the shoulders and abducting the arms. Asymmetric tonic seizures vary, from a slight rotation of the head to a tonic contraction of all the musculature of one side of the body. Occasionally, tonic seizures terminate with a clonic phase. Eyelid retraction, staring, mydriasis, and apnea are commonly associated with the motor activity and may be the most prominent features. The seizures may cause falls and injuries.

Tonic seizures are typically activated by sleep and may occur repetitively throughout the night. They are much more frequent during non-REM sleep than during wakefulness and usually do not occur during REM sleep. During tonic seizures, the patient is unconscious, although arousal from light sleep may occur. Because these seizures can be very brief, they often go undetected. Tonic seizures are usually brief, lasting from a few seconds to 1 minute, with an average duration of about 10–20 seconds. In seizures lasting longer than a few seconds, impairment of consciousness is usually apparent. Postictal impairment, with confusion, tiredness, and headache, is common. The degree of postictal impairment is usually related to the duration of the seizure.

Atonic seizures begin suddenly and without warning and cause the patient, if standing, to fall quickly to the floor. Because the lack of tone may be complete, the child has no means of self-protection, and injuries often occur. The attack may be fragmentary and lead to dropping of the head with slackening of the jaw or dropping of a limb. In atonic seizures, a loss of electromyographic activity occurs. Consciousness is impaired during the fall, although the patient may regain alertness immediately on hitting the floor.

Although tonic and atonic seizures can occur at all ages and, therefore, are not as age-dependent as are infantile spasms, they typically begin during childhood. Atonic seizures are common in Lennox–Gastaut syndrome, but they are usually less frequent than tonic and myoclonic seizures.

3. Electroencephalographic Phenomena

The interictal EEG of patients with tonic seizures is usually quite abnormal, consisting of slowing of the background, with multifocal spikes, sharp waves, and bursts of irregular spike-and-wave activity. The ictal EEG manifestations of tonic seizures usually consist of bilateral synchronous spikes of 10 to 25 Hz of medium to high voltage, with a frontal accentuation. Simple flattening or desynchronization may also occur. Occasionally, multiple spike-and-wave or diffuse slow activity may occur during a tonic seizure.

Atonic seizures are usually associated with rhythmic spike-and-wave complexes varying from slow (1 to 2 Hz) to more-rapid, irregular spike activity or multiple spike-and-wave activity. In myoclonic–astatic seizures, the EEG pattern consists of bilaterally synchronous, regular, or irregular 2- to 3-Hz spike-and-wave activity, and the background activity exhibits an excess of monomorphic theta activity.

4. Basic Mechanisms

Although tonic and atonic seizures are classified as generalized seizures, in some patients, a focal onset to the ictus can be detected that rapidly generalizes to involve diffuse cortical structures. Tonic seizures often begin in the frontal lobe, which accounts for the intense motor activity seen during these seizures. Because of the sudden loss of muscle tone, it has been surmised that atonic seizures involve brainstem structures.

5. Differential Diagnosis

Tonic seizures are usually not difficult to diagnose. Sometimes children with very severe encephalopathies have episodes of opisthotonic posturing that may resemble tonic seizures. Recording an episode usually helps distinguish the two events; tonic seizures are associated with spike–wave discharges or a discharge of rapid spikes, whereas no epileptiform discharges should be seen during opisthotonic posturing.

Paroxysmal choreoathetosis refers to a rare, usually familial disorder characterized by episodic attacks of severe dystonia, choreoathetosis, or both. Two types have been described: *paroxysmal dystonic choreoathetosis of Mount and Reback* and *paroxysmal kinesigenic choreoathetosis*. In paroxysmal dystonic choreoathetosis, the patient has a sudden onset of severe, often painful dystonia that may affect the arms, legs, or trunk and speech. Consciousness is not impaired during the attacks, which last from minutes to hours and are often precipitated by alcohol, caffeine, excitement, stress, or fatigue. The disorder is inherited through an autosomal-dominant pattern. Paroxysmal kinesigenic choreoathetosis is characterized by the sudden assumption of dystonic posturing or choreoathetosis. The kinesigenic attacks are usually shorter in duration than the dystonic form and are frequently induced by sudden movements or a startle. These attacks can occur hundreds of times daily.

Atonic seizures on occasion may be confused with pallid infantile syncope (which is discussed in Chapter 9). *Spasmus nutans* refers to a disorder occurring in toddlers that is characterized by head tilt, head nodding, and nystagmus, which is often asymmetric. The head nodding may be confused with atonic seizures. Spasmus nutans is usually a self-limiting condition, disappearing after a period of 4 months to several years.

6. Etiology

As with infantile spasms, virtually any disorder that can lead to brain damage may result in tonic and atonic seizures. Common etiologies include hypoxic–ischemic encephalopathy, head injuries, encephalitis, strokes, congenital brain anomalies, and metabolic disturbances.

7. Management

As with infantile spasms, the laboratory studies needed are determined largely by the history and physical examination. Every child with tonic or atonic seizures should have an EEG and neuroimaging. A normal EEG is very unusual in patients with atonic and tonic seizures and should suggest another diagnosis. MRI is useful in screening for congenital brain anomalies, congenital infections, and metabolic disturbances. Patients without an adequate explanation for the seizures should also have metabolic screening, including urine and serum amino acid screening, serum ammonia, organic acid, lactate, pyruvate, and liver-function tests. A spinal-fluid examination should include glucose (which should be compared with a serum glucose level), protein, and cell count. Cerebrospinal fluid amino acids, pyruvate, and lactate should be obtained in children when metabolic disease is suspected.

8. Treatment

Treatment of tonic and atonic seizures presents the clinician with a difficult task. Complete seizure control is rarely achieved. Because of the intractable nature of the seizures and their mixed types, a tendency exists to give the child numerous antiepileptic drugs. This polypharmaceutical approach rarely results in good seizure control and usually causes toxic reactions—fatigue, nausea, and ataxia—from the cumulative effect of the drugs. Valproic acid, felbamate, lamotrigine, the benzodiazepines, and topiramate have been efficacious in some patients. The ketogenic diet should also be considered if antiepileptic drugs are not effective (see Chapter 10 for details).

9. Prognosis

The vast majority of children with atonic and tonic seizures have the Lennox–Gastaut syndrome. In general, this syndrome is associated with a poor prognosis.

C. Lennox–Gastaut Syndrome

The Lennox–Gastaut syndrome is characterized by a mixed seizure disorder of which tonic seizures are a major component, as well as a slow spike-and-wave EEG pattern. The syndrome always begins in childhood and is often accompanied by mental retardation. The syndrome usually has onset between infancy and age 7 years. It is reviewed in detail in Chapter 6.

III. GENERALIZED/IDIOPATHIC OR SYMPTOMATIC EPILEPSIES

A. Benign Myoclonic Epilepsy of Infancy

Benign myoclonic epilepsy in infancy is characterized by the occurrence of brief myoclonic seizures occurring in otherwise normal infants and toddlers between the ages of 4 months and 3 years. The myoclonic seizures are always brief and usually involve the arms and head, but not the legs. The frequency and intensity of the seizures is variable. Other seizure types do not develop.

The interictal EEG in the condition is usually normal. Myoclonic jerks are associated with generalized spike-and-wave or polyspike-and-wave activity. The frequency of the discharges is greater than 3 Hz, and discharges usually last 1 to 3 seconds. Some bursts of spike-and-wave activity occur rarely during the awake state without any accompanying clinical changes. Photosensitivity occurs in some of the patients. Some patients have generalized spike-and-wave discharges only during sleep. Sleep organization appears to be normal.

B. Severe Myoclonic Epilepsy of Infancy or Dravet Syndrome

Severe myoclonic epilepsy in infancy, also termed Dravet syndrome, is a disorder that typically begins during the first year of life as a febrile seizure that is either generalized or unilateral. The febrile seizures tend to be long and recurrent. Between 1 and 4 years of age, myoclonic seizures develop. Partial seizures often occur as well. Psychomotor development is typically delayed from the second year of life, and ataxia, corticospinal tract dysfunction, and nonepileptic myoclonus may occur. The epilepsy is very resistant to all forms of treatment, and the children are mentally retarded.

At the time of the first febrile seizure, the EEG is usually normal and without any paroxysmal abnormalities. Between ages 1 and 2 years, the myoclonic seizures begin. The myoclonus can be massive, involving whole muscles, particularly the axial ones, or be barely discernible. The jerks can be isolated or occur in flurries. On EEG monitoring, generalized spike-and-wave or polyspike-and-wave activity is seen during the seizures. When absence seizures occur, they are also associated with generalized spike-and-wave activity. The generalized discharges increase during drowsiness. Focal and multifocal spikes and sharp waves are also seen. De novo truncating mutations of the *SCN1A* gene on chromosome 2p24 in coding for the neuronal voltage-gated sodium channel α_1 subunit have been found in severe myoclonic epilepsy in infancy. Interestingly, inherited missense mutations of the same gene will result in generalized epilepsy, febrile seizures plus (GEFS+) (see Chapter 8).

C. Myoclonic–Astatic Epilepsy Syndrome

Atonic attacks may be associated with myoclonic jerks before, during, or after the atonic seizure. This combination has been described as myoclonic–astatic seizures, also known as Doose syndrome. In this syndrome, astatic (defined as the inability to stand) seizures occur suddenly, without warning, and the child collapses onto the floor as if his or her legs had been pulled out from under. No apparent loss of consciousness accompanies these seizures. At times, the astatic seizures are so short that only a brief nodding of the head and slight flexion of the knees is seen. The myoclonic seizures in this disorder are characterized by symmetric jerking of the arms and shoulders, with simultaneous nodding of the head. Some myoclonic jerks are violent, with the arms flung upward; some are so mild that they are easier to feel than to see. A combination of myoclonic and astatic seizures is frequently observed. In these children, the loss of postural tone is immediately preceded by myoclonic jerks—hence the term *myoclonic–astatic seizures*.

The onset of the disorder takes place between the first and fifth years of age and occurs in boys more frequently than in girls. With few exceptions, the mental and motor development of the children is normal before the onset of the disorder. However, in some children, the prognosis is unfavorable, and dementia may occur. Absence status is reported to play a role in the pathogenesis of the dementia.

IV. SEIZURES NOT NECESSARILY REQUIRING A DIAGNOSIS OF EPILEPSY: FEBRILE CONVULSIONS

Febrile convulsions usually occur between ages 6 months and 5 years. Febrile convulsions are reviewed in Chapter 8.

REFERENCES

1. Chiron C, Dumas C, Jambaque I, et al. Randomized trial comparing vigabatrin and hydrocortisone in infantile spasms due to tuberous sclerosis. *Epilepsy Res* 1997;26:389–395.
2. Claes S, Devriendt K, Lagae L, et al. The X-linked infantile spasms syndrome (MIM 308350) maps to xp11.4-xpter in 2 pedigrees. *Ann Neurol* 1997;42:360–364.
3. Curatolo P, Bombardieri R, Verdecchia M, et al. Intractable seizures in tuberous sclerosis complex: from molecular pathogenesis to the rationale for treatment. *J Child Neurol* 2005;20:318–325.
4. Dulac O, Plouin P, Schulmberger E. Infantile spasms. In: Wyllie E, ed. *The treatment of epilepsy: principles and practice.* Philadelphia: Lippincott Williams & Wilkins, 2001:415–452.
5. Egli M, Mothersill I, O'Kane M, et al. The axial spasm: the predominant type of drop seizure in patients with secondary generalized epilepsy. *Epilepsia* 1985;26:401–415.
6. Holmes GL, Stafstrom CE. Tuberous sclerosis complex and epilepsy: recent developments and future challenges. *Epilepsia* 2007;48:617–630

7. Koul R, Chacko A, Ganesh A, et al. Vigabatrin associated retinal dysfunction in children with epilepsy. *Arch Dis Child* 2001;85(6): 469–473.

8. Farrell K. Symptomatic generalized epilepsy and the Lennox-Gastaut syndrome. In: Wyllie E, ed. *The treatment of epilepsy: principles and practice.* Philadelphia: Lippincott Williams & Wilkins, 2001:525–536.

9. Holmes GL. Myoclonic, tonic, and atonic seizures in children. *J Epilepsy* 1988;1:173–195.

10. Ikeno T, Shigematsu H, Miyakoshi M, et al. An analytic study of epileptic falls. *Epilepsia* 1985;26:612–621.

11. Kalviainen R, Nousiainen I. Visual field defects with vigabatrin: epidemiology and therapeutic implications. *CNS Drugs* 2001; 15(3):217–230.

12. Koul R, Chacko A, Ganesh A, et al. Vigabatrin associated retinal dysfunction in children with epilepsy. *Arch Dis Child* 2001;85(6): 469–473.

13. Kramer V, Sue WC, Mikati M. Hypsarrhythmia: frequency of variant patterns and correlation with etiology and outcome. *Neurology* 1997;48:197–203.

14. Mackay MT, Weiss SK, Adams-Webber T, et al. Practice parameter: medical treatment of infantile spasms: report of the American Academy of Neurology and the Child Neurology Society. *Neurology* 2004;62(10):1668–1681.

15. Mikati MA, Lepejien GA, Holmes GL. Medical treatment of patients with infantile spasms. *Clin Neuropharmacol* 2002;25: 61–70.

16. Rantala H, Patkonen T. Occurrence, outcome and prognostic factors of infantile spasms and Lennox-Gastaut syndrome. *Epilepsia* 1999;40:286–289.

17. Scheffer IE, Wallace R, Mulley JC, et al. Clinical and molecular genetics of myoclonic-astatic epilepsy and severe myoclonic epilepsy in infancy (Dravet syndrome). *Brain Dev* 2001;23: 732–735.

18. Serratosa JM. Myoclonic seizures. In: Wyllie E, ed. *The treatment of epilepsy: principles and practice.* Philadelphia: Lippincott Williams & Wilkins, 2001:405–414.

19. Sugawara T, Mazaki-Miyazaki E, Fukushima K, et al. Frequent mutations of SCN1A in severe myoclonic epilepsy in infancy. *Neurology* 2002;58(7):1122–1124.

20. Thiele EA. Managing epilepsy in tuberous sclerosis complex. *J Child Neurol* 2004;19:680–686.

Epilepsies with Childhood Onset (1 to 12 Years)

The groups of epilepsy syndromes and the specific epilepsy syndromes with onset during childhood (1 to 12 years) and accompanying seizure types are listed in Table 6-1.

I. SYMPTOMATIC AND PROBABLY SYMPTOMATIC FOCAL EPILEPSIES

Symptomatic focal epilepsies can occur at any age. Three seizure types occur with these epilepsies: simple partial (focal); complex partial (psychomotor, temporal lobe); and tonic–clonic (grand mal). The clinical and electroencephalographic (EEG) features of these three seizure types are reviewed in Chapter 2; management and prognosis are reviewed in Chapter 3. Differential diagnostic entities to consider in children and adults when diagnosing these seizure types are listed in Chapter 3 and reviewed in Chapter 9.

Depending on locus of onset, five symptomatic and probably symptomatic epilepsy syndromes have been recognized (Table 6-1). Clinical and EEG features, management, and prognosis of these five syndromes are reviewed in Chapter 3.

II. IDIOPATHIC FOCAL EPILEPSIES

Partial seizures may be a significant component of three important syndromes: benign childhood epilepsy with centrotemporal spikes, early-onset benign childhood occipital epilepsy, and late-onset occipital epilepsy.

A. Benign Childhood Epilepsy with Centrotemporal Spikes (BCECTS, Rolandic Epilepsy)

1. Definitions and Etiology

BCECTS is an important, distinct epileptic syndrome occurring in childhood that is characterized by nocturnal tonic–clonic seizures of probably focal onset and diurnal simple partial seizures arising from the lower rolandic area of the cortex. The EEG pattern is characteristic, consisting of midtemporal–central spikes. The clinician must be aware of this syndrome because evaluation and prognosis differ considerably from those of other focal seizure disorders.

BCECTS is limited to the pediatric age group. Seizures begin between the ages of 2 and 12 years, although more typically, the child is between 5 and 10 years of age. Seizures of BCECTS remit spontaneously and do not occur after 16 years of age. The developmental and neurologic examination is usually normal.

The disorder is usually familial. Fifty percent of close relatives (siblings, children, and parents of the probands) demonstrate the EEG abnormality between the ages of 5 and 15 years. Before 5 and after 15 years of age, penetrance is low, and few patients demonstrate the abnormality. Only 12% of patients who inherit

Table 6-1.   Groups of epilepsy syndromes and specific epilepsy syndromes with onset during childhood (1–12 years) and accompanying seizure types

I. Symptomatic and probably symptomatic focal epilepsies
  A. Mesial temporal lobe epilepsy syndromes (SPS, CPS, TCS)
  B. Lateral temporal lobe syndromes (SPS, CPS, TCS)
  C. Frontal lobe epilepsy syndromes (SPS, CPS, TCS)
  D. Parietal lobe epilepsy syndromes (SPS, CPS, TCS)
  E. Occipital lobe epilepsy syndromes (SPS, CPS, TCS)
II. Idiopathic focal epilepsies
  A. Benign childhood epilepsy with centrotemporal spikes (SPS, CPS, TCS)
  B. Early-onset benign childhood epilepsy (SPS with autonomic symptoms)
  C. Late-onset occipital childhood epilepsy (SPS with visual symptoms)
III. Idiopathic generalized epilepsies
  A. Childhood absence epilepsy (ABS, TCS)
  B. Juvenile absence epilepsy (ABS, TCS)
  C. Juvenile myoclonic epilepsy (MYO, TCS, ABS)
  D. Epilepsy with tonic–clonic seizures on awakening (TCS)
  E. Epilepsy with random tonic–clonic seizures (TCS)
  F. Epilepsy with myoclonic–astatic seizures (MYO, ATO)
IV. Epileptic encephalopathies
  A. Lennox–Gastaut syndrome (TON, TCS, MYO, ABS, ATO)
  B. Landau–Kleffner syndrome
V. Progressive myoclonus epilepsies
  A. Progressive myoclonus seizures (MYO, TCS, CLO)
VI. Seizures not necessarily requiring a diagnosis of epilepsy
  A. Febrile seizures (TCS, TON)
  B. Reflex seizures (SPS, CPS, TCS, MYO, ABS)

ABS, absence seizure; ATO, atonic seizure; CLO, clonic seizure; CPS, complex partial seizure (psychomotor, temporal lobe); MYO, myoclonic seizure; SPS, simple partial (focal) seizure; TCS, tonic–clonic (grand mal) seizure; TON, tonic seizure.

the EEG abnormality have clinical seizures. The EEG trait of midtemporal–central spikes has been linked to chromosome 15q14. However, the inheritance of the epilepsy appears to have a multifactorial inheritance.

2. Seizure Phenomena

The syndrome also is termed *benign rolandic epilepsy* because of its characteristic feature, partial seizures involving the region around the lower portion of the central gyrus of Rolando. Although a nocturnal tonic–clonic seizure is the most dramatic and common mode of initial presentation, diurnal simple partial seizures may also demand a neurologic evaluation.

The characteristic features of daytime seizures include (a) somatosensory stimulation of the oral–buccal cavity, (b) speech arrest, (c) preservation of consciousness, (d) excessive pooling of saliva, and (e) tonic or tonic–clonic activity of the face. Less often, the somatosensory sensation spreads to the face or arm. On rare occasions, a typical jacksonian march of tonic or tonic–clonic activity occurs.

Although the somatosensory aura is quite common, this history is frequently not elicited, especially in young patients. Motor phenomena during the daytime attacks are usually restricted to one side of the body and include tonic, clonic, or tonic–clonic events. These attacks most frequently involve the face, although the arm and leg may be involved. Although seizures rarely generalize during wakefulness, the sensory or motor phenomena may change sides during the course of the attack. Arrest of speech may initiate the attack or occur during its course. Consciousness is rarely impaired during the daytime attacks. After the seizure, the child may feel numbness, pins and needles, or "electricity" in his or her tongue, gums, and cheek on one side. Postictal confusion and amnesia are unusual after seizures in BCECTS. In nocturnal seizures, the initial event is typically clonic movements of the mouth with salivation and gurgling sounds from the throat. Secondary generalization of the nocturnal seizure is common. The initial focal component of the seizure may be quite brief.

The seizures may occur both during the day and during the night, although in most children, seizures are most common during sleep. Daytime and nocturnal seizures are both brief. The frequency of seizures in BCECTS is typically low, and for status epilepticus to develop is unusual.

3. Electroencephalographic Phenomena

BCECTS is characterized by a distinctive EEG pattern. The characteristic interictal EEG abnormality is a high-amplitude, usually diphasic spike with a prominent, following slow wave. The spikes or sharp waves appear singly or in groups at the midtemporal (T3, T4) and central (rolandic) region (C3, C4) (Fig. 6-1). The spikes may be confined to one hemisphere or occur bilaterally. Rolandic spikes usually occur on a normal background.

Occasional records show generalized spike–wave discharges, usually during sleep. Most children with BCECTS who have spike–wave discharges during sleep do not have typical absence seizures.

Sleep usually increases the number of spikes. Because approximately 30% of children with BCECTS have spikes only during sleep, an EEG should be obtained during sleep from children suspected to have the syndrome. Sleep states are usually normal in BCECTS.

4. Management

If the patient has a clinical history and the EEG characteristics of BCECTS and a normal neurologic examination, further workup is not necessary. If the neurologic examination is abnormal or the EEG demonstrates abnormalities other than the typical epileptiform discharge, further evaluation with magnetic resonance imaging (MRI) is recommended.

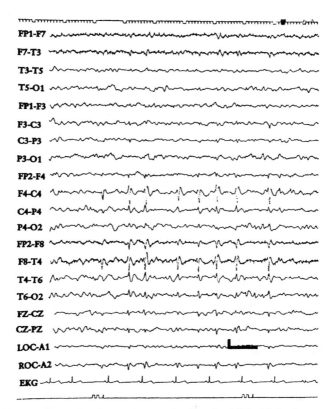

Fig. 6-1.   Example of centrotemporal spikes in child with benign childhood epilepsy. Note that spikes are present in both the right central (C4) and right mid-temporal (T4) areas. EKG, electrocardiogram.

Because of the benign nature of BCECTS, many physicians may choose not to treat the first or second seizure. If treatment is initiated, the seizures are usually controlled with a single antiepileptic drug. Drugs used for partial seizures (e.g., phenobarbital, phenytoin, carbamazepine, oxcarbazepine, and valproic acid) are usually effective.

The EEG is not a good predictor of recurrence risk. Most patients can be tapered off medications after 1 to 2 years of seizure control, regardless of whether the EEG normalizes.

5. Prognosis

The prognosis of BCECTS is generally good, with the majority of children going into remission by the teenage years. However, in a small percentage of patients with BCECTS, deficits in verbal memory or language skills develop. Children with BCECTS should be monitored closely for school performance.

B. Childhood Epilepsy with Occipital Paroxysms (CEOP)

1. Definition

Two distinct forms of CEOP are found. The early-onset type, or Panayiotopoulos syndrome, occurs in young children with a peak of onset at 5 years. The late-onset, or Gastaut, type has an age at onset of around 8 to 9 years. Both syndromes are associated with occipital spikes.

2. Seizure Phenomena

The early-onset type, or Panayiotopoulos syndrome, is characterized by ictal vomiting and deviation of the eyes, often with impairment of consciousness and progression to generalized tonic–clonic seizures. The seizures are infrequent and often solitary, but in around one third of the children, the episodes evolve into partial status epilepticus. Two thirds of the seizures occur during sleep. The late-onset, or Gastaut, type consists of brief seizures with mainly visual symptoms, such as elementary visual hallucinations, illusions, or amaurosis, followed by hemiclonic convulsions. Postictal migraine headaches occur in half of the patients.

3. Electroencephalographic Phenomena

The interictal EEG in both conditions is characterized by normal background activity and well-defined occipital discharges. The occipital spikes are typically high in voltage (200 to 300 mV) and diphasic, with a main negative peak followed by a relatively small positive peak and a negative slow wave. The discharges may be unilateral or bilateral and are increased during non–rapid eye movement sleep. An important feature in this syndrome is the prompt disappearance with eye opening and reappearance 1 to 20 seconds after eye closure.

4. Differential Diagnosis

Patients with CEOP should be differentiated from children with occipital spikes occurring during both eye opening and eye closure. These children are usually younger than 4 years of age. Only approximately half of the children in studies with occipital spikes have seizures. Unlike CEOP, these children typically do not have visual phenomena or postictal headaches.

Additional words of caution regarding occipital spikes are necessary. The syndrome of CEOP requires more than the EEG finding of occipital spikes for diagnosis. As is the case with centrotemporal spikes, a reactive occipital spikes pattern does not develop in all children with seizures. Occipital spikes are seen in other disorders. Children with myoclonic, absence, and photosensitive epilepsies may have similar EEG findings, but they are not classified as having benign occipital epilepsy (BOE). Occipital spikes also can be seen in young children with visual disorders, Sturge–Weber syndrome, epilepsy with bilateral occipital calcification, late infantile neuronal ceroid lipofuscinosis, and other occipital structural lesions.

5. Prognosis

The prognosis in the early-onset (Panayiotopoulos) type is excellent, and it typically resolves within several years of onset. The prognosis in the late-onset (Gastaut) form is variable. Although most patients have a benign course, seizure control may be difficult in some patients. Although seizures may continue into adulthood, many children outgrow their seizures.

III. IDIOPATHIC GENERALIZED EPILEPSIES

A. Childhood Absence Epilepsy and Juvenile Absence Epilepsy

1. Seizure Types

Typical absence seizures (Fig. 6-2), myoclonic, and generalized-onset tonic–clonic seizures may occur in these syndromes. The clinical and EEG features of these seizure types are reviewed in Chapter 2.

2. Other Features

In childhood absence epilepsy (pyknolepsy), the frequency of absence seizures is high, with seizures occurring up to several hundred times per day. The condition appears to be inherited in an autosomal-dominant pattern with incomplete penetrance. In juvenile absence epilepsy, the seizure frequency is much lower. In juvenile myoclonic epilepsy, myoclonic and generalized tonic–clonic seizures also are seen, and for children with the syndrome to have many absence seizures is unusual. Childhood absence epilepsy usually begins between the age of 3 years and puberty; juvenile absence epilepsy and juvenile myoclonic epilepsy begin during or after puberty. Although generalized tonic–clonic seizures can occur in both syndromes, the incidence is higher in children with juvenile absence seizures than with the childhood form.

The syndrome of *epilepsy with myoclonic absences* is characterized by absences accompanied by severe bilateral, rhythmic clonic, and sometimes tonic, activity. The myoclonic movements involve mainly the muscles of the shoulders, arms, and legs. The muscles of the face are less frequently involved. Typically, a rhythmic and striking jerking of the shoulders, head, and arms is seen. Tonic contractions occur in the shoulder and deltoid muscles and result in elevation of the arms. The disorder typically begins between 5 to 10 years of age and affects boys more frequently than girls. Seizures are frequent and less responsive to medication than are those of childhood absence epilepsy. Mental deterioration and evolution to Lennox–Gastaut syndrome (LGS) may occur.

An allelic association of juvenile absence epilepsies with a kainate-selective GluR5 receptor on chromosome 21q22.1 has been reported. Linkage to another locus, 8q24, has recently been confirmed in a large family with absence and generalized tonic–clonic seizures.

3. Management

Patients with suspected absence seizures do not require an extensive evaluation. Children who have typical absence seizures, with

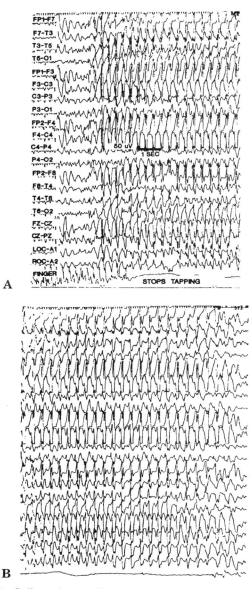

Fig. 6-2. Spike-and-wave discharge with frequency of 3 Hz in child with typical absence seizures. Note that child quits tapping with finger shortly after onset of the spike-and-wave discharge (A). The child began tapping again shortly after the spike-and-wave discharge stopped (B).

consistent ictal and interictal EEG features, and normal intelligence and neurologic examinations require no further diagnostic tests. Patients who have abnormal neurologic examinations or a history of developmental delay, or who have focal slowing or consistently focal spikes on the EEGs, should have an imaging study, preferably an MRI.

Antiepileptic drugs are recommended for all children with adequate documentation of absence seizures. Although not life threatening, absence seizures may lead to poor school performance and accidents. Because even brief bursts of generalized spike-and-wave discharge can affect cognitive function and responsiveness, trying to control the seizures as quickly as possible with minimal drug toxicity is prudent.

Because absence seizures are brief and often subtle, their frequency can be grossly underestimated by parents. Each follow-up evaluation by the physician should include 3 to 5 minutes of hyperventilation. Activation of a seizure by hyperventilation indicates that the patient is not under optimal control, regardless of the history supplied by the patient and parents.

Accidental injury is common with absence seizures and usually occurs after antiepileptic drug treatment is started. Injury-prevention counseling is indicated. Bicycle accidents pose a special risk, and helmet use, as with all children, should be mandatory.

4. Treatment

The drugs of choice for treatment of typical absence seizures are ethosuximide, lamotrigine, and valproic acid. All of these drugs are effective in the treatment of typical absence seizures, and a previously untreated patient has a better than 70% chance of significant reduction or total elimination of seizures. Lamotrigine and valproic acid also have efficacy for tonic–clonic seizures (sometimes associated with absence seizures), but ethosuximide does not. A single drug should be chosen and, after appropriate laboratory studies, administered according to the guidelines in Chapter 11, Table 11-2.

Most clinicians begin therapy with ethosuximide, primarily because of the rare, but severe, hepatotoxicity and pancreatitis associated with valproic acid and the risk of lamotrigine-associated rashes. Lamotrigine and valproic acid are considered the drugs of choice in the patient who has both absence and tonic–clonic seizures. Clonazepam also demonstrates efficacy in absence seizures, but it is usually reserved for refractory cases because of the relatively high incidence of drowsiness and behavioral side effects.

The combination of ethosuximide or lamotrigine and valproic acid may be more effective than either drug alone, although drug interactions do occur, requiring monitoring of clinical toxicity and serum drug levels.

The duration of therapy is variable, although a general rule is to taper patients off therapy after 2 seizure-free years. The EEG is very helpful in this situation because persistence of generalized spike-and-wave discharge indicates that the likelihood of recurrence of the seizures is high. It is important that hyperventilation is performed during the EEG.

5. Prognosis

In general, children with absence seizures do well, with a significant proportion (65% in one study) going into remission before adulthood. Childhood absence seizures often remit by puberty, whereas juvenile absence seizures may persist into the late teenage years. Although absence seizures rarely develop in adults, childhood-onset absences may continue into adulthood. Children with juvenile myoclonic epilepsy are more likely to continue to have absence seizures into adulthood. Likewise, myoclonic absences have a poor prognosis. Favorable prognostic signs for outgrowing absence seizures are no family history of epilepsy, normal EEG background activity, normal intelligence, and absence of absence status epilepticus, myoclonic seizures, or tonic–clonic seizures. Nearly 90% of children with these characteristics remit. As a general rule, onset of generalized tonic–clonic seizures before absence seizures carries a poorer prognosis than does the reverse. In one study, in 15% of children with absence seizures, juvenile myoclonic epilepsy later developed.

Patients with atypical absences have a less favorable outlook. Children with atypical absences and the LGS often have frequent and refractory seizures, and status epilepticus is common. The course and prognosis of epilepsy with myoclonic absences is variable but less favorable than that with childhood absence epilepsy.

B. Juvenile Myoclonic Epilepsy, Epilepsy with Tonic–Clonic Seizures on Awakening, and Epilepsy with Random Tonic–Clonic Seizures

Juvenile myoclonic epilepsy, epilepsy with tonic–clonic seizures on awakening, and epilepsy with random tonic–clonic seizures may begin before the age of 12 years. However, these epilepsy syndromes typically begin after the age of 12 years and therefore are reviewed in Chapter 7.

C. Epilepsy with Myoclonic–Astatic Seizures

This syndrome is reviewed in Chapter 5.

IV. EPILEPTIC ENCEPHALOPATHIES

A. Lennox–Gastaut Syndrome

1. Definitions

The LGS is characterized by a mixed seizure disorder (of which tonic seizures are a major component) and by a slow spike-and-wave EEG pattern. The syndrome always begins in childhood and is often accompanied by mental retardation. The incidence of LGS is estimated at 0.3 in 1,000 live births.

The child with the LGS typically has a mixture of seizure types. The most frequently occurring are tonic, tonic–clonic, myoclonic, atypical absences, and head drops, which represent a form of atonic, tonic, or myoclonic seizure. The syndrome is characterized by very frequent seizures, usually occurring multiple times daily. Atypical absence seizures often are unnoticed by patients and parents and may be best confirmed by simultaneous EEG/video recording.

2. Seizure Phenomena

Tonic seizures are among the most frequently occurring seizure types in this syndrome. They are typically activated by sleep and may occur repetitively throughout the night. They are much more frequent during non-REM sleep than during wakefulness and do not occur during REM sleep. In the LGS, tonic seizures are usually brief, lasting from a few seconds to 1 minute, with an average duration of about 10 seconds. The seizures may throw the patient off balance, and they are responsible for many of the falls observed in children with this syndrome. Eyelid retraction, staring, mydriasis, and apnea are commonly associated and may be the most prominent features. During tonic seizures, the patient is unconscious, although arousal from light sleep may occur. Because the seizures are often very brief, they usually go undetected.

3. Electroencephalographic Phenomena

The hallmark of the EEG finding in the LGS is the slow spike-and-wave discharge superimposed on an abnormal, slow background. The slow spike-and-wave or sharp-and-slow-wave complexes consist of generalized discharges occurring at a frequency of 1.5 to 2.5 Hz (Fig. 6-3). The morphology, amplitude, and repetition rate may vary both between bursts and during paroxysmal bursts of spike-and-wave activity; asymmetries of the discharge frequently occur. The area of maximum voltage, although variable, is usually frontal or temporal in location. Sleep frequently increases the frequency of the discharges, whereas hyperventilation and photic stimulation rarely activate these discharges.

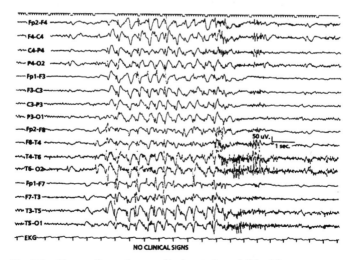

Fig. 6-3.   Slow spike-and-wave discharge in a child with Lennox–Gastaut syndrome. Compare the frequency and morphology with those in Fig. 6-2. EKG, electrocardiogram.

During non-REM sleep, slow spike-and-wave discharges may be replaced by multiple spike-and-wave discharges, whereas in REM sleep, the paroxysmal activity decreases markedly. The typical EEG manifestation of tonic seizures is the occurrence of fast-rhythm discharges of 10 to 20 Hz of progressively increasing amplitude, at times followed by a few slow waves or spike waves. In atonic seizures, the EEG pattern is most frequently a fast, recruiting discharge, but bursts of slow spike–wave complexes or high-amplitude 10-Hz discharges are sometimes recorded. During myoclonic seizures, the EEG demonstrates bursts of irregular spike–wave activity. Atypical absence seizures are associated with slow (less than 2.5 Hz), often asymmetric, and irregular spike-and-wave activity.

4. Treatment

Treatment of LGS presents the clinician with a formidable task. Complete seizure control is rarely achieved. Because of the intractable nature of the seizures and their mixed types, a tendency exists to give the child numerous drugs. This polypharmaceutical approach rarely results in good seizure control and usually causes toxic reactions—fatigue, nausea, and ataxia—from the cumulative effect of the drugs. Valproic acid, phenytoin, felbamate, lamotrigine, topiramate, and the benzodiazepines are most commonly used to treat this syndrome.

Valproic acid has the advantage of being a broad-spectrum drug with effectiveness against all of the common seizure types in the syndrome. This, coupled with the lack of sedative side effects, has prompted widespread use of the drug in this syndrome. However, because of its association with hepatotoxicity, the drug must be used cautiously in children, particularly those younger than 2 years.

Lamotrigine and topiramate have also been reported to be effective in reducing seizure frequency. Both drugs are well tolerated by children. However, lamotrigine may result in rashes, particularly if the drug is added to valproic acid. Topiramate has been associated with weight loss, acidosis, renal stones, and cognitive impairment, particularly at high doses. Total seizure control is rarely achieved with either drug.

Felbamate was the first drug proven to be effective in a placebo-controlled study in the treatment of the LGS. The drug was found to be effective in a number of seizure types, including atonic or drop attacks, but it was found to be associated with aplastic anemia and hepatotoxicity and is now reserved for patients for whom other forms of therapy have failed.

Phenytoin can be useful in the treatment of tonic and atonic seizures, although it rarely is helpful in atypical absence seizures. The benzodiazepines, such as clonazepam, also have a broad spectrum of action, but they are hindered by the high incidence of adverse side effects, such as fatigue, irritability, and cognitive impairment. In addition, in a large number of patients, tolerance to the antiepileptic effect of the drug develops.

Despite the goal of seizure control with a single drug, most children with LGS are taking multiple drugs. Although the efficacy of combination therapy has not been evaluated well, occasionally polytherapy is useful in controlling seizures. The combination of lamotrigine and valproic acid has been very effective in the treatment of some children with LGS.

Overall, the literature supports the consensus view that the ketogenic diet improves seizure control to a remarkable degree in some children. One third to one half of children with LGS appear to have an excellent response to the ketogenic diet, in terms of a marked or complete cessation of seizures, or reduction in seizure severity. An improvement in alertness and behavior has also been reported on the diet, although this has never been subjected to scientific scrutiny. Another one third of children have a partial or incomplete response, with some reduction in seizure frequency or severity, and the remaining one third to one half do not seem to benefit from the diet. Although the difficulties of initiating and maintaining the diet are substantial, parents and children readily adapt to the rigors of the diet if it is effective in reducing seizure frequency.

Significant problems associated with the diet include weight loss, lethargy, renal stones, hemolytic anemia, hypoproteinemia, renal tubular acidosis, and elevation of hepatic enzymes. The ketogenic diet is discussed in detail in Chapter 10.

5. Prognosis

Mental retardation is present before onset of the seizures in 20% to 60% of patients. Some patients, those whose seizures have idiopathic or cryptogenic etiologies, have normal IQ scores or developmental histories before the onset of their seizures. However, cryptogenic etiology does not ensure a good outcome after seizures begin. The proportion of retarded patients increases with age because of the deterioration that frequently occurs in LGS, although a few rare patients escape mental retardation. Fluctuations in cognitive abilities may occur in LGS patients and correlate, to some degree, with the intensity of EEG abnormalities. Behavioral problems are also common in LGS, ranging from hyperactivity to frank psychotic and autistic behavior. Abnormalities of the neurologic examination are common in the disorder.

Although the natural course of the disorder is a decreasing frequency of atonic, myoclonic, and atypical absence seizures with increasing age, often an increase in generalized tonic–clonic seizures and an emergence of partial seizures occurs. Only a few children undergo seizure remission.

B. Landau–Kleffner Syndrome

1. Definition and Clinical Features

The Landau–Kleffner syndrome (LKS) is a rare childhood disorder consisting of an acquired aphasia and epileptiform discharges involving the temporal or parietal regions of the brain.

Although a considerable amount of variation exists in the disorder, the typical history is of developing an abrupt or gradual loss of language ability and inattentiveness to sound, with onset during the first decade of life. This interruption in communication skills is generally closely preceded, accompanied, or followed by the onset of seizures, an abnormal EEG, or both. Receptive dysfunction, often referred to as *auditory agnosia*, may be the dominant feature early in the course of the disorder. In some children, the disorder progresses to a point at which the child cannot even recognize sounds. In addition to the aphasia, many of the children have behavioral and psychomotor disturbances, often appearing autistic. The neurologic examination, other than the mental status examination, is usually normal.

The clinical course of LKS is variable, and the long-term outcome of the aphasia is quite unpredictable, although the epilepsy and EEG abnormalities frequently regress or disappear over time. Some patients with the syndrome have an abnormal EEG, but seizures never develop.

A condition related to LKS is epilepsy with continuous spike–wave discharges during sleep (CSWDS). The disorder has also been called *electrical status epilepticus during sleep* (ESES). However, ESES is an EEG diagnosis, and the principal criterion is that the occurrence of generalized spike-and-wave activity is the dominant pattern during sleep, occupying no less than 85% of the total slow-wave sleep time. CSWDS is a clinical syndrome encompassing both the clinical features and the EEG findings. CSWDS begins during early childhood, peaking between 4 and 5 years of age. The child may have partial, generalized tonic–clonic, or myoclonic seizures. Seizures may occur during sleep or in the awake state.

Significant similarities can be seen between LKS and CSWDS, suggesting that the two disorders are part of the spectrum of seizure-related aphasia. Both disorders are associated with cognitive impairment, particularly language, and behavioral disturbances.

2. Electroencephalographic Phenomena

No specific EEG pattern is associated with LKS. Most commonly, repetitive spikes, sharp waves, and spike-and-wave activity are seen in the temporal region or parietal–occipital regions bilaterally. Sleep usually activates the record, and in some cases, the abnormality is seen only in sleep recordings. The distinguishing feature of CSWDS is the continuous bilateral and diffuse slow spike–wave activity persisting through all of the slow-sleep stages. The spike–wave index (total minutes of all spike–waves multiplied by 100 and divided by the total minutes of non-REM sleep without spike–wave activity) ranges from 85% to 100%.

3. Basic Mechanisms

Although the pathogenesis of the language disorder in these patients is not known, the epileptiform activity noted on the EEG may result in subclinical seizures. Speech deficits may be explained by either disruption of normal connections or an excessive inhibitory reaction to epileptiform discharges. Speech usually does not improve in the syndrome unless the EEG improves. However, if the aphasia is simply the result of ongoing epileptiform activity, it seems strange that most antiepileptic drugs are ineffective. Furthermore, the severity of the aphasia does not always have a close correlation with the degree of EEG abnormality or clinical seizures.

Another viewpoint is that the epileptiform activity is an epiphenomenon and simply reflects an underlying cortical abnormality.

Even if the EEG parallels speech recovery, this does not prove that epileptiform activity causes aphasia. The decreased epileptiform activity during speech recovery may simply reflect resolution of the injury to the speech areas.

4. Etiology

Neuroradiologic examinations are usually normal in LKS, and, in most cases, the paroxysmal discharges recorded during wakefulness and sleep do not seem to be promoted by a detectable structural epileptogenic lesion. However, a handful of patients with the syndrome have had tumors, neurocysticercosis, vasculitis, and encephalitis.

5. Treatment

Treatment of LKS and CSWDS can be frustrating. Unless objective evidence of changes in speech is found by an impartial, blinded observer, separating a placebo effect from drug-related improvement is difficult. Standard antiepileptic drugs such as valproic acid and lamotrigine can sometimes both reduce seizure frequency and improve language and cognitive function.

Recently, success has been found with high-dose diazepam treatments in CSWDS. Children are given a test dose of diazepam, 0.7–1.0 mg/kg, in the hospital setting during overnight EEG monitoring and oxygen-saturation monitoring. If the EEG shows an improvement after the diazepam, the child is prescribed 0.5 to 0.7 mg/kg of diazepam given at bedtime for 4 to 6 weeks. At that point, an EEG is obtained, and the drug tapered over several weeks. Children who respond with an improvement in the EEG and language function are then monitored periodically to assess for relapses. Children who do not improve either on the EEG or clinically will be prescribed a different therapy.

Administration of corticosteroids resulted in improved speech, suppression of seizures, and normalization of the EEG in several small series of children. However, experience with corticosteroid treatment is inadequate to provide strict treatment guidelines. The authors usually treat children with LKS and CSWDS with 2 mg/kg/d of prednisone for 2 months. At that time, the prednisone is slowly tapered until the child is taking 0.5 mg/kg every other day. If corticosteroids are beneficial, this dosage is usually maintained for 6 to 8 months. If treatment has not been effective, the drug is discontinued. In cases of relapse, the dose is increased and maintained for a longer period.

Subpial cortical transections have been reported to be useful in patients with LKS. However, like treatment with steroids, this procedure has not been studied in any controlled manner.

6. Prognosis

The outcome in both LKS and CSWDS is variable. Recovery of language in LKS is highly dependent on age at onset of the syndrome, with the best recovery seen in children with early onset. Likewise, in CSWDS, outcome varies from full recovery to continued speech and cognitive impairment. Most patients with CSWDS have some amelioration in their cognition and behavioral disorders over time.

V. PROGRESSIVE MYOCLONUS ENCEPHALOPATHIES

A. Progressive Myoclonus Epilepsy

1. Clinical Features

Progressive myoclonus epilepsy (PME) encompasses a group of disorders in which myoclonus is a major component. In addition, the patients typically have generalized tonic–clonic or clonic seizures, mental deterioration culminating in dementia, and a neurologic syndrome that almost always includes cerebellar dysfunction. The myoclonus involves a combination of segmental, arrhythmic, asynchronous, asymmetric myoclonus and massive myoclonia. In addition to cerebellar symptoms, common neurologic deficits involve visual, pyramidal, extrapyramidal systems, and partial seizures, particularly beginning in the occipital region.

Conditions in which PME is seen include Unverricht-Lundborg disease (Baltic myoclonus), sialidosis, Gaucher disease (glucocerebroside β-glucosidase deficiency), mitochondrial encephalomyelopathy with ragged-red fibers (MERRF), Lafora disease, and neuronal ceroid lipofuscinosis (NCL). Unverricht-Lundborg disease is caused by mutations in the gene encoding cystatin B (*CSTB*), a cystine protease inhibitor. Lafora disease is caused by mutations in the *EPM2A* gene mapped to chromosome 6q23-25. The infantile form of NCL is caused by mutations in the *LCN1* gene resulting in a deficiency of palmitoylprotein thioesterase. The late infantile form of NCL is caused by a mutation in the *CLN2* gene causing a deficiency of the lysosomal protease tripeptidyl-peptidase. Juvenile NCL is caused by a deficiency of a lysosomal membrane protein called battenin. MERRF is caused by a point mutation in the mitochondrial gene for tRNA. Sialidosis type II is caused by a mutation of *NEU1* resulting in a marked deficiency of the activity of lysosomal α-neuraminidase.

Progressive myoclonus epilepsy usually entails relentless deterioration of neurologic functions and increasing severity of the myoclonus and seizures. Almost all patients are severely ataxic, demented, wheelchair-bound, or bedridden. The exceptions are patients with Unverricht–Lundborg disease and sialidosis, both of which may occur with minimal or absence of dementia. For a review of these disorders, the reader is referred to Berkovic and Benbadis (2).

2. Electroencephalographic Features

Even though their etiologies are different, many of the PMEs share similar EEG findings. Typically, the alpha activity slows and is eventually replaced by theta- and delta-range frequencies. Epileptiform activity consists of bilateral synchronous spikes, polyspikes, spike-and-wave, or polyspike-and-wave complexes. When focal spikes are present, they are most commonly seen in the occipital region. During the awake state, the myoclonus may or may not be associated with spikes or spike-and-wave activity. During sleep, spike-and-wave discharges may decrease. The major exceptions to this rule are the sialidoses and neuronal ceroid lipofuscinosis.

Although visual evoked potentials and brainstem auditory evoked potentials are usually normal in the PMEs, somatosensory evoked potentials may be abnormal, demonstrating giant responses.

3. Management

Although myoclonic seizures can be seen in some benign syndromes, they are also associated with a number of malignant conditions. Because of this, children with myoclonic seizures should be closely evaluated.

Once the diagnosis is established, children should have an MRI seeking congenital anomalies, infections, and metabolic disturbances. Unless an etiology for the seizures is clear, patients should have metabolic screening that includes urine and serum amino acids, ammonia, lactate, pyruvate, organic acids, and liver-function tests. Spinal-fluid examination should include glucose (which should be compared with the serum glucose level), protein, and cell count. Cerebrospinal fluid amino acids, pyruvate, and lactate should be tested in children when metabolic disease is suspected. If a question of a mitochondrial encephalopathy exists, DNA testing for specific deletions and a muscle biopsy evaluating structure of the mitochondria should be performed.

4. Treatment

Myoclonic seizures may be difficult to control. Valproic acid and the benzodiazepines are probably the most effective antiepileptic drugs used in this syndrome. Some anecdotal evidence indicates that topiramate and zonisamide may be effective for PME. The ketogenic diet should also be considered if drugs are not effective (see Chapter 10 for details). Phenytoin, carbamazepine, gabapentin, lamotrigine, and vigabatrin can sometimes exacerbate myoclonic seizures.

5. Prognosis

Children with PME do poorly; those with benign myoclonic epilepsy and juvenile myoclonic epilepsy do much better.

VI . SEIZURES NOT NECESSARILY REQUIRING A DIAGNOSIS OF EPILEPSY

A. Febrile Seizures

See Chapter 8.

B. Reflex Seizures

See Chapter 8.

REFERENCES

1. Bare MA, Clauser TA, Strawsburg RH. Need for electroencephalogram video confirmation of atypical absence seizures in children with Lennox-Gastaut syndrome. *J Child Neurol* 1998; 13:498–500.
2. Berkovic SF, Benbadis S. Absence seizures. In: Wyllie E, ed. *The treatment of epilepsy: principles and practice.* Philadelphia: Lippincott Williams & Wilkins, 2001:345–356.

3. Berkovic SF, Benbadis S. Childhood and juvenile absence epilepsies. In: Wyllie E, ed. *The treatment of epilepsy: principles and practice*. Philadelphia: Lippincott Williams & Wilkins, 2001: 485–490.
4. Bien CG, Widman G, Urbach H, et al. The natural history of Rasmussen's encephalitis. *Brain* 2002;125(pt 8):1751–1759.
5. Caraballo R, Cersosimo R, Medina C, et al. Panayiotopoulos-type benign childhood occipital epilepsy: a prospective study. *Neurology* 2000;55(8):1096–1100.
6. Eriksson AS, Nergardh A, Hoppu K. The efficacy of lamotrigine in children and adolescents with refractory generalized epilepsy: a randomized, double-blind, crossover study. *Epilepsia* 1998;39: 495–501.
7. Farrell K. Symptomatic generalized epilepsy and the Lennox-Gastaut syndrome. In: Wyllie E, ed. *The treatment of epilepsy: principles and practice*. Philadelphia: Lippincott Williams & Wilkins, 2001:525–536.
8. Landau WM, Kleffner FR. Syndrome of acquired aphasia with convulsive disorder in children. *Neurology* 1957;7:523–530.
9. Loiseau P. Idiopathic and benign partial epilepsies. In: Wyllie E, ed. *The treatment of epilepsy: principles and practice*. Philadelphia: Lippincott Williams & Wilkins, 2001:475–484.
10. Motte J, Trevathan E, Arvidsson JFV, et al. Lamotrigine for generalized seizures associated with the Lennox-Gastaut syndrome. *N Engl J Med* 1997;337:1807–1812.
11. Neubauer BA, Fiedler B, Himmelein B, et al. Centrotemporal spikes in families with rolandic epilepsy: linkage to chromosome 15q14. *Neurology* 1998;51:1608–1612.
12. Nordli D, DeVivo CC. The ketogenic diet. In: Wyllie E, ed. *The treatment of epilepsy: principles and practice*. Philadelphia: Lippincott Williams & Wilkins, 2001:1001–1006.
13. Panayiotopoulos CP. Benign childhood epileptic syndromes with occipital spikes: new classification proposed by the International League Against Epilepsy. *J Child Neurol* 2000;15(8):548–552.
14. Penry JK, Porter RJ, Dreifuss FE. Simultaneous recording of absence seizures with videotape and electroencephalography. *Brain* 1975;98:427–440.
15. Rantala H, Patkonen T. Occurrence, outcome and prognostic factors in infantile spasms and Lennox-Gastaut syndrome. *Epilepsia* 1999:40:286–289.
16. Sander T, Hildmann T, Kretz R, et al. Allelic association of juvenile absence epilepsy with a GluR5 kainate receptor gene (GRIK1) polymorphism. *Am J Med Genet* 1997;74:416–421.
17. Serrotosa JM. Myoclonic seizures. In: Wyllie E, ed. *The treatment of epilepsy: principles and practice*. Philadelphia: Lippincott Williams & Wilkins, 2001:395–404.
18. Tassinari CA, Rubboli G, Volpi L, et al. Encephalopathy with electrical status epilepticus during slow sleep or ESES syndrome including the acquired aphasia. *Clin Neurophysiol* 2000; 111(suppl 2):S94–S102.
19. Tatum W, Genton P, Bureau M, et al. Less common epilepsy syndromes. In: Wyllie E, ed. *The treatment of epilepsy: principles and practice*. Philadelphia: Lippincott Williams & Wilkins, 2001:551–575.

20. Tuchman RF, Rapin I. Regression in pervasive developmental disorder: seizure and epileptiform electroencephalogram correlates. *Pediatrics* 1997;99:560–566.
21. Westmoreland BF. The EEG findings in extratemporal seizures. *Epilepsia* 1998;39(suppl 4):1–8.
22. Wirrell EC, Camfield CS, Camfield PR, et al. Long-term prognosis of childhood absence epilepsy: regression or progression to juvenile myoclonic epilepsy. *Neurology* 1996;47:912–918.
23. Wirrell EC, Camfield CS, Dooley JM, et al. Accidental injury is a serious risk in children with typical absence seizures. *Arch Neurol* 1996;53:929–932.
24. Zara F, Bianchi A, Avanzini G, et al. Mapping of genes predisposing to idiopathic generalized epilepsy. *Hum Mol Genet* 1995;4:1201–1207.

Epilepsies with Juvenile and Adult Onset (12 Years and Older)

The groups of epilepsy syndromes and the specific epilepsy syndromes with juvenile and adult onset (12 years and older) and accompanying seizure types are listed in Table 7-1.

I. SYMPTOMATIC AND PROBABLY SYMPTOMATIC FOCAL EPILEPSIES

Symptomatic focal epilepsies can occur at any age. Three seizure types are associated with these epilepsies: simple partial (focal); complex partial (psychomotor, temporal lobe); and tonic–clonic (grand mal). The clinical and electroencephalographic (EEG) features of these three seizure types are reviewed in Chapter 2; management and prognosis are reviewed in Chapter 3. Differential diagnostic entities to consider in children and adults in the diagnosis of these seizure types are listed in Chapter 3 and reviewed in Chapter 9.

Depending on locus of onset, five types of symptomatic focal epilepsy syndromes have been recognized (Table 7-1). Clinical and EEG features and management and prognosis of these five types are reviewed in Chapter 3.

II. IDIOPATHIC GENERALIZED EPILEPSIES

A. Juvenile Absence Epilepsy

Childhood and juvenile absence epilepsy are reviewed in detail with childhood epilepsies in Chapter 6. Only special features of this epilepsy in adults are presented here.

Childhood and juvenile-onset absence epilepsies persist into adulthood in 30% to 50% of patients and may be difficult to control. Absence seizures may be overlooked during childhood and first come to medical attention in the late teens or early twenties (e.g., after joining the military, going to college, or starting a job). Absence seizures must be clearly differentiated from complex partial seizures, because both may first be seen with lapses of consciousness and automatisms (see Chapter 9). The treatment of absence seizures differs from that of complex partial seizures. Hyperventilation is useful for producing clinical and EEG manifestations of absence seizures in patients of all ages.

Absence seizures may be difficult to control in adults who fail to "outgrow" them. The combination of ethosuximide and valproic acid is sometimes effective when monotherapy fails.

Approximately one third to one half of patients with absence seizures experience tonic–clonic seizures at some time during their lives. Unlike absence seizures, tonic–clonic seizures persist past the teens in the majority of patients. Because of the high incidence of tonic–clonic seizures in juvenile absence seizures,

I. Symptomatic and probably symptomatic focal epilepsies
    A. Mesial temporal lobe epilepsy syndromes (SPS, CPS, TCS)
    B. Lateral temporal lobe epilepsy syndromes (SPS, CPS, TCS)
    C. Frontal lobe epilepsy syndromes (SPS, CPS, TCS)
    D. Parietal lobe epilepsy syndromes (SPS, CPS, TCS)
    E. Occipital lobe epilepsy syndromes (SPS, CPS, TCS)
II. Idiopathic generalized epilepsies
    A. Juvenile absence epilepsy (ABS, TCS)
    B. Juvenile myoclonic epilepsy (MYO, TCS, ABS)
    C. Epilepsy with tonic–clonic seizures on awakening (TCS)
    D. Epilepsy with random tonic–clonic seizures (TCS)
III. Progressive myoclonus epilepsies
IV. Seizures not necessarily requiring a diagnosis of epilepsy
    A. Alcohol/drug related (TCS)
    B. Eclampsia (TCS)
    C. Seizures with special modes of precipitation (SPS, CPS, TCS, MYO, ABS)

ABS, absence seizure; CPS, complex partial (psychomotor, temporal lobe) seizure; MYO, myoclonic seizure; SPS, simple partial (focal) seizure; TCS, tonic–clonic (grand mal) seizure.

some physicians start all such patients on valproic acid as the first drug.

Absence status epilepticus is more common in adults than in children. Clinical, EEG, and management aspects of absence status epilepticus are described in Chapter 12.

B. Juvenile Myoclonic Epilepsy
1. Definition and Clinical Features

Juvenile myoclonic epilepsy (JME) is a syndrome of myoclonic and tonic–clonic seizures with typical onset at 12 to 18 years of age (range, 8 to 30 years). It is the most common cause of primarily generalized myoclonic and tonic–clonic seizures in adults. Other synonyms for this syndrome are impulsive petit mal and syndrome of Janz.

The characteristic symptom is sudden, mild-to-moderate jerks of the shoulders and arms that occur shortly after awakening. No disturbance of consciousness is noticeable. Jerks also may occur when the patient is falling asleep or at any time. Approximately 90% of patients also have tonic–clonic seizures, which also tend to occur shortly after awakening in the morning. In approximately half of patients, the myoclonic seizures precede the tonic–clonic seizures and vice versa. Absence seizures occur in 10% to 30% of patients. The absence seizures usually begin before the other seizure types and are relatively infrequent, brief, and not associated with myoclonic jerks or automatisms. The accumulated evidence supports JME and the subclinical EEG abnormality (fast spike–wave trait) as having complex inheritance, or in some cases, autosomal dominant with variable penetrance.

2. Electroencephalographic Features

Interictal EEGs in untreated persons show bilateral, symmetric, synchronous, and diffuse polyspike- and slow-wave complexes with a frequency of 4 to 6 Hz (Fig. 7-1). During myoclonias, 6- to 16-Hz polyspikes lead to higher voltage-recruiting patterns at the start of tonic–clonic seizures. No close phase correlation is apparent between EEG spikes and jerks. During absence seizures, the 4- to 6-Hz discharges may slow to 3 Hz and occur as polyspike–wave or spike–wave activity. Frequently, patients are photosensitive.

3. Diagnosis

A history of myoclonic seizures, tonic–clonic seizures, or both on awakening suggests the diagnosis of JME. The myoclonic and absence seizures are often ignored by the patient, and the physician should always inquire about myoclonic seizures on awakening and absence seizures in a teenager or young adult first seen with tonic–clonic seizures. The family history is positive for seizures in half of patients. The diagnosis is confirmed by EEG. Intelligence is in the normal range. Neurologic examination and imaging studies are normal.

4. Differential Diagnosis

Juvenile myoclonic epilepsy must be differentiated from other myoclonic epilepsies of childhood, progressive myoclonic epilepsies, epilepsy with grand mal seizures on awakening, epilepsy with random tonic–clonic seizures, and juvenile absence epilepsy. Note that in JME, myoclonic seizures, absence seizures, and tonic–clonic seizures on awakening can occur in the same patient at different times.

A number of rare myoclonic epilepsies occur earlier in life than JME: myoclonic absence epilepsy, myoclonic–astatic epilepsy, early childhood myoclonic epilepsy, and benign or severe myoclonic epilepsy in infants (see Chapters 5 and 6 and ref. 9).

A number of rare, progressive myoclonic epilepsy syndromes exist in adults, characterized by progressive neurologic deterioration, dementia, and ataxia (see Chapter 6); JME has none of these characteristics.

Epilepsy with grand mal seizures on awakening is closely related to JME (see the following section, II.C), but myoclonic and absence seizures are not present. In epilepsy with random tonic–clonic seizures, the tonic–clonic seizures occur at times other than on awakening, and myoclonic and absence seizures are absent.

In juvenile absence epilepsy, myoclonic seizures are absent, and the tonic–clonic seizures occur randomly (i.e., not just on awakening). The interictal EEG findings of juvenile absence epilepsy (3-Hz spike–wave, usually exacerbated by hyperventilation, seldom photosensitive) are different from those in JME (4- to 6-Hz polyspike–wave, seldom exacerbated by hyperventilation, often photosensitive).

5. Management

Patients should be warned to avoid circumstances that can precipitate JME: sleep deprivation, early awakening, alcohol intake,

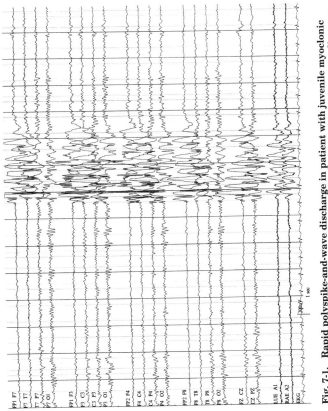

Fig. 7-1. Rapid polyspike-and-wave discharge in patient with juvenile myoclonic epilepsy. No clinical symptoms occurred during discharge. EKG, electrocardiogram.

fatigue, and flickering lights (in some patients). Valproic acid, lamotrigine, and levetiracetam can be effective in controlling all three seizure types in JME although in rare patients, lamotrigine may exacerbate myoclonic seizures. When additional seizure control is needed, phenytoin is effective for the tonic–clonic seizures of JME; ethosuximide is effective for the absence seizures; and clonazepam is effective for the myoclonic seizures. Carbamazepine may be effective for the tonic–clonic seizures, but it may make absence and myoclonic seizures worse. Uncontrolled studies suggest that topiramate may be effective for all three seizure types. (This indication has not been approved by the U.S. Food and Drug Administration.) Dosing directions for the drugs in children and adults are given in Chapter 11.

6. Prognosis

The seizures usually can be completely controlled with medication. JME tends to be a lifelong trait, and drugs seldom can be discontinued without recurrence of seizures.

C. Epilepsy with Tonic–Clonic Seizures on Awakening

Epilepsy with tonic–clonic seizures on awakening is similar to JME, with onset occurring mostly during the second decade of life. The tonic–clonic seizures occur exclusively or predominantly (more than 90% of the time) after awakening, regardless of the time of day, or in a second-seizure peak in the evening period of relaxation. Myoclonic and absence seizures do not occur. As with JME, a genetic predisposition has been noted, and evidence exists that both epilepsies are linked to the JME-1 locus of chromosome 6.

The EEG shows generalized spike–wave patterns and may show photosensitivity. The associated tonic–clonic seizures respond to valproic acid, phenytoin, or carbamazepine administered as directed in Chapter 11.

D. Epilepsy with Random Tonic–Clonic Seizures

This syndrome also has onset during the second decade. Myoclonic or absence seizures are not present. Tonic–clonic seizures may occur any time (not just after awakening). A familial tendency for this disorder exists, but it is not linked to the JME-1 locus of chromosome 6. The seizures respond to valproic acid, phenytoin, or carbamazepine, administered as directed in Chapter 11.

III. PROGRESSIVE MYOCLONUS EPILEPSIES
See Chapter 6.

IV. SEIZURES NOT NECESSARILY REQUIRING A DIAGNOSIS OF EPILEPSY

A. Alcohol/Drug Related (Tonic–Clonic)
See Chapter 8.

B. Eclampsia (Tonic–Clonic)
See Chapter 8.

C. Reflex Epilepsies (Simple Partial, Complex Partial, Tonic–Clonic, Myoclonic, Absence)

See Chapter 8.

REFERENCES

1. Annegers JF. The epidemiology of epilepsy. In: Wyllie E, ed. *The treatment of epilepsy: principles and practice*. Philadelphia: Lippincott Williams & Wilkins, 2001:131–138.
2. Commission on Classification and Terminology of the International League Against Epilepsy. Proposal for revised clinical and electroencephalographic classification of epileptic seizures. *Epilepsia* 1981;22:489–501.
3. Engel J. A proposed diagnostic scheme for people with epileptic seizures and with epilepsy: report of the International League Against Epilepsy Task Force on Classification and Terminology. *Epilepsia* 2001;42:1212–1218.
4. Gastaut H. Generalized convulsive seizures without local onset. In: Vinken PJ, Bruyn GW, eds. *Handbook of clinical neurology, vol 15: The epilepsies*. Amsterdam: Elsevier, 1974:107–129.
5. Greenburg DA, Dufner M, Resor S, et al. The genetics of generalized epilepsies of adolescent onset: differences between juvenile myoclonic epilepsy and epilepsy with random grand mal and with awakening grand mal. *Neurology* 1995;45:942–946.
6. Hauser WA, Hesdorffer DC. Remission, intractability, mortality, and comorbidity of seizures. In: Wyllie E, ed. *The treatment of epilepsy: principles and practice*. Philadelphia: Lippincott Williams & Wilkins, 2001:139–148.
7. Janz D. The idiopathic generalized epilepsies of adolescence with childhood and juvenile age of onset. *Epilepsia* 1997;39:4–11.
8. Serratosa JM. Juvenile myoclonic epilepsy. In: Wyllie E, ed. *The treatment of epilepsy: principles and practice*. Philadelphia: Lippincott Williams & Wilkins, 2001:491–508.
9. Serratosa JM. The progressive myoclonus epilepsies. In: Wyllie E, ed. *The treatment of epilepsy: principles and practice*. Philadelphia: Lippincott Williams & Wilkins, 2001:509–537.

Seizures Not Necessarily Requiring a Diagnosis of Epilepsy

The specific seizure syndromes not requiring a diagnosis of epilepsy are listed in Table 8-1.

I. FEBRILE SEIZURES

A. Definition

A febrile seizure is a seizure disorder that occurs in children between 6 months and 5 years of age, in association with a fever but without evidence of intracranial infection. The first febrile seizure in the majority of children occurs before 3 years, with the average age at onset between 18 and 22 months. Most studies have demonstrated a higher incidence in boys.

B. Seizure Phenomena

Febrile seizures may be of any type, although they are usually generalized tonic–clonic or tonic. Febrile seizures are classified as complex if the seizure duration is longer than 15 minutes, if more than one seizure occurs in 24 hours, or if focal features are present.

C. Electroencephalographic Phenomena

Electroencephalography (EEG) has not been found to be useful in the evaluation of a child with febrile seizures. Although some controversy remains, most authorities believe that the EEG is a poor predictor of either febrile or afebrile seizure recurrence. Approximately one third of patients with febrile seizures have an abnormal EEG when the record is obtained within a week of the seizure. The most common abnormality is occipital slowing, but generalized spike-and-wave and focal spikes may occur. However, this epileptiform activity is not predictive of the eventual development of epilepsy. The American Academy of Pediatrics does not recommend the use of routine EEG in patients with febrile seizures.

D. Management

The physician must first identify whether an underlying illness exists that requires immediate, specific treatment. The most urgent diagnostic decision is whether to do a lumbar puncture. One of the earliest signs of meningitis may be a seizure that, like a febrile seizure, is usually short and generalized tonic–clonic. (Although meningitis typically results in meningismus, in patients younger than 2 years, clinical signs of meningitis may be minimal or absent.)

In the absence of specific clinical indications, the literature yields little evidence indicating that other tests are helpful in determining etiology of seizures associated with fever. Skull films,

Table 8-1. Seizures not necessarily requiring a diagnosis of epilepsy

---

I. Febrile seizures (TCS, TON)
II. Alcohol related (TCS)
III. Drug related (TCS)
IV. Eclampsia (TCS)
V. Reflex seizures (SPS, CPS, TCS, MYO, ABS)

ABS, absence seizure; CPS, complex partial (psychomotor, temporal lobe) seizure; MYO, myoclonic seizure; SPS, simple partial (focal) seizure; TCS, tonic–clonic (grand mal) seizure; TON, tonic seizure.

serum glucose, calcium, blood urea nitrogen, and electrolytes are of low yield and are not routinely recommended. Brief, single, self-limited febrile seizures from which the child fully recovers are seldom caused by conditions such as hypoglycemia or toxins. Unless the physical examination points to a possible structural lesion, a computed tomographic scan or magnetic resonance imaging is not warranted in the evaluation of febrile seizures. Because the EEG is of questionable value after febrile seizures, routine EEGs are not necessary.

E. Treatment

Most experts agree that no preventive therapy is indicated for the child who has experienced a first or even a second febrile seizure. In practice parameters provided by the American Academy of Pediatrics, it is stated that the potential adverse effects of prophylactic therapy are not commensurate with the benefit. Children who experience complex febrile seizures, characterized by partial or prolonged seizures and concomitant neurologic developmental abnormality, are more likely to have recurrent seizures. These patients are frequently considered to have epilepsy initially triggered by fever and are more often treated with long-term antiepileptic drug therapy.

For children who experience frequent or prolonged febrile seizures, treatment with oral diazepam (0.3 mg/kg every 8 hours) during the febrile illness will reduce the likelihood of a seizure. However, parents may not be aware that the child has a fever until a seizure occurs. In addition, diazepam can lead to significant lethargy and possibly mask signs of a serious illness such as meningitis. Most physicians no longer use oral diazepam as prophylactic therapy. Diazepam rectal gel (Diastat) can be administered at the onset of a febrile seizure in a child with a history of prolonged seizures. See Chapter 11 for dosage recommendations.

F. Prognosis

Febrile seizures are associated with a very low mortality rate. When deaths do occur, they are almost always secondary to the agent causing the fever or to an antecedent neurologic disorder. In addition, the incidence of acquired motor or intellectual abnormalities after a febrile seizure is low.

Although relatively few children who experience febrile seizures develop epilepsy, recurrences of febrile seizures are commonplace. In the National Collaborative Perinatal Project, approximately one third of the children had at least one recurrence, and one half of those who had one recurrence had an additional attack.

Recurrence risk is not uniform for all children with febrile seizures. The most important factor appears to be age at onset of the first febrile seizure. The younger the child at the first attack, the more likely are further febrile seizures. Children who experience their first seizure at younger than 13 months have a greater than a 2:1 chance of developing further febrile seizures. This compares with a risk of approximately 20% in patients who have their first febrile seizure after age 32 months. Three fourths of recurrence takes place within 1 year of the first febrile seizure, and 90% within 2 years.

Although children who have one or more febrile seizures are at higher risk than the normal population for the development of epilepsy, the risk is quite small. A large epidemiologic study in the United States examined the frequency of afebrile seizures in 1,706 children who had experienced at least one febrile seizure and were followed up to the age of 7 years. At least one afebrile seizure had occurred by the age of 7 in 3% of the patients with febrile seizures. Two percent of the group had two or more afebrile seizures by age 7 and would be considered to have epilepsy. Of 39,179 children who had never been reported to experience a febrile seizure, 0.5% had epilepsy by age 7 years. The risk for developing epilepsy, therefore, was 4 times higher in the group that had febrile seizures.

The risk of developing unprovoked seizures is increased by several factors: neurodevelopmental anomalies, complex febrile seizures, recurrent febrile seizures, brief duration of fever before initial seizure, and family history of epilepsy.

Prolonged febrile seizures have been implicated as a predisposing factor for the development of temporal lobe epilepsy and mesial temporal sclerosis, a pathologic condition of hippocampal sclerosis and atrophy with loss of neurons in the CA1 region and the *end-folium* region (CA3/CA4), but with relative sparing of the CA2 region (see Chapter 3). In most children with prolonged febrile seizures, temporal lobe epilepsy does not develop. Whether febrile status epilepticus plays a causal role in mesial temporal sclerosis is not clear but is now undergoing study.

A large epidemiologic study found that children who had febrile convulsions (simple or complex) performed as well as other children in terms of their academic progress, intellect, and behavior at 10 years.

G. Generalized Epilepsy with Febrile Seizures Plus

This syndrome (GEFS+) most often manifests with childhood onset (median age, 1 year) of multiple febrile seizures. Unlike typical febrile seizures, seizures with fever may persist beyond years 1 through 5, and afebrile seizure may also occur. Seizures usually cease by mid-childhood (median age, 11 years). Other phenotypes may include absence, myoclonic, atonic, or myoclonic–astatic seizures (see ref. 23 for details). This seizure type is inherited in an autosomal-dominant pattern with 50% to 60% penetrance and has been linked to multiple loci including: 2q24 (*SCN1A* and

SCN2A), 19q13 (*SCN1B*), and 5q31 (*GABRG2*). The genes on 2q24 and 19q13 produce subunits of the voltage-gated sodium channels, whereas the gene on 5q31 codes for the γ_2 subunit of the γ-aminobutyric acid (GABA)$_A$ receptor. The sodium channel is composed of an α subunit and one or more regulatory β subunits, and mutations of the subunits typically result in an increase in Na$^+$ currents and an increase in excitability. Phenotypes also vary across families because of different mutations and differences in other genetic and environmental cofactors.

As example of the varying phenotype associated with the sodium channel mutations is severe mycolonic epilepsy of infancy (SMEI), also called Dravet, a devastating disorder characterized by severe myoclonic seizures and mental regression. Mutations in *SCN1A* have been found in SMEI (Dravet syndrome), and most mutations are spontaneous. In 30% to 70% of SMEI patients, truncating and missense mutations in (*SCN1A*) have been identified. The majority of patients have truncating mutations that are predicted to be loss-of-function alleles. Recent evidence suggests that the Na$^+$ channels with mutations are expressed preferentially on interneurons. The loss of function of Na$^+$ channels in interneurons would be expected to lead to a severe lack of effective inhibition in the children and may account for the severe seizure phenotype. In addition to Dravet syndrome, some infants with other forms of early childhood epilepsy have *SCN1A* mutations (10).

II. ALCOHOL-RELATED EPILEPSY SYNDROMES

Most alcohol-related seizures are caused by alcohol withdrawal. However, one must be aware that alcoholics are at risk of having several other medical conditions that may present as seizures (see section **II.E**). Moreover, alcohol-withdrawal seizures frequently are accompanied by other symptoms and signs of alcohol withdrawal (anxiety, insomnia, irritability, nausea, tremor, tachycardia, hypertension, fever, hyperreflexia, and hallucinations) and may progress to delirium tremens. Alcoholism affects all social classes; 50% of alcoholics have attended college and hold managerial or professional positions.

A. Clinical Features of Alcohol-withdrawal Seizures

Patients usually are chronic alcoholics 30 years of age or older (Table 8-2). Ninety percent of alcohol-withdrawal seizures occur 7 to 48 hours after cessation of drinking, and 50% occur 13 to 24 hours after drinking has ceased. Thus some alcohol often is still present in the plasma at the time of the seizure, and the patient's breath may have the odor of alcohol on arrival at the hospital. Alcohol-withdrawal seizures can occur up to 7 days after stopping drinking. Clinical examination frequently reveals tremulousness and some myoclonic jerks of the extremities. Seizures typically are generalized-onset tonic–clonic. Seizures may be single (40%) or multiple (usually two to four). The time between the first and last seizure usually is less than 6 hours. If untreated, in one third of patients, full-blown delirium tremens develops, and in a small number, tonic–clonic status epilepticus.

Table 8-2. Features of seizures associated with alcohol use

Seizure category	Age at Onset	Acute Intoxication	First 48 hr of Withdrawal	Seizures after Prolonged Abstinence	Interictal EEG	Photic Sensitivity	Treatment
Acute seizures (electrolyte disturbance, hypoglycemia, meningitis)	Any age	Yes	Yes	No	Abnormal (slow)	Absent	Specific
Withdrawal seizures ("rum fits," alcoholic epilepsy)	30+ (90%)	No	Yes	No	90% normal	50% photomyoclonic (photomyogenic) or photoconvulsive	Lorazepam or diazepam and abstinence
Epilepsy after alcoholism, diazepam,	Any age	Infrequently	Yes	Yes	Usually abnormal (epileptiform patterns or slowing)	50% photomyoclonic (photomyogenic) or photoconvulsive	Lorazepam or maintenance antiepileptic drugs, and abstinence

EEG, electroencephalography.

III. DRUG-RELATED EPILEPSY SYNDROMES

A. Recreational Drug-induced Seizures

Amphetamines, cocaine, phencyclidine, and combinations of these drugs are the most common causes of recreational drug-induced seizures. Seizures are independent of route of administration and may occur in first-time or long-term abusers.

1. Amphetamines, Cocaine, and Phencyclidine

A. INTRODUCTION AND MECHANISMS OF ACTION. Amphetamines include amphetamine sulfate (Benzedrine), dextroamphetamine (Dexedrine), and methamphetamine (Methedrine, referred to as *ice*). Amphetamines are sympathetic stimulants that act through norepinephrine- and dopamine-mediated systems. Amphetamines may be smoked or taken orally.

Cocaine is a powerful sympathetic and central nervous system (CNS) stimulant and an effective local anesthetic. The sympathomimetic effects result from blocking the reuptake of the neurotransmitters norepinephrine, acetylcholine, serotonin, and dopamine by presynaptic neurons. Cocaine may be smoked (crack) or taken by nasal, oral, or intravenous routes. Cocaine frequently is cut with other drugs of abuse (amphetamines, opiates, phencyclidine).

Phencyclidine (PCP, angel dust) is a powerful sympathetic stimulant and psychotomimetic that may produce CNS stimulation or depression, depending on dosage. At high doses, it also has cholinergic properties. Phencyclidine may be smoked or taken by the nasal, oral, or intravenous routes.

B. CLINICAL FEATURES. These three drugs have many similarities in clinical features and treatment, because all three are sympathetic stimulants that also can cause CNS stimulation.

Minor toxic manifestations include tachypnea, tachycardia (occasionally, bradycardia with cocaine), mild hypertension, dry mouth, dizziness, chest pains, palpitations, abdominal cramps, nausea, diarrhea, mydriasis, diaphoresis, flushing, hyperactivity, hyperreflexia, irritability, confusion, apprehension, and hallucinations.

Major toxic manifestations include severe hypertension (may be associated with intracranial hemorrhage); tachyarrhythmias (may progress to ventricular tachycardia or fibrillation); severe hyperthermia (may lead to coagulopathies, rhabdomyolysis, or renal failure); seizures (tonic–clonic); acidosis; delirium; psychosis; coma; and myocardial ischemia or infarction. Hypotension or circulatory collapse (sometimes fatal) may occur because of cardiac arrhythmias, myocardial infarction, or catecholamine depletion.

Special features of cocaine intoxication include respiratory depression (often preceded by a tonic–clonic seizure, may lead to sudden death) and prominent cardiac toxicity (sensitizes the myocardium to epinephrine and norepinephrine, has a direct cardiotoxic effect, and causes coronary artery spasm).

Special features of phencyclidine intoxication include the triad of altered mental status (agitation, confusion, violent or bizarre behavior, psychosis, catatonia, stupor, coma); hypertension; and horizontal or vertical nystagmus. Bronchial hypersecretion, bronchospasm, or dystonic reactions also may occur.

C. MANAGEMENT. Most stimulant-related seizures are single tonic–clonic seizures. Multiple or focal seizures suggest additional drug use or an underlying seizure disorder.

Seizures are managed immediately with intravenous lorazepam or diazepam. Adequate doses should be administered to terminate seizures and to diminish agitation, reduce hypertension, and slow tachycardia. Repetitive or prolonged seizures require the administration of a loading dose of phenobarbital or phenytoin after the procedures described in Chapter 7. General anesthesia with pentobarbital may be necessary in persistent seizures. Patients with seizures should be evaluated for intracranial hemorrhage or other new CNS lesions and for rhabdomyolysis.

Other aspects of management include provision of a cool and quiet environment, gastric decontamination, sedation, and treatment of other manifestations, including arrhythmias, hypertension, hypotension, respiratory depression, hyperthermia, chest pain, behavioral disturbances, uncontrollable motor activity, and (for phencyclidine) dystonic reactions and bronchospasm. For these topics, the reader is referred to a textbook of emergency medicine, such as Howell's (see references).

2. Opiates

Although opiates generally cause CNS depression, overdose with meperidine (Demerol) or propoxyphene (Talwin) may cause seizures. Naloxone hydrochloride is used to reverse the CNS effects (including seizures) of opiate intoxication. Propoxyphene overdose may require larger than average doses.

B. Nonrecreational Drug-induced Seizures

A long list of drugs prescribed for valid indications may precipitate seizures (Table 8-3).

Antidepressants and antipsychotics draw special consideration because of the not-infrequent association of epilepsy with depression or psychosis. The use of these drugs in persons with epilepsy is reviewed in Chapter 10.

High-dose intravenous penicillin may induce refractory status epilepticus, especially in patients with structural brain lesions. In this situation, the penicillin should be stopped immediately. Theoretic and empiric evidence indicates that phenobarbital reverses penicillin-induced seizures because of opposing actions on chloride channels.

C. Sedative–hypnotic Drug-withdrawal Seizures

1. Description and Mechanism of Action

The usual drugs to cause withdrawal seizures are the sedative–hypnotic classes of drugs: barbiturates, benzodiazepines, and nonbarbiturate sedative–hypnotic agents. The mechanism of action and clinical features of seizures caused by withdrawal from these drugs are similar to those of alcohol-withdrawal seizures.

2. Clinical Features

Onset of symptoms is dependent on the duration of action and elimination half-life of the drug. Short-acting agents (e.g., alpra-

**Table 8-3.   Safe and unsafe drugs in patients
with porphyria**

Safe Drugs	Unsafe Drugs
Acetaminophen	Barbiturates
Acetazolamide	Carbamazepine
Allopurinol	Chloramphenicol
Aminoglycosides	Chlordiazepoxide
Amitriptyline	Diphenhydramine
Aspirin	Enalapril
Atropine	Ergot compounds
Bromides	Erythromycin
Bupivacaine	Ethanol
Chloral hydrate	Flucloxacillin
Chlorpromazine	Flufenamic acid
Codeine	Griseofulvin
Corticosteroids	Hydrochlorothiazide
Diazepam	Imipramine
Gabapentin	Lisinopril
Heparin	Methyldopa
Insulin	Metochlopromide
Meclizine	Nifedipine
Meperidine	Oral contraceptives
Morphine	Pentazocine
Penicillins (see *Unsafe Drugs* for exceptions)	Phenytoin
Procaine	Piroxicam
Prochlorperazine	Pivampicillin
Promethazine	Progesterone
Propoxyphene	Pyrazinamide
Propranolol	Rifampin
Propylthiouracil	Sulfonamides
Quinidine	Theophylline
Streptomycin	Valproic acid
Temazepam	Verapamil
Tetracycline	
Thyroxine	
Trifluoperazine	
Warfarin	

From Eisenschenk S, Gilmore RL. Seizures associated with nonneurological
medical conditions. In: Wyllie E, ed. *The treatment of epilepsy: principles and
practice*. Philadelphia: Lippincott Williams & Wilkins, 2001:657–670, with
permission.

zolam) may show withdrawal features within 24 hours; long-
acting agents (e.g., diazepam, phenobarbital) may not show withdrawal features for 7 days or longer. Symptoms include weakness,
insomnia, restlessness, anorexia, apprehension, headache, anxiety, and irritability. Signs include tremor, fever, diaphoresis,
dehydration, tachycardia, postural hypotension, dyspnea, and

hyperreflexia. More serious findings include myoclonus, seizures (may progress to status epilepticus), hyperpyrexia, hallucinations, and delirium.

3. Management

A. BARBITURATE OR NONBARBITURATE SEDATIVE–HYPNOTIC DEPENDENCE. Tolerance to sedative or hypnotic drugs is confirmed by administering 200 mg of pentobarbital intramuscularly or *per os.* Absence of sedation after 1 hour confirms tolerance. The patient's daily habitual dose is estimated by history. This dose of the abused drug (or an equivalent dose of phenobarbital, up to 500 mg/d) is administered initially by using a t.i.d. regimen, and then gradually discontinued. The following dosages are equivalent to 30 mg of phenobarbital: 100 mg of pentobarbital; 500 mg of chloral hydrate; 350 mg of ethchlorvynol; 250 mg of glutethimide; 250 mg of methaqualone.

B. BENZODIAZEPINE DEPENDENCE. The patient is restarted on a daily dose of benzodiazepine (or an equivalent dose of phenobarbital up to 500 mg per day) by using a t.i.d. regimen and then gradually discontinued. The following dosages are equivalent to 30 mg of phenobarbital: 10 mg diazepam or 100 mg chlordiazepoxide.

D. Other Drug-withdrawal Seizures

Suddenly stopping opiates, amphetamines, or cocaine may induce tonic–clonic seizures. Suddenly stopping an antiepileptic drug in a patient with epilepsy may precipitate seizures of the patient's usual type, status epilepticus, or both.

IV. ECLAMPSIA

A. Definition

Preeclampsia (toxemia gravidarum) is a pregnancy-induced disorder consisting of proteinuria and edema after week 20 of gestation. The disorder is complex and may involve multiple organ systems with resultant pulmonary edema, oliguria, disseminated intravascular coagulopathy, and hepatic hemorrhages. Neurologic problems include headache, confusion, hyperreflexia, visual hallucinations, and even blindness. Eclampsia is the occurrence of convulsions, not caused by any coincidental neurologic disease such as long-standing epilepsy or intracranial structural lesions, in a woman who has the criteria for preeclampsia. The timing of seizures does not correlate with the severity of preeclampsia, and seizures may occur even when few signs of preeclampsia are present.

The causes of preeclampsia/eclampsia are poorly understood, and why seizures occur with the condition is not clear. Some evidence suggests primary roles for endothelial damage, increased platelet aggregation and platelet consumption, and hypertension in the pathogenesis of the disorder. Pathologic examination of the brain has revealed diffuse cerebral edema; subarachnoid, subcortical, and petechial hemorrhages; and small infarctions of multiple areas in the brain.

B. Seizure Phenomena

The seizures may be partial or secondarily generalized; they may appear before, during, or after childbirth. Although they are most common within the first postpartum day, some patients may experience them for as long as a month after delivery.

C. Electroencephalographic Phenomena

EEGs are usually abnormal with focal or diffuse slowing and epileptiform activity. The epileptiform activity can be focal, multifocal, or generalized.

D. Treatment

Magnesium sulfate has been a standard treatment for both preeclampsia and eclampsia. Magnesium blocks the NMDA channel, a subtype of the glutamate receptor. Therefore magnesium blockade might work as both an anticonvulsant and neuroprotectant through this mechanism. Magnesium sulfate might also act as a calcium antagonist, preventing cerebral vasoconstriction and subsequent epileptogenic cortical injury. Although magnesium is not an effective treatment in other forms of epilepsy, its role in the treatment of seizures secondary to eclampsia has now been demonstrated. However, magnesium sulfate is not without problems. It has a short half-life and can lead to sedation in the mother and hypotonia, hyporeflexia, and lethargy in the newborn.

Other drugs used in the treatment of seizures in eclampsia include phenytoin, nimodipine, diazepam, and lorazepam. Phenytoin is particularly useful because it is effective in stopping the seizures and has minimal effects on the infant. As for status epilepticus, a loading dose of 20 mg/kg can be given, with maintenance doses started 24 hours later. Nimodipine has been shown to be inferior to magnesium sulfate for prevention of eclampsia.

V. REFLEX SEIZURES

In reflex seizures, seizures are regularly elicited by some specific stimulus or event. As the term is commonly used, *reflex seizures* include cases in which the stimulus does not invariably produce a seizure, in which spontaneous seizures may occur, or in which both are true.

Animal studies indicate that reflex seizures may be caused by hyperexcitable neurons (on a structural or biochemical basis) in either primary receptive areas or in their efferent connections. Entry of a stimulus activates these hyperexcitable neurons.

The types of stimuli that can evoke seizures are visual (most common), thinking, music, eating, reading, exercise, proprioception, praxis, somatosensory, and others.

A. Reflex Seizures with Visual Triggers

Visual reflex seizures are divided into two major groups, depending on whether seizures are induced by flickering light.

1. Seizures Induced by Flickering Light

A distinct group of patients with photosensitive epilepsy has seizures provoked by flickering lights and demonstrate on the

EEG an epileptiform discharge elicited by a strobe light. The photoconvulsive response is characterized by spike-and-wave and multiple spike-and-wave complexes that are bilaterally synchronous, symmetric, and widespread. These may be contrasted with spikes that are time-linked with photic stimulation and confined to the occipital region, which may be a normal finding. The photoconvulsive response may be self-limited and cease during stimulation or continue beyond the stimulation. Seizures evoked by photic stimulation are usually primarily generalized: generalized tonic–clonic, absence, or myoclonic seizures. Although patients with partial seizures may have photoconvulsive responses during the EEG, it is unusual for a partial seizure to be provoked by photic stimulation. Generalized epileptiform discharges during photic stimulation correlate with generalized seizures, whereas focal discharges are more commonly associated with partial seizures.

Photosensitive seizures can be classified into two major groups: (a) pure photosensitive seizures, in which clinical seizures occur only when the patient is exposed to the photic stimulus, and (b) photosensitive seizures, in which spontaneous seizures occur in addition to those induced by light stimulation. Precipitating stimuli that can produce a seizure include television and video games, sunlight reflected from water, sunlight viewed through leaves of trees in a breeze or while driving along tree-lined streets, discotheque lights, and faulty fluorescent lighting. Photosensitive epilepsy usually appears around puberty, with the mean age at onset of 14 years. Some patients experience pleasant sensations during photosensitive seizures and self-induce such seizures by engaging in activities such as rapidly waving their hands in front of their eyes or purposefully staring at blinking lights.

2. Seizures Not Induced by Flicker

Absence, myoclonus, or, more rarely, tonic–clonic seizures may occur in response to patterns (pattern-sensitive seizures). Such patterns typically are striped and include common objects such as a television screen at short distances, striped clothing or drapes, and escalator steps. Eye closure may produce absence or myoclonic seizures in some persons. Some persons with pattern-sensitive seizures or seizures induced by eye closure deliberately induce seizures because of pleasurable sensations associated with seizures.

B. Reflex Seizures Induced by Nonvisual Stimuli
1. Seizures Induced by Thinking

Some patients have myoclonic, absence, or tonic–clonic seizures induced by specific thinking tasks. Such tasks include card or board games, mental arithmetic, manipulation of spatial information, and complex decision making. Often, more than one trigger, spontaneous seizures, or both are present. Interictal EEGs are usually normal or show photosensitivity (25%). Ictal EEGs show generalized spike-and-wave patterns. Age at onset is in the teens, with a male preponderance.

2. Musicogenic Seizures

Some patients have simple partial seizures, complex partial seizures, or both, in response to music (often a specific piece). Emotional reactions mediated by limbic structures may play a role. Spontaneous seizures may also occur. Interictal EEGs show sharp and slow activity in temporal leads, more often on the right side.

3. Eating Seizures

Simple or complex partial seizures, or both, may be induced by the sight or smell of food or by gastric distention after eating food. Such patients usually have focal symptomatic epilepsy originating in the temporolimbic area. Sensory, autonomic, or emotional inputs to this area during eating appear to activate seizures.

4. Reading Seizures and Language-induced Seizures

Reading (usually prolonged), speaking, or writing may induce a typical seizure pattern of jaw jerks or clicks followed by a generalized convulsion if the inducing activity is not stopped. Absence of jaw jerks or presence of spontaneous seizures, or both, may occur. The interictal EEG usually is normal. Ictal EEGs may show focal (temporoparietal) or generalized discharges.

5. Exercise-induced Seizures

Such seizures can arise after several minutes of vigorous exercise. The clinical seizures occur as complex partial seizures of temporal lobe type. Left temporal sharp or slow seizures may be seen on the interictal EEG.

6. Proprioceptive Input (Movement-induced Seizures)

Sudden, unexpected stimuli may produce lateralized tonic seizures in patients with lesions in the supplementary motor area or mesial frontal cortex (startle epilepsy). A second syndrome consists of attacks induced by active or passive movement without startle.

7. Praxis-induced Seizures

Myoclonic, absence, or tonic–clonic seizures may be induced by performing certain tasks such as typing. EEGs obtained simultaneously with the seizures show bilateral spikes or spike–waves, often with a central predominance. Many patients have other types of generalized seizures, including juvenile myoclonic epilepsy.

8. Seizures Triggered by Somatosensory Stimulation

Touching or rubbing parts of the body may induce partial seizures, often with localized sensory symptoms. These seizures occur in patients with postrolandic lesions and are treated with drugs for partial seizures.

9. Other Types of Reflex Epilepsies

Seizures have been reported in association with touch, tooth brushing, walking, defecation, hot water, and vestibular stimulation.

C. Management of Reflex Seizures

Management of reflex seizures offers three options: (a) avoidance of trigger, (b) desensitization therapy, and (c) antiepileptic drugs. Avoidance of the trigger is effective in some, but not all, patients. Television epilepsy can be helped by increasing distance from the television, by using a small screen in a well-lit room, and by use of a remote control to avoid the need to approach the television closely. Desensitization therapy has been successfully applied to many forms of reflex epilepsy. Valproic acid and lamotrigine are the drugs of choice for reflex epilepsies with absence, myoclonic, or tonic–clonic seizures. Partial seizures are treated with oxcarbazepine, carbamazepine, or phenytoin.

REFERENCES

1. American Academy of Pediatrics, Committee on quality Improvement Subcommittee on Febrile Seizures. Practice parameter: long-term treatment of the child with simple febrile seizures. *Pediatrics* 1999;103:1307–1308.
2. Belfort MA, Anthony J, Saade GR, et al. A comparison of magnesium sulfate and nimodipine for prevention of eclampsia. *N Engl J Med* 2003;348:304–311.
3. D'Onofrio G, Tathlev NK, Ulrich AS, et al. Lorazepam for the prevention of recurrent seizures related to alcohol. *N Engl J Med* 1999;340:915–919.
4. Duchowny M. Febrile seizures in childhood. In: Wyllie E, ed. *The treatment of epilepsy: principles and practice.* Philadelphia: Lippincott Williams & Wilkins, 2001:601–608.
5. Dulac O. Use of antiepileptic drugs in children. In: Levy RH, Mattson RH, Meldrum BS, et al., eds. *Antiepileptic drugs.* 5th ed. Philadelphia: Lippincott Williams & Wilkins, 2002: 119–131.
6. Eisenschenk S, Gilmore RL. Seizures associated with nonneurological medical conditions. In: Wyllie E, ed. *The treatment of epilepsy: principles and practice.* Philadelphia: Lippincott Williams & Wilkins, 2001:657–670. (Has reviews of eclampsia and drug- and alcohol-related seizures.)
7. Farwell JR, Lee YJ, Hirtz DG, et al., eds. Phenobarbital for febrile seizures: effects on intelligence and on seizure recurrence. *N Engl J Med* 1990;322:364–369.
8. Gilliam FG, Chiappa RH. Significance of spontaneous epileptiform abnormalities associated with photoparoxysmal response. *Neurology* 1995;45:453–456.
9. Goldfrank LR, Flomenbaum NE, Lewin NA, et al., eds. *Toxicologic emergencies.* East Norwalk, CT: Appleton & Lange, 1997.
10. Harkin LA, McMahon JM, Iona X, et al. The spectrum of SCN1A-related infantile epileptic encephalopathies. *Brain* 2007;130:843–852.
11. Hirtz DG, Nelson KB. The natural history of febrile seizures. *Annu Rev Med* 1983;34:453–471.
12. Howell JM. *Emergency medicine.* Philadelphia: Saunders, 1998.
13. Iwasaki N, Nakayama J, Hamano K, et al. Molecular genetics of febrile seizures. *Epilepsia* 2002;43(suppl 9):32–35.
14. Kaplan PW, Repke JT. Eclampsia. *Neurol Clin* 1994;12:565–582.

15. Leone M, Bottacchi E, Beghi E, et al. Alcohol use is a risk factor for a first generalized tonic-clonic seizure. *Neurology* 1997;48: 614–620.
16. Lucas MJ, Leveno KJ, Cunningham FG. A comparison of magnesium sulfate with phenytoin for prevention of eclampsia. *N Engl J Med* 1995;333:201–205.
17. O'Dell C, Shinnar S, Ballaban-Gil KR, et al. Rectal diazepam gel in the home management of seizures in children. *Pediatr Neurol* 2005;33:166–172.
18. Porter RJ, Mattson RH. Alcohol and drug abuse. In: Engel J, Pedley TA, eds. *Epilepsy: a comprehensive textbook*. Philadelphia: Lippincott-Raven, 1997:2629–2635.
19. Roman NP, Colton T, Labazzo J, et al., eds. A controlled trial of diazepam administered during febrile illnesses to prevent recurrence of febrile seizures. *N Engl J Med* 1993;329:79–84.
20. Ryan SG. Ion channels and the genetic contribution to epilepsy. *J Child Neurol* 1999;14:58–66.
21. Singh R, Scheffer IE, Crossland K, et al. Generalized epilepsy with febrile seizures plus: a common childhood onset genetic epilepsy syndrome. *Ann Neurol* 1999;45:75–81.
22. Stein RJ, Chudnofsky CR. *Emergency medicine*. Boston: Little, Brown, 1994.
23. Strum JW, Fedi M, Bercovic SF, et al. Exercise-induced temporal lobe epilepsy. *Neurology* 2002;59:1246–1248. (A video is available with this reference. See article for details.)
24. Tarkka R, Paakko E, Pyhtinen J, et al. Febrile seizures and mesial temporal sclerosis: no association in a long-term follow up study. *Neurology* 2003;60:215–218.
25. Verity CM, Greenwood R, Golding J. Long-term intellectual and behavioral outcomes of children with febrile convulsions. *N Engl J Med* 1998;338:723–728.
26. Wallace RH, Scheffer IE, Barnett S, et al. Neuronal sodium-channel alpha1-subunit mutations in generalized epilepsy with febrile seizures plus. *Am J Hum Genet* 2001;68:859–865.
27. Weiser HG, Hungerbuhler H, Siegel AM, et al. Musicogenic epilepsy: review of the literature and case report with single photon emission computed tomography. *Epilepsia* 1997;38:200–207.
28. Wolf P. Behavioral therapy. In: Engel J, Pedley TA, eds. *Epilepsy: a comprehensive textbook*. Philadelphia: Lippincott-Raven, 1997: 1359–1364.
29. Zifkin B, Anderman F. Epilepsy with reflex seizures. In: Wyllie E, ed. *The treatment of epilepsy: principles and practice*. Philadelphia: Lippincott Williams & Wilkins, 2001:537–550.

9

Diagnosis and Differential Diagnosis

Diagnostic tasks in epilepsy management include establishing a seizure diagnosis and an etiologic diagnosis and identification of precipitating factors. This is accomplished by a combination of history taking, physical examination, electroencephalography (EEG), and laboratory examinations. Common differential diagnostic problems are reviewed at the end of this chapter.

I. SEIZURE DIAGNOSIS

The first step in managing a patient for whom a diagnosis of epilepsy is possible is establishing definitively whether the patient has epilepsy. Patients who are erroneously diagnosed with epilepsy will be unnecessarily subjected to many inconveniences, including medication that may produce serious side effects, expensive laboratory tests, loss of a driver's license, and possible loss of employment. Specific differential-diagnostic entities that must be differentiated from seizures are discussed in section **IX**.

If a patient has epilepsy, accurately determining which type(s) of epileptic seizure the patient has is crucial, so that he or she can be given correct therapy. The diagnosis of seizure type should be made according to the International Classification of Epileptic Seizures, reviewed briefly in Chapter 1 and in detail in Chapter 2. The specific epilepsy syndrome should also be identified, as treatment of a given seizure type may vary among the specific epilepsy syndromes. For example, tonic–clonic seizures as part of mesial temporal lobe epilepsy are often treated differently from tonic–clonic seizures as part of juvenile myoclonic epilepsy.

II. ETIOLOGIC DIAGNOSIS

Epilepsy is a symptom, not a disease. A seizure can be a symptom of old or recent cerebral trauma, a brain tumor, a brain abscess, encephalitis, meningitis, a metabolic disturbance, drug intoxication, drug withdrawal, and many other disease processes. It is imperative that the underlying cause of a patient's seizure be identified and treated, so that a reversible cerebral disease process is not overlooked, and seizure control can be facilitated.

III. PRECIPITATING FACTORS

In addition to determining the underlying cause(s) of a patient's seizure disorder, identifying and managing factors that precipitate seizures in a given individual, such as anxiety, sleep deprivation, and alcohol withdrawal (Fig. 9-1), also are important. Management of such precipitating factors reduces seizure frequency and the patient's need for medication.

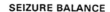

SEIZURE BALANCE

Seizure Control

Adequate Amount of AED in Blood
Adequate Sleep and Rest   Correct AED
Fluid and   Good Nutrition
Electrolyte Balance   Alcohol Abstinence
Low Anxiety Level

Trauma/Illness/Fever   Hyperventilation
Lack of Sleep
Photosensitivity
Increased Emotional Stress
Hormonal Changes
Fluid & Electrolyte Imbalance
Alcohol/Drugs

Seizure Precipitants
(Triggers)

Fig. 9-1.   Factors promoting seizure control and factors precipitating seizures. AED, antiepileptic drug.

IV. HISTORY

The best way to diagnose which type of seizure a patient has is actually to observe a seizure, although the physician usually does not have the opportunity to do so. Often, the most important differential-diagnostic information is contained in the history gathered from the patient, reliable observers, or both. Family members and friends of the patient should be encouraged to try to videotape the events, when possible.

The history for seizure diagnosis should include exact details of events before, during, and after the seizure, obtained from the patient and observers. Partial seizure symptoms and signs (motor, sensory, autonomic, psychic); alteration of consciousness; automatisms; tonic movements, clonic movements, or both; tongue biting; incontinence; and postictal behavior are important details. The duration, time of occurrence (e.g., on awakening, when drowsy, during sleep), and frequency of seizures also are important. For example, tonic–clonic seizures occurring during the first few hours of sleep are usually secondarily generalized, whereas tonic–clonic seizures occurring on awakening are usually primarily generalized. Past or current occurrence of other seizure types (especially myoclonic or absence) often is not volunteered by the patient and should be specifically solicited. Specific questions regarding entities that may be confused with seizures are discussed later, in section **IX**.

The history for etiology should include questions regarding family history of epilepsy, head trauma, birth complications, febrile convulsions, middle ear and sinus infections (which may erode through bone and cause cerebral focus), alcohol or drug abuse, and symptoms of malignancy.

The history for precipitating factors should include factors such as fever, anxiety, sleep deprivation, menstrual cycle, alcohol, hyperventilation, flickering lights, or television (Fig. 9-1).

V. PHYSICAL EXAMINATION

Although neuroimaging has supplanted the neurologic examination in the eyes of some, the value of the examination should not be underestimated. A detailed physical and neurologic examination can frequently point to the etiology of the epilepsy. The physical examination should be directed toward uncovering evidence of past or recent head trauma; infections of the ears and sinuses; congenital abnormalities (e.g., hemiatrophy, stigmata of tuberous sclerosis); focal or diffuse neurologic abnormalities; stigmata of alcohol or drug abuse; and signs of malignancy. Subtle but "hard" findings may be useful in uncovering evidence of focal brain dysfunction indicative of symptomatic focal epilepsy. Such findings include facial asymmetry, asymmetry of thumb size (indicates contralateral cerebral damage during infancy or childhood), drift or pronation of outstretched hands, dystonic posture when walking on sides of feet, or naming difficulty (left temporal dysfunction). Finally, 3 minutes of vigorous hyperventilation usually produces absence seizures in untreated absence seizure patients.

VI. ELECTROENCEPHALOGRAPHY

The EEG is a helpful diagnostic tool in the investigation of a seizure disorder. It confirms the presence of abnormal electrical activity, gives information regarding the type of seizure disorder, and discloses the location of the seizure focus. Both routine (paper tracing) and digital recording techniques are in regular use. In some instances, the routine EEG is normal, although the patient has seizures or is suspected of having them. Under these circumstances, the study is repeated after the patient is deprived of sleep (4 hours or less of sleep the night before the study), and special (e.g., temporal or sphenoidal) leads also may be used. This procedure is helpful in bringing out the abnormality in many cases, especially if discharges arise from the temporal lobe.

If the history unequivocally points to a seizure disorder, the patient should be treated despite normal waking and sleep-deprived EEGs. The usual EEG study samples only roughly 1 hour of time and is normal in a significant percentage of patients with epilepsy. In cases in which whether a patient has seizures is uncertain or the seizure type cannot be determined despite a careful history, physical examination, and routine waking and sleep-deprived EEGs, the diagnosis often can be established by prolonged monitoring of the EEG.

VII. LABORATORY EXAMINATION (INCLUDING NEUROIMAGING)

Usually, the following laboratory tests should be performed in evaluating the cause of a newly diagnosed seizure disorder: metabolic screen, EEG recording in waking and sleep states, and magnetic resonance imaging (MRI) or computed tomographic (CT) scan. MRI is preferred over CT because of its greater sensitivity and specificity for identifying small lesions. A toxic screen should be performed if alcohol or drug abuse or withdrawal is suspected. A lumbar puncture (for opening pressure, cell counts, protein, glucose, cytology, culture, and serology) should be performed if infection or malignancy is suspected.

The American Academy of Neurology has published practice parameters for neuroimaging (NI) studies (MRI, CT) of patients having a first seizure. Emergency NI (scan immediately) should be performed when a health care provider suspects a serious structural lesion. Clinical studies have shown a higher frequency of life-threatening lesions in patients with new focal deficits, persistent altered mental status (with or without intoxication), fever, recent trauma, persistent headache, history of cancer, history of anticoagulation, or suspicion of acquired immunodeficiency syndrome.

Urgent NI (scan is included in the disposition or is performed before disposition when follow-up of the patient's neurologic problem cannot be ensured) should be considered for patients who have completely recovered from their seizure and for whose seizures no clear-cut cause (e.g., hypoglycemia, hyponatremia, tricyclic overdose) has been identified to help determine a possible structural source. Because adequate follow-up is needed to ensure a patient's neurologic health, urgent NI may be obtained before disposition when timely follow-up cannot be ensured.

Additionally, for patients with first-time seizure, emergency NI should be considered if the patient is older than 40 years or has had partial-onset seizures.

MRI and CT are the two imaging techniques used in routine diagnosis and management of epilepsy. A number of specialized imaging studies are used for localizing seizure-producing lesions for purposes of surgical resection. These studies include single-photon emission CT (SPECT), positron emission tomography (PET), proton magnetic resonance spectroscopy, and magnetoencephalography (MEG). These specialized tests are discussed in Chapter 10.

VIII. SYNTHESIS OF DATA

By combining history, physical examination, and EEG information, the health care provider should be able to determine (a) whether the patient's events are seizures and (b) the patient's seizure type(s) according to the International Classification of Epileptic Seizures (see Chapter 2, Table 2-1). If this cannot be done, additional history (e.g., additional witnesses) or additional EEG (e.g., long-term EEG monitoring) information, or both, should be obtained. If all possible information has been gathered and the diagnosis remains uncertain, the health care provider usually is forced to act on the basis of available history. If the history strongly suggests a recurrent seizure type, a therapeutic trial of antiepileptic medication appropriate for the seizure type is usually begun. If the history does not strongly suggest recurrent seizures, observation without medication is the usual plan. Management of a patient having a single seizure is discussed in Chapter 10.

Seizure type combined with additional information from history, physical examination, EEG, and laboratory tests often allows determination of the patient's specific epilepsy syndrome according to the International Classification of Epilepsies and

Table 9-1. Differential diagnosis of epilepsy at various ages

A. All ages
  1. Epilepsy vs. migraine
  2. Epilepsy vs. syncope
  3. Epilepsy vs. Ménière disease
  4. Epilepsy vs. episodic dyscontrol (rage attacks)
  5. Epilepsy vs. psychogenic seizure
  6. Absence seizures vs. complex partial seizures
B. In children
  1. Epilepsy vs. movement disorder (tic, chorea, tremor)
  2. Epilepsy vs. cyanotic breath-holding spell
  3. Epilepsy vs. pallid infantile syncope
  4. Epilepsy vs. prolonged Q-T syndrome
  5. Epilepsy vs. sleep disturbance (night terrors, sleepwalking)
  6. Epilepsy vs. abdominal migraine vs. intraabdominal disease
  7. Epilepsy vs. episodic dyscontrol
C. In adults
  1. Epilepsy vs. transient ischemic attack
  2. Epilepsy vs. transient global amnesia

Epileptic Syndromes. This determination assists with selection of therapy and counseling regarding prognosis and familial occurrence.

IX. DIFFERENTIAL DIAGNOSIS OF EPILEPSY
The common differential diagnostic problems associated with epilepsy at various ages are shown in Table 9-1.

A. All Ages
1. Epilepsy Versus Migraine
A. COMMON FEATURES. Episodic occurrence, headache, sensory (visual, paresthesias) or motor (weakness) aura, loss of consciousness (basilar migraine), and focal slowing on EEG are all common features of both epilepsy and migraine. Both disorders are common, and they can occur in the same patient.

B. FEATURES SUGGESTING EPILEPSY. Absent or less severe headache, bilateral and nonpulsatile; paroxysmal activity on interictal and ictal EEG (spikes, sharp waves, spike–waves); and persistent slowing on interictal EEG are features suggesting epilepsy.

C. FEATURES SUGGESTING MIGRAINE. Severe unilateral, pulsatile headache; nausea and vomiting; photophobia; family history of migraine; and EEG slowing only during or immediately after an attack are features suggesting migraine.

D. OTHER. The neurologic auras of migraine may occur with or without headache. A large and conflicting literature exists on the EEG in migraine. Patients with only migraine may have paroxysmally abnormal EEGs. Abdominal epilepsy and abdominal migraine are discussed in section **IX.B.6**.

E. DIFFERENTIAL DIAGNOSIS. The differential diagnosis is listed in Table 9-2.

Table 9-2.   **Migraine versus temporal lobe epilepsy**

	Migraine	Temporal Lobe Epilepsy
Aura duration	2–5 min	5–30 sec
Aura type	Visual phenomenon most common	Aura often difficult to define and consists of fear, detachment, or abdominal sensation
Impairment of consciousness	Usually none except in complex partial seizures	Impaired consciousness in complex partial seizure
Postictal impairment	No postictal impairment	Postictal impairment in complex partial seizure
EEG	Interictal and ictal EEG usually normal or shows nonspecific findings	Interictal and ictal EEG usually abnormal.

2. Epilepsy Versus Syncope

A. DEFINITIONS. Syncope, or fainting, is the sudden loss of muscle tone, collapse of posture, and loss of consciousness associated with a decrease in systemic blood pressure. Syncopal attacks begin with a clouding of consciousness accompanied by vertigo, nausea, and a waxy pallor of the skin. The attack usually lasts approximately 10 seconds.

Syncope can occur because of one of two mechanisms: autonomic failure and neural mediation. In autonomic failure, sympathetic efferent activity is chronically impaired, so that vasoconstriction is deficient. On standing, blood pressure always decreases (i.e., orthostatic hypotension), and syncope or presyncope occurs. In neurally mediated syncope, the failure of symptomatic efferent vasoconstriction traffic (and hypotension) occurs episodically in response to a trigger. Between syncopal episodes, the patients have normal blood pressure and orthostatic responses.

Convulsive syncope has an onset similar to that of a typical syncopal attack. However, the onset is followed by a tonic spasm in which the back, head, and lower limbs are bent backward and the fists are clenched. This is often accompanied by mydriasis, nystagmus, drooling of saliva, and incontinence. The patient may bite his or her tongue, although this is rare.

The patient who falls to the floor quickly recovers from a faint when the blood pressure is reestablished. If the person is unable to reach the supine position, as when fainting occurs in a chair or in a phone booth, cerebral circulation is reestablished more slowly. Under these conditions, convulsive syncope is more likely to occur.

B. DIFFERENTIAL DIAGNOSIS. See Table 9-3.

Table 9-3. Seizure versus syncope

Clinical Feature	Syncope	Seizure
Age at onset	Adult or child	Adult or child
Posture	Depends on initial condition or posture (erect)	Any posture
Muscle tone	Flaccid	Increased in tonic–clonic and some absence and complex partial seizures
Duration	10 sec	1–2 min (tonic–clonic); 1–3 min (complex partial); <15 sec (absence)
Sleep	Rarely occurs in sleep (but may if cardiac in origin)	May occur during sleep, on awakening, or after sleep deprivation
Incontinence	Rarely	Often
Tongue biting or injury	Not likely with hypotonia	May occur during tonic phase
Skin color	Pale	Flushed
Respirations	Slow unless syncope is caused by hyperventilation	Apnea; gasping
Perspiration	Cold, clammy	Hot, sweaty
Electroencephalogram during event	Nonspecific slow	Specific paroxysms
Electroencephalogram	Normal	Paroxysmal activity between events
Electrocardiogram	May show arrhythmia, PVCs, asystole, or other abnormality	Usually normal
Family history	Of syncope (sometimes)	Positive for seizure (sometimes)

PVC, premature ventricular contraction.

C. **OTHER.** Loss of postural tone, along with loss of consciousness, may cause falls that mimic syncope in absence, atonic, and complex partial seizures. Prolonged EEG monitoring, prolonged electrocardiographic monitoring, or both is indicated when a differential diagnosis cannot be made on the basis of the criteria listed in Table 9-3. One channel of a prolonged EEG recording can be devoted to electrocardiographic monitoring.

3. Epilepsy Versus Ménière Disease

A. **COMMON FEATURES.** Episodic vertigo, tinnitus, or both can occur in epilepsy and in Ménière disease. Interictal EEG is abnormal in 25% of Ménière disease patients (temporal slowing).

B. **FEATURES SUGGESTING EPILEPSY.** Other symptoms of simple partial or complex seizures of lateral temporal origin (altered consciousness, language disorders, visual misperceptions) and sharp waves or spikes on interictal EEG suggest a diagnosis of epilepsy.

C. **FEATURES SUGGESTING MÉNIÈRE DISEASE.** Hearing loss suggests a diagnosis of Ménière disease.

4. Epilepsy Versus Episodic Dyscontrol (Rage Attacks)

A. **DEFINITIONS.** The episodic dyscontrol syndrome is characterized by recurrent attacks of uncontrollable rage, aggression (verbal or physical), or both. Of particular note, attacks typically have an identifiable precipitant, although the severity of the precipitant typically does not justify the severity of the attack. The syndrome is usually seen in teenagers and young adults, but it can be seen in younger children and older adults. Many patients have an irritable personality between attacks. In many patients, neurologic impairment is evident on neurologic examination. In particular, evidence may be seen of ventromedial frontal lobe impairment because this area is involved in measuring behavioral response to environmental stimuli. The diagnosis is based on the history provided by patients, relatives, and onlookers. The patient's attacks occur suddenly and can be explosive and characterized by uncontrollable behavior, consisting of verbal aggression and even physical violence, such as kicking, gouging, scratching, spitting, hitting, and biting. In girls and women, the violence is frequently verbal and consists of obscene, profane language. Patients often display remarkable strength and speed in their attacks. During the attacks, the patients often appear temporarily psychotic, and after the attacks, amnesia, fatigue, and, occasionally, remorse may occur. Finally, for episodic dyscontrol syndrome and real partial seizures to exist in the same patient is not uncommon because both are consequences of brain damage (especially in head-injury patients).

B. **DIFFERENTIAL DIAGNOSIS.** See Table 9-4.

5. Epilepsy Versus Psychogenic Seizures

A. **EXTENT OF PROBLEM.** Psychogenic seizures are more common than is generally realized. The incidence is estimated at three per 100,000, and the prevalence is estimated at 300,000 to 400,000 cases in the United States. Of persons referred to epilepsy centers for medically refractory epilepsy, 10% to 30% have psychogenic seizures. Some patients with psychogenic seizures also have "real" seizures, making management particularly complex.

Table 9-4. Epilepsy versus episodic dyscontrol (rage attacks)

Clinical Data	Episodic Dyscontrol	Epilepsy[a]
Precipitating factors	Almost always	Occasionally
Warning	No	May have aura
Violence	Frequently; often person-directed	Rarely; almost never person-directed
Stereotype of attacks	Variable	Usually stereotyped
Incontinence	Rarely	Occasionally
Self-injury	Occasionally	Occasionally
Amnesia for event	Often	Usually for part of event
Postictal symptoms	Frequently exhausted, confused	Usually tired, disoriented, confused
Interictal behavioral abnormalities	Frequently	Occasionally
Response to antiepileptic drugs	Variable	Variable
Electroencephalogram		
Interictal	Frequently abnormal	Frequently abnormal
Ictal	No change	Epileptiform discharges

[a]Complex partial seizures.

B. DEFINITION. Psychogenic seizures are episodes of altered movement, emotion, sensation, or experience that are similar to those caused by epilepsy but have purely emotional causes. Psychogenic seizures may mimic any seizure type, but tonic–clonic and complex partial are the most common types mimicked. Psychogenic seizures may be deliberate, willed acts (malingering) to gain a desired end. Prisoners and persons receiving compensation for seizures sometimes fall into this category. Psychogenic seizures may also be subconscious acts. Persons with limited intelligence and persons with a history of physical or sexual abuse may use psychogenic seizures as a "cry for help." Persons with normal intelligence may use psychogenic seizures to control their environments.

C. DIFFERENTIAL DIAGNOSIS. See Table 9-5.

D. OTHER. In patients having both psychogenic and "real" seizures, the psychogenic seizures have the features listed for that category in Table 9-5. The "real" seizures have the features listed for that category in the same table. The best differential diagnostic test is to record a typical attack with EEG and video-monitoring. Use of suggestion during photic stimulation or hyperventilation may produce a psychogenic seizure. Clinical features

Table 9-5.   **Epilepsy versus psychogenic seizures**

	Epilepsy	Psychogenic Seizures
Setting	Neutral	Emotionally charged
Stereotype of attacks	Stereotyped, with minor variations among attacks	Sometimes rigidly stereotyped; sometimes variable and affected by environment
Pace	Abrupt onset and end of attack	Gradual buildup and prolonged resolution
Eyes	Open	Closed tightly
Tongue biting, incontinence, postictal confusion	Often present, side of tongue	May be present, tip of tongue
Self-injury	Common	Rare
Incontinence	Sometimes	Infrequent
Breathing	Stertorous (if generalized tonic–clonic) postictal	Normal or hyperventilation postictal
Family history	Family history of typical epileptic phenomena	May have epilepsy in family
Memory of event	Fragmentary recall or no recall of event	Indifference, apparent amnesia for event
Attitude toward event	Desire to know about attack, to replace lost time (ego-alien)	Denial of details and unwillingness to consider motivational determinants
Motivation	Secondary gain usually lacking	Secondary gains often identifiable
Interictal electroen-cephalogram	Abnormal (most)	Normal (63%–73%)
General features		
Specific precipitant	Rare	Common (often stress)
Onset	Usually short	Often gradual
Patient's control	Inability to respond to or abort attack	Ability to respond to or abort attack
Eyes	Open	Forcefully closed
Injury	Common	Less common
Urination	May occur	May occur
Defecation	May occur	May occur

continued

Table 9-5. *Continued*

	Epilepsy	Psychogenic Seizures
Tonic–clonic seizure	Onset with vocalization and tonic phase	Side-to-side neck movements
Mouth	Open during tonic phase	Closed during tonic phase
Followed by	Synchronous clonic movements, flaccid coma	Nonsynchronous movements, pelvic thrusting
Duration	≤2 min	Prolonged motor activity No rigidity Vocalization throughout attack Variable duration
Complex partial seizure	Onset with epigastric sensation: special senses sensation; behavioral changes: unilateral sensory or motor symptoms	Onset with behavioral changes, hyper-ventilation, headache, dizziness
Vocalization	Onset with motionless stare	Complex
Duration	Simple, often repetitive	Variable
	1–3 min	Directed violence

can be carefully observed. The EEG is abnormal during all tonic–clonic seizures, 90% of complex partial seizures, and only 50% of simple partial seizures.

Evidence has been reported suggesting that recall under hypnosis may be a method with high specificity and sensitivity for differentiating psychogenic from "real" seizures.

Serum prolactin levels are reliably (91%) elevated after tonic–clonic seizures, but not after psychogenic or complex partial seizures. A sample must be obtained within 10 minutes of the seizure and again in 90 to 120 minutes (control). An elevation of 2.5 times over control suggests a tonic–clonic seizure.

E. TREATMENT. No controlled trials of treatment for psychogenic seizures have been made. Treatment methods include psychodynamic therapy, family therapy, hypnosis, psychotropic medications for coexisting disorders such as depression or anxiety, and some combination of these.

6. Absence Seizures versus Complex Partial Seizures

A. COMMON FEATURES. Intermittent loss of consciousness, sometimes with automatisms, is a common feature of absence seizures and complex partial seizures. Both seizure types occur in children and in adults.

Table 9-6.   **Absence versus complex partial seizures**

	Absence Seizures	Complex Partial Seizures
Age at onset	Childhood	Any age; relatively rare in childhood
Aura	None	Common
Seizure Duration	Seconds	Minutes
Alertness	Out of contact	Out of contact
Automatisms	Simple or complex	Simple or complex
Staring	Yes	Yes
Speech	Never formed; patient sometimes hums	Incoherent, dysphasic, or none
Postictal confusion	Never	Often
Amnesia for attack	Yes	Yes, some islands of memory
Precipitation by hyperventilation	Often	Rarely
Precipitation by photic stimulation	Sometimes	Very rarely
Electroencephalogram	3-Hz spike–wave	Temporal slowing or sharp activity

B. **DIFFERENTIAL DIAGNOSIS.** See Table 9-6.

C. **OTHER.** Diagnosing physicians display a mistaken tendency to call lapses of consciousness in children *absence seizures* and lapses in consciousness in adults *complex partial seizures*. Both seizure types occur in both age groups.

B. In Children

1. Epilepsy versus Movement Disorder (Tic, Chorea, Tremor, Stereotypies)

A. **DEFINITIONS.** On occasion, movement disorders such as tics and chorea may be confused with partial motor seizures. In children, tics involve primarily the head, neck, and shoulders and consist of complex movements such as facial grimacing, eye blinking or rolling, head nodding or turning, and shrugging of the shoulders. Tics can usually be suppressed, at least temporarily, by an effort of will, whereas seizures cannot. In chorea, the movements occur randomly, usually in multiple muscle groups, whereas seizures are usually characterized by repetitive, stereotyped movements affecting the same muscle groups. Seizures do not have the characteristic, continuous flow of movements that is so distinctive of chorea. Tremors can usually be differentiated from seizures by the smooth to-and-fro movements associated with tremors, which are more abrupt and have distinct intervals between each movement. Stereotypies consist of complex movements such as twirling, head banging, and hand flapping. Stereotypies are typically seen in children with autistic spectrum disorder and can usually be readily distinguished from seizures. If a doubt exists about the diagnosis, video-EEG monitoring can be useful.

2. Epilepsy versus Cyanotic Breath-holding Spells

A. DEFINITIONS: Such spells typically begin with some type of event distressing to the child, either frustration, fright, or minor injuries, such as mild blows, cuts, bumps, or spankings. The elements of unexpectedness and surprise are often present. The child then begins vigorously to cry. After the first few cries, the child suddenly gasps, holds his or her breath, and becomes cyanotic, most prominently around the lips. The child then becomes rigid, loses consciousness, and may assume an opisthotonic posture. Shortly thereafter, the child loses muscle tone and remains limp until normal breathing is restored. The child regains composure rapidly, and the marked lethargy and confusion seen after a generalized tonic or tonic–clonic seizure usually do not occur. Usually, the period of breath-holding is brief and may be associated with a very brief period of cyanosis. However, if the apnea results in significant hypoxia, a brief generalized tonic–clonic seizure may ensue. Even when the child has a convulsion as a component of the breath-holding attack, the postictal phase is very brief. Most breath-holding episodes last 1 minute or less.

The majority of children begin having breath-holding spells between the ages of 6 and 18 months. However, for breath-holding spells to have their onset in the first weeks of life is not rare. Approximately 5% of children have the onset of breath-holding attacks after 2 years of age. The children usually have normal neurologic and developmental examinations.

B. DIFFERENTIAL DIAGNOSIS. See Table 9-6.

3. Epilepsy versus Pallid Infantile Syncope

A. DEFINITIONS. Pallid infantile syncope, also termed *reflex anoxic seizures, vagal attacks*, or *white breath-holding*, are less common than cyanotic breath-holding attacks. Like cyanotic breath-holding attacks, pallid infantile syncope is precipitated by a stressful situation, such as unexpected pain. A few seconds after the provocation, the child suddenly falls limply to the ground. Crying before the loss of consciousness may or may not be present. The child then quickly regains consciousness, or in more severe cases, convulsions may occur. Although cyanosis may occur, it is not as prominent as during cyanotic breath-holding spells. Pallor and cold sweats may precede the loss of consciousness. Although not always obvious to the observer, the child usually does not breathe during the initial phase of the attack. As with cyanotic breath-holding attacks, children usually recover quickly from pallid infantile syncope.

The age range for pallid infantile syncope is broader than for cyanotic breath-holding spells, varying from 3 months to 14 years, with a median age of 4 years. The disorder is especially common between the ages of 12 and 18 months, when the onset of walking is associated with frequent falls.

At one time, ocular compression was commonly performed to aid in the diagnosis of pallid infantile syncope and breath-holding attacks. During ECG and EEG monitoring, pressure on the ocular globe was applied. Asystole of 2 seconds or greater duration occurred in more than half of children with pallid infantile syncope and in one fourth of those with cyanotic breath holding. In cases in which asystole lasted 10 seconds or more, a typical anoxic seizure followed a period of unconsciousness with decerebrate posturing and extension of all limbs. Although some laboratories continue to use this procedure, most clinicians rely on the history for the diagnosis. Table 9-7 lists the differentiating features of cyanotic breath-holding, pallid infantile syncope, and generalized tonic–clonic seizures.

B. DIFFERENTIAL DIAGNOSIS. See Table 9-6.

4. Epilepsy versus Prolonged Q-T Syndrome

Prolonged Q-T syndrome can mimic idiopathic epilepsy. This is a serious disorder that can lead to ventricular fibrillation or tachycardia. Any child with unexplained episodes of loss of consciousness should have an electrocardiogram; this test is especially important if the family history is positive or if the loss of consciousness was induced by exercise, fright, or excitement.

5. Epilepsy versus Sleep Disturbance (Night Terrors, Sleepwalking)

A. COMMON FEATURES (WITH COMPLEX PARTIAL SEIZURES). Recurrence in sleep, prominent fear and autonomic phenomena (night terrors), automatic behavior, and amnesia for the event are common features of epilepsy and of sleep disturbance.

B. FEATURES SUGGESTING NIGHT TERRORS. Onset between 4 and 12 years of age, typical spell beginning 1 to 2 hours after falling asleep (stages 3 and 4 sleep), terrified scream, appearing panic-stricken and confused, tachypnea, diaphoresis, dilated pupils often present, fearful for up to 15 minutes before falling back to sleep without difficulty, and normal EEG suggest a diagnosis of night terrors.

C. FEATURES SUGGESTING SLEEPWALKING. Typical spell beginning 1 to 2 hours after falling asleep (stages 3 and 4 sleep); walking about in a trance and carrying out purposeful activity such as dressing, opening doors, and eating; somniloquy or sleep talking that may occur independently or with sleepwalking; and normal EEG suggest a diagnosis of sleepwalking.

D. FEATURES SUGGESTING COMPLEX PARTIAL SEIZURES. Occurrence of seizures shortly after going to bed at night or in the early morning hours (stages 1 or 2 sleep); other clinical features of complex partial seizures; and sharp waves or spikes on interictal EEG suggest a diagnosis of complex partial seizures.

6. Abdominal Epilepsy versus Abdominal Migraine Versus Intraabdominal Disease

A. COMMON FEATURES. Recurrent abdominal pain with vomiting and other autonomic signs and symptoms and childhood occurrence are common features of abdominal epilepsy, abdominal migraine, and intraabdominal disease.

B. FEATURES SUGGESTING EPILEPSY. Other clinical features of simple or complex partial seizures (may not be present); sharp waves or spikes on interictal EEG; and response to antiepileptic drugs suggest a diagnosis of epilepsy.

Table 9-7. Differentiation of breath-holding attacks and pallid infantile syncope from generalized tonic or tonic–clonic seizures

Clinical Data	Cyanotic Breath-holding	Pallid Infantile Syncope	Seizures: Tonic–clonic or tonic
Age	6 mo–6 yr	12–18 mo; highly variable	Any age
Precipitating factors	Almost always	Almost always	Occasionally
Family history	Frequently positive for breath-holding	Frequently positive for syncope	Frequently positive for seizures
Sequence of events	Crying→apnea→loss of consciousness	Upset→pallor→loss of consciousness	Aura→loss of consciousness
Heart rate during ocular compression	Bradycardia or no change	Marked bradycardia or asystole	Physiologic tachycardia
Postictal symptoms	Usually none	Usually none	Always with generalized tonic–clonic seizure; usually brief symptoms with tonic seizure
Electroencephalogram			
Interictal	Normal	Normal	Usually abnormal
Ictal	Slowing	Slowing	Epileptiform activity

C. FEATURES SUGGESTING MIGRAINE. Other clinical features of migraine (may not be present); family history of migraine; and response to antimigraine drugs suggest a diagnosis of migraine.

D. OTHER/INTRAABDOMINAL DISEASE. Most children with recurrent abdominal pain do not have epilepsy or migraine. Other causes should be sought vigorously.

7. Staring Attacks versus Absence or Complex Partial Seizures

A. DEFINITIONS. Children with staring episodes are often referred for evaluation by concerned parents or teachers. Staring attacks can be due to daydreaming in normal children or a "shutting down" behavior by children with autistic spectrum disorder. It is unusual for children with absence or complex partial seizures to have staring as the only manifestation of a seizure. Hyperventilation in an untreated child with absence seizures is highly likely to induce an attack. Staring attacks usually last less than 30 seconds, whereas the average complex partial seizure lasts several minutes.

C. In Adults

1. Epilepsy versus Transient Ischemic Attacks

A. COMMON FEATURES. Both partial seizures and transient ischemic attacks often begin at 50 years of age or older. Transient sensory, motor, speech, vestibular, or memory symptoms may occur with either. Both typically last only a few minutes.

B. FEATURES SUGGESTING EPILEPSY. Onset of seizures at a younger age suggests epilepsy (although this is not uncommon in elderly patients). So does the presence of other signs or symptoms of partial seizures (motor, sensory, autonomic, or psychic); alteration of consciousness; automatisms; postictal confusion; hemianopic; scotomatous; or positive (lights, colors) visual symptoms; duration of seizure less than 3 minutes; and focal spikes or slowing on interictal EEG.

C. FEATURES SUGGESTING A TRANSIENT ISCHEMIC ATTACK. Duration longer than 3 minutes (may be briefer); monocular blindness; signs or symptoms suggesting carotid artery distribution deficit (hemiparesis, hemisensory loss, neglect of one side, aphasia); signs or symptoms suggesting vertebral artery distribution deficit (vertigo, diplopia, dysphagia, dysarthria, deafness, drop attacks); cardiovascular risk factors (may be present in older patient with seizures); carotid bruit or decreased pulse (may be present in older patient with seizures); and normal interictal EEG suggest diagnosis of a transient ischemic attack.

2. Transient Global Amnesia

Transient global amnesia usually occurs in patients older than 50 years. Onset of amnesia is sudden, and the amnesia lasts for several hours. Patients are alert with fluent speech but are confused. Recurrent attacks may occur in up to 25% of patients. Debate as to whether these attacks are of vascular origin, seizure origin, or both is ongoing. Such patients usually are not treated with antiepileptic drugs unless paroxysmal activity is found on the EEG.

REFERENCES

1. American Academy of Neurology Quality Standards Subcommittee. Practice parameter: neuroimaging in the emergency patient presenting with seizure: summary statement. *Neurology* 1996;47:280–291.
2. American Clinical Neurophysiology Society. Indications for obtaining an electroencephalogram. *J Clin Neurophysiol* 1998; 15:76–77.
3. Barnett HJM, Mohr JP, Stein BM, et al., eds. *Stroke: pathophysiology, diagnosis and management*, 2nd ed. New York: Churchill Livingstone, 1998.
4. Benbadis SR, Johnson K, Anthony K, et al. Induction of psychogenic nonepileptic seizures without placebo. *Neurology* 2000; 55:1904–1905.
5. Breningstall G. Breath holding spells. *Pediatr Neurol* 1996;14: 91–97.
6. Carpay JA, deWeed AW, Schimsheiner RJ, et al. The diagnostic yield of a second EEG after partial sleep deprivation: a prospective study in children with newly diagnosed seizures. *Epilepsia* 1997;38:595–599.
7. Commission on Classification and Terminology of the International League Against Epilepsy. Proposal for revised clinical and electroencephalographic classification of epileptic seizures. *Epilepsia* 1981;22:489–501.
8. Devinsky O. Nonepileptogenic psychogenic seizures: quagmires of pathophysiology, diagnosis and treatment. *Epilepsia* 1999;39: 458–462.
9. Devinsky O, Sauchez-Villasenor F, Vasquez B, et al. Clinical profile of patients with epileptic and non-epileptic seizures. *Neurology* 1996;46:1530–1533.
10. Engel J Jr. A proposed diagnostic scheme for people with epileptic seizures and with epilepsy: report of International League Against Epilepsy Task Force on Classification and Terminology. *Epilepsia* 2001;42:796–803.
11. Grafman J, Schwab K, Waren D, et al. Frontal lobe injuries, violence, and aggression. *Neurology* 1996;46:1231–1238.
12. Gumnit RJ. Psychogenic seizures. In: Wyllie E, ed. *The treatment of epilepsy: principles and practice*. Philadelphia: Lippincott Williams & Wilkins, 2001:699–704.
13. Hirtz D, Ashwal S, Berg A, et al. Practice parameter: evaluating first nonfebrile seizure in children: report of the Quality Standards Committee of the American Academy of Neurology, Child Neurology Society, and the American Epilepsy Society. *Neurology* 2000;55:616–623.
14. Kramer G. Epilepsy and EEG. *Epilepsia* 2000;41(suppl 3):1–74.
15. Kuyk J, Spinhoven P, Van Dyck R. Hypnotic recall: a positive criterion in the differential diagnosis between epileptic and pseudoepileptic seizures. *Epilepsia* 1999;40:485–491.
16. Lesser RP. Psychogenic seizures. *Neurology* 1996;46:1499–1507.
17. Miller JW, Petersen RC, Metter EJ, et al. Transient global amnesia. *Neurology* 1987;37:733–737.
18. Nuwer M. Assessment of digital EEG, quantitative EEG, and EEG brain mapping: report of the American Academy of Neurology and the American Clinical Neurophysiology Society. *Neurology* 1997;49:277–292.

19. Pellock J. Other nonepileptic paroxysmal disorders. In: Wyllie E, ed. *The treatment of epilepsy: principles and practice.* Philadelphia: Lippincott Williams & Wilkins, 2001:705–716. (Excellent review of entities that can be confused with seizures.)

20. Rosenow F, Wyllie E, Kotagal P, et al. Staring spells in children: descriptive features distinguishing epileptic and nonepileptic events. *J Pediatr* 1998;133:660–663

21. Shields RW. Neurocardiogenic syncope. *J Clin Neurophysiol* 1997; 14:169–209.

22. Szafkarski JP, Ficker DM, Cahill WT, et al. Four year incidence of psychogenic nonepileptic seizures in adults in Hamilton County, OH. *Neurology* 2000;55:1561–1563.

23. Thompson JL, Ebersole JS. Inpatient/outpatient EEG monitoring. *J Clin Neurophysiol* 1999;16:91–140.

24. Wong PKH. Digital EEG. *J Clin Neurophysiol* 1998;15:457–492.

Management

I. ESTABLISH DIAGNOSIS

The first step in managing epilepsy is to correctly determine seizure type, epileptic syndrome, etiology, and precipitating factors. This process is described in Chapter 9.

II. IDENTIFY AND ADDRESS PSYCHOLOGICAL AND SOCIAL PROBLEMS

Seizures are a relatively rare phenomenon for most patients. The psychological consequences of having epilepsy, however, are present all the time. Loss of one's driver's license, employment, self-esteem, and position in one's peer group are all potential problem areas that may cause more suffering than the seizures themselves. Furthermore, the anxiety associated with these psychological problems may precipitate seizures in some patients. That the patient will experience psychological problems as a consequence of having epilepsy must be anticipated. The health care provider also must be prepared to assist the patient by carefully explaining the nature of the medical problems and the effect the problems will have on driving and employment by providing emotional support, by giving the patient an opportunity to talk through his or her problems, and by referring the patient to various resources available to assist the epilepsy patient (e.g., social workers, epilepsy societies, vocational counselors). For more details, see Chapter 15.

III. PRINCIPLES OF PHARMACOLOGIC THERAPY

A. Begin Monotherapy with Drug of Choice

Once the exact type of seizure has been determined, the physician should initiate monotherapy (single-drug therapy) with the drug that has shown the best combination of high efficacy and low toxicity in comparative studies of drugs for the patient's seizure type (Table 10-1). If a patient has more than one type of seizure, therapy should begin with the drug of choice for the combination of seizure types present (Table 10-1). Reasons for selection of specific drugs as drugs of choice for specific seizure types are given in section **IV**.

The single-drug approach for initial treatment is preferred because monotherapy with an appropriately selected drug pushed to the adequate dosing rate controls seizures in 60% to 90% of patients, and polytherapy (therapy with more than one drug) exposes the patient to several unnecessary risks. Factors that appear to be associated with failure of monotherapy include persistent noncompliance, drug allergy, large or progressive brain lesions, partial seizures, more than one type of seizure, neuropsychiatric handicaps, and high pretreatment seizure frequency.

The risks of unnecessary polytherapy are many. Chronic toxicity is associated with the use of any antiepileptic drug. Polytherapy may include barbiturates, which are associated with

Table 10-1.   Antiepileptic drugs of choice

Seizure Type	Drug(s) of First Choice[a]	Drug(s) of Second Choice[a]	Alternative Drug(s)[a]
Partial (simple, complex, secondarily generalized tonic–clonic)	Carbamazepine Oxcarbazepine Phenytoin	Gabapentin Lamotrigine Levetiracetam Topiramate Valproic acid	Phenobarbital Primidone Tiagabine Zonisamide
Primarily generalized tonic–clonic	Phenytoin Valproic acid	Carbamazepine Lamotrigine Topiramate	Phenobarbital Primidone
Absence	Ethosuximide Valproic acid	Lamotrigine Valproate	Clonazepam

[a]Listed alphabetically within groups.

high risk for cognitive and behavioral toxicity. Other risks of unnecessary polytherapy include drug allergy, drug interactions, exacerbation of seizures, noncompliance, costs, and the inability to evaluate the effectiveness of individual antiepileptic drugs.

B. Push the First Drug Tried

The first drug tried for a seizure disorder is usually among the least-toxic drugs available, and the physician must be certain that the maximal possible therapeutic effect has been obtained from the first drug before adding other drugs. Therapy usually begins with a so-called average dosage of antiepileptic drug. If the seizures are controlled with this average dosage and no serious side effects appear, no further changes are necessary. If the seizures are not controlled with this dosage and no serious drug toxicity occurs, the dosage of the drug should be systematically increased until the seizures are controlled or until side effects preclude further dosage increase.

The drug plasma concentration should be determined if a patient's seizures are not controlled by an average or high drug dosage. Many correctable causes of lower than expected drug plasma concentration exist, including inadequate dosing rate, noncompliance, poor absorption, drug interactions, generic drug substitutions, pregnancy, and patient error. To substitute or to add a more toxic drug because the patient has a low plasma concentration of the first drug is a serious error. A drug cannot be said to be ineffective until it is documented that the seizures are not controlled with a high therapeutic plasma concentration of the drug, unless drug toxicity precludes reaching such concentrations.

The therapeutic range of drug plasma concentration represents values applicable to average patients. Some patients require higher drug plasma concentrations than the therapeutic range for good seizure control. If a patient has a high therapeutic plasma concentration of a nontoxic drug, poor seizure control, and no drug side effects, the best approach usually is to increase the dosage of the first drug rather than to add a more-toxic second drug.

C. Add Additional Drugs

If the first drug is pushed to its maximal tolerated dosage and seizures still are not controlled, a second antiepileptic drug should be added. In general, adding the second drug and continuing administration of the first drug (at least temporarily) is best because (a) the first drug will provide protection while the plasma concentration of the second drug is being built up, (b) discontinuing the first drug may result in withdrawal activation of the seizure disorder, and (c) evidence exists that two antiepileptic drugs in combination may control seizures in some patients when either drug alone does not.

When a therapeutic plasma concentration of the second drug is obtained, the physician should consider tapering the patient off the first drug because of the many hazards of prolonged polytherapy. The decision to taper the patient off the first drug must be individualized and should take into consideration the antiepileptic effect of the first drug when it is given alone, the side effects of the first drug, and the psychosocial consequences to the patient of having a seizure if discontinuation of the first drug results in loss of complete seizure control. The adverse effects of antiepileptic drugs on behavior and cognition argue that the physician should attempt to minimize the number of these drugs given to children. In adults, the hazards of polytherapy must be weighed against the risk of loss of job or driver's license if discontinuation of the first drug results in a recurrence of seizures. If discontinuation of the first drug is elected, it should be done slowly.

A third drug should not be added until it is documented that seizures cannot be controlled with maximal tolerated doses of the first two drugs tried. Adding a third drug (at least temporarily) is usually better than substituting a third drug for the first or second drug, for reasons similar to those cited earlier for adding, rather than substituting, a second drug. After a therapeutic plasma concentration of the third drug is reached, the physician may elect to discontinue one of the first two drugs, by using the guidelines just outlined.

IV. DRUGS OF CHOICE

A. First-choice Drugs for Simple Partial, Complex Partial, and Secondarily Generalized Tonic–Clonic Seizures

Simple partial (focal); complex partial (psychomotor, temporal lobe); and tonic–clonic (grand mal) seizures are the most common types of seizure disorders and occur at all ages. Note that a tonic–clonic seizure may be focal (partial seizures secondarily generalized) or generalized (primarily generalized) in onset (see Chapter 2). Carbamazepine (Tegretol), phenobarbital, phenytoin (Dilantin), primidone (Mysoline), and valproic acid (Depakote) are the drugs that have been used as initial therapy for simple partial, complex partial, and partial seizures secondarily generalized. These five drugs have been compared in adults in two large Veterans Administration Cooperative studies. Carbamazepine and phenytoin had the best combined efficacy and safety results. Primidone was inferior to the other four drugs for all seizure types because of a significantly higher incidence of intolerable toxicity. More recently, oxcarbazepine (Trileptal) has been compared with carbamazepine, phenytoin, and valproic acid. All drugs had similar efficacy, but oxcarbazepine has the fewest side effects.

Carbamazepine, oxcarbazepine, and phenytoin are the three drugs of choice for partial seizures and for partial seizures secondarily generalized in adults, based on the following: (a) carbamazepine, oxcarbazepine, and phenytoin have fewer side effects than phenobarbital or valproic acid, regardless of seizure type; (b) carbamazepine and phenytoin are more effective than phenobarbital or valproic acid for complex partial seizures; (c) no statistically significant differences were seen in efficacy when carbamazepine, oxcarbazepine, and phenytoin were compared; and (d) monotherapy with carbamazepine, oxcarbazepine, or phenytoin produces a satisfactory long-term result in approximately 60% to 80% of patients. Gabapentin, lamotrigine, and topiramate are not approved by the U.S. Food and Drug Administration (FDA) for initial therapy of partial seizures. Lamotrigine is approved for conversion to monotherapy for partial seizures.

In children, comparative studies have demonstrated that carbamazepine, phenytoin, and valproic acid are equally efficacious. Phenobarbital and primidone also are efficacious, but side effects, such as irritability, hyperactivity, and lethargy, limit these drugs to second-line therapy. In general, carbamazepine is preferred over phenytoin because of the erratic absorption in children, resulting in fluctuating blood levels and cosmetic side effects such as gingival hypertrophy and hirsutism. Because it is sometimes difficult to distinguish between partial seizures and primarily generalized seizures in infants, valproate may be an appropriate first choice in some children.

Gabapentin, lamotrigine, levetiracetam, oxcarbazepine, topiramate, tiagabine, and zonisamide all have been tested as adjunctive therapy for refractory partial seizures in children, with promising results.

B. Second-choice Drugs for Simple Partial, Complex Partial, and Secondarily Generalized Tonic–Clonic Seizures

No definitive trials have been published establishing the drug of second choice for patients whose first-choice drug (carbamazepine, oxcarbazepine, or phenytoin) has failed a trial. Probably the most common practice is to add or substitute another first-choice drug based on the results of initial therapy studies. This practice has been questioned because (a) carbamazepine and phenytoin have complex drug interactions when taken together, and (b) all three drugs have the same mechanism of action.

Three older drugs (phenobarbital, primidone, valproic acid) and seven new drugs (gabapentin, lamotrigine, levetiracetam, oxcarbazepine, tiagabine, topiramate, zonisamide) have been used as alternative drugs in patients failing to respond to carbamazepine, oxcarbazepine, or phenytoin. The advantages and disadvantages of these drugs are summarized in Table 10-2 and the review by Cramer et al. (12). Phenobarbital and primidone have fallen from favor because of the high incidence of cognitive/behavioral side effects and drug interactions. Although used by many experts, valproic acid is not more effective than newer agents in adults and shows more problems with serious toxicity, nuisance toxicity, and drug interactions.

Few comparative studies of the new antiepileptic drugs are available. The information here and in Table 10-2 is based on separate studies in adults using varying methods. The results of these studies may not be strictly comparable and may not apply to children.

Gabapentin and levetiracetam have no serious drug toxicity, little nuisance toxicity, and no drug interactions. Lamotrigine is well tolerated by many patients and has few drug interactions with non-antiepileptic drugs. Topiramate has the highest reported responder rate and few drug interactions. Tiagabine has the lowest responder rate, several side effects, multiple drug interactions, and inconvenient administration. Topiramate and zonisamide can cause kidney stones.

The opinion of many experts is that the efficacy-to-toxicity ratios for valproic acid may be more favorable in children than in adults.

C. Drugs for Primarily Generalized Tonic–Clonic Seizures

For primarily generalized tonic–clonic seizures, carbamazepine, phenytoin, and valproic acid are all effective as initial therapy. Topiramate is effective as adjunctive therapy for primarily generalized tonic–clonic seizures. Valproic acid has efficacy against absence and myoclonic seizures (sometimes associated with primarily generalized tonic–clonic seizures), whereas carbamazepine and phenytoin do not. Absence seizures may worsen in some patients taking carbamazepine or phenobarbital. Valproic acid is the drug of first choice for persons with primarily generalized tonic–clonic seizures with absence seizures, myoclonic seizures, or both. Lamotrigine, gabapentin, levetiracetam, oxcarbazepine, tiagabine, and zonisamide have shown promise against primarily generalized tonic–clonic seizures in a limited number of studies.

D. Antiepileptic Drugs of Choice for Absence Seizures

Ethosuximide, valproic acid, and clonazepam are the three drugs used to treat absence seizures (Table 10-1) and are equally effective for that purpose. Ethosuximide has the fewest side effects and is the first-choice drug for uncomplicated absence seizures. For patients with tonic–clonic seizures, myoclonic seizures, or both, in addition to absence seizures, valproic acid is the drug of first choice (ethosuximide has no efficacy for tonic–clonic or myoclonic seizures). Lamotrigine has been reported to be effective

Table 10-2. Adjunctive medications for partial seizures

	Responder Rate[a,b]	No Serious Toxicity	No Nuisance Toxicity	No Drug Interactions	Administration
Gabapentin	30%–40%	+	±	+	t.i.d.
Lamotrigine	30%–40%	−	±	±	b.i.d.
Levetiracetam	30%–40%	+	+	+	b.i.d.
Oxcarbazepine	30%–50%	±	±	±	b.i.d.
Phenobarbital	?[c]	+	−	−	q.d.
Primidone	?[c]	+	−	−	t.i.d.
Tiagabine	20%–30%	−	−	−	b.i.d. or t.i.d.
Topiramate	40%–50%	−	−	+	b.i.d.
Valproic acid	30%–40%	−	−	−	b.i.d. or t.i.d.
Zonisamide	30%–40%	−	−	−	b.i.d.

[a]Percentage of patients having a ≥50% reduction in partial seizure frequency.
[b]Based on separate studies using varying methods in adults. Results may not be strictly comparable and may not apply to children.
[c]Not determined in a modern controlled study.

for absence and primarily generalized tonic–clonic seizures (it is not yet approved by the FDA for these indications) and is used by some experts for the combination of absence and tonic–clonic seizures. Clonazepam is not a favored therapy because of side effects (drowsiness, hyperactivity); tolerance to antiabsence effect; and equivocal efficacy against tonic–clonic seizures.

V. SINGLE SEIZURE

Epilepsy, by definition, is recurring spontaneous seizures. Epilepsy must begin with a first seizure, but not all first seizures mean the beginning of epilepsy. Three fourths of persons with an isolated seizure never have another.

A single first seizure may be caused by (a) external events affecting the brain in patients susceptible to seizures (e.g., drug toxicity, drug withdrawal, sleep deprivation); (b) somatic disease that transiently affects a normal brain (e.g., hypoglycemia, hypoxia, syncope, hyponatremia); (c) a neurologic disease injuring the brain (e.g., head injury, stroke, neoplasm); and (d) a first seizure as part of symptomatic or idiopathic epilepsy. Etiologies (a) and (b) are not indicative of recurring spontaneous seizures and do not require long-term antiepileptic drug treatment. Etiologies (c) and (d) are associated with a risk of recurring spontaneous seizures.

Factors increasing risk for recurring seizures in adults include (a) evidence of structural lesion (strongest predictor); (b) abnormal electroencephalogram (EEG); (c) partial seizure type; (d) family history; and (e) postictal motor paralysis. Persons with no risk factors have only a 15% chance of a second seizure within 2 years. Persons with two or more risk factors have a 100% chance of seizure recurrence within 2 years.

Antiepileptic drug therapy with therapeutic blood levels has been shown to reduce the risk of seizure recurrence after a first seizure. Persons with two or more risk factors probably should be treated. Treatment may not be obligatory in other patients, but they should be warned of the risk of recurrent seizures (especially in the next 2 years) and advised to take appropriate precautions.

The American Academy of Neurology has a position statement for management of first seizures in children and adolescents. Risk factors for recurring seizures in children include (a) symptomatic etiology of the seizures, (b) epileptiform activity on the EEG, (c) occurrence during sleep, and (d) partial seizure type. The American Academy of Neurology concludes

1. Treatment with an antiepileptic drug is not indicated for the prevention of the development of epilepsy.

2. Treatment with an antiepileptic drug may be considered in circumstances where the benefits of reducing the risk of a second seizure outweigh the risks of pharmacologic and psychosocial side effects.

VI. DRUG INTERACTIONS

Four forms of clinically important drug interactions have been found with antiepileptic drugs: (a) induction of biotransformation of coadministered drug; (b) inhibition of biotransformation of coadministered drug; (c) displacement from protein-binding sites of coadministered drug; and (d) pharmacodynamic interactions (both drugs affect common receptor sites, drug plasma concentration unchanged). Drug interactions may be bidirectional (i.e., each drug is affected by the presence of the other drug), and one drug may have more than one type of drug interaction with the other. The mechanistic and clinical aspects of antiepileptic drug interactions have been reviewed in depth elsewhere (30).

Common drug interactions between antiepileptic drugs and between antiepileptic drugs and other types of drugs are reviewed in Chapter 11. Other, less common drug interactions have been reported. Whenever an additional drug of any type is to be added to a patient's antiepileptic drug regimen, consulting a listing of possible drug interactions, such as that of Hansten and Horn (see ref. 19), is prudent.

VII. COMPLIANCE

As many as 70% of persons with epilepsy omit some doses of antiepileptic drug. As many as 50% of persons with epilepsy admit to having had seizures after omitting doses of antiepileptic drugs. Risk factors for noncompliance include long use of antiepileptic drugs, high number of doses taken per day, and high number of pills taken per day. These facts call for simplifying the antiepileptic drug regimen wherever possible and regular monitoring of antiepileptic drug plasma concentration.

VIII. ANTIEPILEPTIC DRUG PLASMA CONCENTRATION DETERMINATIONS (BLOOD LEVELS)

A. Definitions

Drug plasma concentration refers to the amount of drug (by weight) dissolved in a unit volume of plasma. *Blood level* is often used as a synonym for drug plasma concentration.

B. Units

The units for antiepileptic drug plasma-concentration determinations most widely used in the United States are weight-per-volume units, such as micrograms per milliliter (μg/mL). In Europe and many other areas of the world, molar units are used. The most widely used molar unit is micromoles (μmol).

C. Indications for Determining Antiepileptic Drug Plasma Concentration

1. Poor Seizure Control

Poor seizure control is the most frequent indication for obtaining antiepileptic drug plasma-concentration determinations. Use of such determinations may decrease by as much as 50% the number of patients whose seizures are poorly controlled when compared with use of empiric determination techniques.

When a patient's seizures are not controlled with an average dosage of an antiepileptic drug appropriate for the type of seizure being treated, the plasma concentration of the drug should be determined. The first drug used in treating a given patient's seizure disorder is usually chosen because it has the best efficacy-to-toxicity ratio for the patient. Many causes may exist for a lower-than-expected drug plasma concentration, and these causes can often be identified and corrected.

2. Initiation of Drug Therapy, Dosage Adjustment, Change of Drug Formulation (Generic Substitution), Change in Concomitant Medication

When initiation of drug therapy, dosage adjustment, a change of drug formulation (generic substitution), or a change in concomitant medication is being considered, determining the plasma concentration of the antiepileptic drug to determine whether it is within the desired range is wise. Sufficient time must be allowed for the steady-state plasma concentration to be attained after any change in drug regimen (see Chapter 11, Table 11-1).

3. Evaluation of Antiepileptic Drug Intoxication

Antiepileptic drug plasma-concentration determinations can assist in evaluating antiepileptic drug intoxication in at least two ways. First, many antiepileptic drugs produce similar toxic symptoms (e.g., drowsiness, ataxia, diplopia). If a patient is taking more than one drug, antiepileptic drug plasma-concentration determinations can determine which drug is present in supratherapeutic concentration in the plasma and therefore is presumably responsible for the patient's toxic symptoms. Second, knowledge of a drug's plasma concentration and elimination half-life can enable the physician to make an educated guess at how long the drug causing intoxication must be withheld before therapy may be resumed at a lower dosing rate.

4. Documentation of Continued Compliance

Patients whose seizures are controlled have a great tendency to begin omitting some of their medication. One estimate is that patients who are seizure free omit one pill per day for every 6 months they are seizure free. Antiepileptic drug plasma concentrations should be determined every 6 to 12 months in patients whose seizures are controlled to detect noncompliance and prevent recurrence of seizures.

5. Pregnancy

During pregnancy, multiple pharmacokinetic changes may result in a net decrease in plasma concentration of antiepileptic drugs. Total (protein bound plus free or non–protein bound) plasma concentration usually decreases to a greater extent than free plasma concentration. See Chapter 13 for further details.

6. Other Diseases

Routine monitoring of antiepileptic drug plasma concentrations is recommended in the presence of other disease that can alter the absorption, distribution, protein binding, biotransformation, or excretion of antiepileptic drugs. Determination of free plasma concentration is useful in conditions in which protein binding may be altered (pregnancy, renal failure, liver failure).

D. Sampling Conditions

Whenever possible, the blood-sampling time for individual patients should be standardized to ensure comparable conditions. Ideally, the samples should be taken at the end of the longest interval between doses (usually just before the morning dose of drug). In outpatients, the morning dose can be postponed a couple of hours to ensure this. If the drug plasma concentration is adequate at this time, it will be adequate throughout the rest of the day. When toxic symptoms of the drug are suspected during the day, the sample is best drawn at the time of maximal plasma drug level.

The following patient data are necessary for a meaningful evaluation of drug levels: age, weight, sex, diagnosis, indications for analysis, clinical conditions of relevance, concomitant medications, and sampling time in relation to the last drug intake.

E. Interpretation

1. Causes of Low Plasma Concentration

Causes of low plasma concentration include noncompliance, poor absorption, failure to reach steady state, change in drug formulation, rapid metabolism, drug interactions, pregnancy, hypoalbuminemia, renal dysfunction, ingestion of incorrect dose, and laboratory error.

2. Causes of High Plasma Concentration

Causes of high plasma concentration include ingestion of incorrect dose (intentional or unintentional), change in drug formulation, drug interactions, hepatic disease, genetically determined slow metabolism, and laboratory error.

3. Laboratory Error

Unfortunately, laboratory errors are common in the measurement of antiepileptic drug plasma concentration. These are usually due to operator error, not to intrinsic unreliability of the analytic method.

IX. DISCONTINUING THERAPY

Uncontrolled seizures and seizures caused by a progressive neurologic illness (e.g., glioblastoma) are indications for continuing antiepileptic drug therapy indefinitely. Antiepileptic drug therapy usually should be maintained for a minimum of 2 to 3 years in adults after diagnosis of epilepsy, even if the patient has no further seizures. When a patient has been free of seizures for 2 to 3 years with antiepileptic drug therapy, the need for continued therapy can be reevaluated. Discontinuing the medication eliminates long-term drug toxicity and has psychosocial and economic benefits. The risk of seizure recurrence is approximately 25% in patients without risk factors and higher than 50% in patients with risk factors. Approximately 80% of seizure recurrences occur within 4 months of the beginning of drug tapering, and 90% occur within the first year. Driving and other dangerous activities should be prohibited for at least the first 4 months after starting drug discontinuation.

Factors favoring increased risk of seizure recurrence include symptomatic etiology; abnormal EEG; seizure onset at younger than 2 years of age or in adolescence; neurologic abnormalities; and severe epilepsy (need for more than one drug, many seizures, seizures difficult to control). Factors favoring decreased risk of seizure recurrence include idiopathic seizures, normal EEG, seizure onset at 2 to 12 years of age, no neurologic abnormalities, and seizures easily controlled with one drug.

Each decision must be made on an individual basis. A history of seizure frequency and risk factors must be obtained. A routine EEG is highly useful, and a long-term EEG recording is sometimes desirable. The probability of recurrent seizures, the consequences of having another seizure, and the benefits of living without medication must be discussed with the patient; the judgment must be weighted by the needs of the individual.

If discontinuation of antiepileptic therapy is elected, medication should be withdrawn slowly. Elimination of 25% of daily dosage every five elimination half-lives is probably the optimal regimen. In general, more-rapid tapering of therapy may precipitate seizures, and more prolonged withdrawal probably does not reduce the risk of seizure recurrence. Special caution is required when discontinuing benzodiazepines, especially clonazepam.

X. MEDICALLY INTRACTABLE EPILEPSY

Many cases of so-called intractable epilepsy are caused by improper diagnosis of seizure type (resulting in the use of improper antiepileptic drugs), failure to push the drugs used to the maximal dosage, or failure to use all available antiepileptic drugs. Some patients, however, continue to have seizures despite a proper seizure diagnosis and maximal therapy with conventional antiepileptic drugs. Some of these cases of drug-resistant epilepsy may be due to overexpression of the multiple drug–resistance gene. This gene produces P-glycoprotein, a substance that inhibits transport of drugs (including phenytoin) across the blood–brain barrier. Patients with partial seizures should be considered for cortical-resection procedures after failure of three antiepileptic drugs to provide adequate control. The efficacy and safety of such procedures in properly selected patients are well proved. In patients whose seizures are not controlled with conventional drugs and who are not candidates for cortical-resection procedures, four therapeutic options are available: (a) vagus nerve stimulation; (b) less commonly used antiepileptic drugs (Chapter 11); (c) experimental drugs (Chapter 11); (d) experimental surgical procedures (see next section); and (e) behavioral therapies. Such therapies usually are available only at specialized epilepsy centers.

XI. PROPHYLACTIC ANTIEPILEPTIC DRUG THERAPY AFTER HEAD INJURY

It has been the practice at many centers to prescribe antiepileptic drugs after head injuries to prevent the development of seizures. The American Academy of Neurology reviewed this issue and found that prophylactic administration of antiepileptic drugs helps prevent occurrence of seizures during the first 7 days after a severe head injury (prolonged loss on consciousness or amnesia, intracranial hematoma or brain contusion, and/or depressed skull fracture). Prophylactic antiepileptic drug administration beyond 7 days after a severe head injury has not been shown to be effective in preventing development of seizures. There is limited information available on prophylactic antiepileptic drug therapy after mild and moderate head injuries. Seizures may arise by different mechanisms after mild to moderate (as compared with severe) head injuries. Thus data from severe-head-injury studies may not extrapolate to lesser head injuries.

XII. PROPHYLACTIC ANTIEPILEPTIC DRUG THERAPY IN PATIENTS WITH NEWLY DIAGNOSED BRAIN TUMORS

The American Academy of Neurology recommends that prophylactic antiepileptic drug therapy not be given to patients with newly diagnosed brain tumors. Such therapy is not successful in preventing first seizures and exposes the patient to unnecessary side effects. In patients who have had surgery for their tumor, prophylactic antiepileptic drug therapy is recommended for only 7 days.

XIII. BONE-DENSITY MONITORING

Prolonged treatment with antiepileptic drugs has been associated with decreased bone density, which does not correlate well with serum vitamin D levels. Enzyme-inducing antiepileptic drugs (phenytoin, phenobarbital, carbamazepine, primidone); polytherapy; and long duration of therapy are associated with higher risks. However, decreased bone density can occur with noninducers such as valproic acid, topiramate, lamotrigine, gabapentin, clonazepam, or ethosuximide. As yet, no firm guidelines exist for monitoring bone density in persons taking antiepileptic drugs. In lieu of evidence firm guidelines, the authors recommend that all patients with epilepsy taking antiepileptic drugs be administered 1000–1500 mg of calcium and 400 International Units of vitamin D daily.

XIV. SURGERY

Although antiepileptic drug therapy is the treatment of choice for most patients with epilepsy, a significant number of patients with seizures respond to surgical treatment. Deciding whether to do a surgical evaluation is dependent on a clear understanding of the indications and contraindications for epilepsy surgery.

A. Selection of Patients for Referral

1. Indications

Medically intractable seizures are usually defined as persistent seizures despite trials of three or more antiepileptic drugs, alone or in combination (Table 10-3). Each of the drugs should be pushed to the maximal tolerated dosage.

A localized seizure focus found on EEG or magnetic resonance imaging (MRI) suggests that the patient will benefit from one of the cortical resection procedures that have a high success rate and low morbidity (see sections **XVI.C.1** and **2**). However, some

Table 10-3.   Indications and contraindications for epilepsy surgery procedures

Indications	Medically intractable seizures (necessary)
	Seizures significantly reduce quality of life (necessary)
	Localized seizure focus (helpful)
	Biological predictors of seizure persistence (helpful)
Contraindications	Benign, self-limited epilepsy syndromes
	Neurodegenerative and metabolic disorders
	Noncompliance with medication
	Severe family dysfunction
	Psychosis

patients with multifocal epilepsy can benefit from other surgical procedures (see sections **XVI.C.3–5**).

Biologic predictors of seizure persistence include frequent seizures, early seizure onset, secondary generalization, structural lesion, and abnormal neurologic status. The presence of these predictors suggests that the seizures are unlikely to improve with passage of time.

2. Contraindications

Benign, self-limited epilepsy syndromes include benign rolandic epilepsy and benign focal epilepsy of childhood with occipital spikes. These patients can benefit from multiple subpial transections.

In patients with severe family dysfunction or psychosis, surgical reduction in seizure frequency seldom results in a significant improvement in quality of life. The other problems continue to dominate their existence.

3. Timing

A trial of drug at maximal tolerated dosage for 3 to 6 months usually is adequate to determine whether the drug is effective. Trials of three drugs should take 12 to 24 months. If three antiepileptic drugs have failed, epilepsy surgery should be considered immediately for three reasons. First, the longer the patient lives as a disabled person with epilepsy, the more difficult it is to become fully functional after successful epilepsy surgery. Second, evidence suggests that seizures may cause brain damage and worsen a seizure disorder and neuropsychological handicaps. Third, evidence also suggests that seizures may have adverse effects on the developing brain.

B. Presurgical Evaluation

1. Fundamental Concepts

The fundamental concept of surgery in patients with partial epilepsies is to identify the area of seizure onset and determine whether it can be safely resected. Although the most important test is the recording of habitual seizures during EEG monitoring, valuable supporting information can be drawn from the history, neurologic examination, neuropsychological evaluation, and neuroimaging (both anatomic and functional). Each epilepsy center has its own surgical protocol, but general agreement exists that surgery should be performed only with concordance of diagnostic studies as to the location of the epileptic focus.

An accurate description of the clinical manifestations of spontaneous seizures is probably the most important piece of clinical information derived from the history. Although observers usually concentrate on the most dramatic portion of the seizure, it is important to question eyewitnesses closely about the initial phases of the seizure. An aura, no matter how brief, often provides considerable localizing information. In infantile spasms, eye deviation or focal twitching before the spasm indicates that the seizure began focally. Likewise, a history of asymmetries of strength postictally, even if subtle, may provide important localization findings as to seizure onset.

With the widespread use of MRI, the value of the neurologic examination has been reduced. However, asymmetries of strength or reflexes may provide evidence of focal pathology, even in the context of normal neuroimaging.

2. Imaging Studies

High-quality MRI is essential in the evaluation of a patient undergoing a surgical evaluation. The MRI is particularly valuable in detecting mesial temporal sclerosis, tumors, vascular malformations, and cerebral dysgenesis (see Chapter 3). MRI scans should include images in the horizontal, coronal, and sagittal planes by using both T_1- and T_2-weighted images. When mesial temporal lobe sclerosis is suspected, thin coronal cuts perpendicular to the plane of the hippocampus can be helpful. A fluid-attenuated inversion recovery (FLAIR) pulse sequence improves contrast between lesions and CNS. Gadolinium enhancement can assist in finding tumors and vascular malformations. Computer-assisted volume analysis of the temporal lobes may detect asymmetries that are not readily apparent on visual analysis of the scan. The presence of focal abnormalities on the MRI, when they correspond to seizure onset on the EEG, provides powerful localizing information. In general, patients with focal abnormalities on MRI have a more favorable prognosis for successful surgery than do patients with normal MRIs.

Some persons with medically intractable partial seizures have neocortical (extrahippocampal) lesions that do not appear on MRI scans. Other techniques must be used. Single-photon emission CT (SPECT) and positron emission tomography (PET) are used increasingly in the evaluation of these patients with intractable epilepsy. Central to the use of SPECT in the localization of epileptic foci are the observations that ictal hyperperfusion occurs at the site of the epileptic focus, and hypoperfusion is usually seen on the interictal scan. The ictal scan is superior to the interictal scan in the localization of the epileptic focus. The most precise localization is through subtracting of the interictal image from the ictal scan and superimposition on the MRI.

Like SPECT, PET scanning is a noninvasive functional imaging test that has been used to evaluate cerebral metabolic rates.

Although many agents have been labeled with positron emitters, 2-deoxy-2[^{18}F]fluoro-D-glucose (FDG) has been the agent most commonly used in epilepsy. The interictal scan typically demonstrates hypometabolism, whereas a scan obtained during a seizure demonstrates hypermetabolism. PET scanning has been found to be a useful adjunctive test in the evaluation of both children and adults with epilepsy. The PET scan may be superior to MRI in localizing focal areas of cortical dysplasia and other structural abnormalities corresponding to surface-EEG localization of epileptogenic regions. In the hands of experienced investigators, the PET may eliminate or reduce the need for invasive monitoring. However, PET scans are available in only a few centers.

Magnetoencephalography (MEG) performs noninvasive monitoring of magnetic fluxes associated with electrical currents in the brain. The technique allows precise, three-dimensional localization on interictal spikes. In addition, MEG can be very useful in mapping motor, sensory, and language cortex. Unfortunately, MEG is available at only a few medical centers.

3. Neuropsychological Studies

Like the neurologic examination, the neuropsychological evaluation can provide useful localizing information. The focal area in which a seizure begins often also has disturbed neuropsychological function. For example, patients with seizures arising in the dominant temporal lobe may have deficits in verbal memory or language acquisition, whereas deficits in visuospatial memory suggest seizure onset in the nondominant temporal lobe. Significant deficits in both suggest bilateral temporal lobe damage and make surgical resection of one temporal lobe risky (see section **XVI.C.1**, later).

The intracarotid amobarbital test (Wada test) involves performance of neuropsychological testing after a region of the brain has been inactivated with amobarbital delivered through selective intracarotid injection. This injection mimics the effect of surgical removal of the region and allows determination of whether the remaining structures can carry out the tasks being studied. Such testing is important if removal of mesial temporal structures is being considered. Memory requires at least one functioning mesial temporal area. Mesial temporal damage is sometimes bilateral, and removal of one mesial temporal area in a patient with bilateral mesial temporal damage may leave the patient with severe memory deficits. Preoperative testing supplies knowledge of whether the remaining mesial temporal area can sustain memory function. The intracarotid amobarbital test is also routinely used to determine the dominant hemisphere for language. This information assists in planning the extent of surgery that can be safely performed.

Functional MRI is increasingly used to localize language and other cortical localization such as motor function. This technique takes advantage of changes in oxygen extraction during activation of cortex, and it is noninvasive and safer than the Wada test. However, the functional MRI has not yet been shown to adequately lateralize memory and therefore has not totally replaced the Wada. However, with improved technology, it is highly likely that the technique will eventually be the preferred test.

Proton magnetic resonance spectroscopy has been beneficial in the localization of the epileptogenic zone in both temporal and extratemporal epilepsy in some epilepsy centers. The technology of MRI spectroscopy is rapidly evolving, and it is anticipated that more epilepsy centers will start using the technique.

4. EEG

Despite the development of newer imaging techniques, EEG investigation remains the cornerstone for localization of the epileptic foci. Both interictal and ictal epileptiform activity are used in the localization of the epileptic zone. In the early years of epilepsy surgery, interictal discharges recorded with scalp electrodes were the primary means for localization. However, interictal discharges on scalp recording are absent in some patients, poorly localized or bilaterally independent in others, and occasionally falsely localizing. Thus interictal discharges are rarely used as the sole means of localization. The onset of an EEG seizure is considered the most reliable of the localizing signs.

For this reason, most patients undergoing a presurgical evaluation have long-term EEG and video monitoring. The goal of the monitoring is to record several of the patient's habitual seizures. To increase the chances of a seizure, antiepileptic drug dosage may be reduced.

A number of problems may occur that limit the usefulness of the ictal EEG. Artifacts may obscure the EEG seizure, seizures may be poorly localized, or the EEG seizures may follow the onset of the clinical seizure. In instances in which seizures cannot be well localized by using surface electrodes, or when the SPECT, PET, MRI, or neuropsychological data are not concordant with the EEG findings, intracranial electrodes are typically used. Although a variety of different types of intracranial electrodes have been used, the most common types are depth, subdural, and epidural. Depth electrodes consist of thin wires with multiple EEG-recording contacts. Depth electrodes are implanted stereotaxically and can be implanted into a variety of cerebral structures; subdural electrodes are placed over the surface of the brain. Depth electrodes allow accurate recordings from structures located at a distance from the surface and are particularly valuable when the clinician suspects the seizures are arising from the amygdala or hippocampus.

Subdural or epidural electrodes consist of strips or grids of electrodes embedded into a thin sheet of plastic. The plastic sheet is quite pliable and is easily inserted into the subdural or epidural space. Subdural or epidural electrode grids may be helpful in planning a safe, effective resection for patients with an epileptogenic region near functional cortex because the clinician can electrically stimulate the electrodes to map functional cortex. Whereas subdural electrode grids may be slipped under the edges of the open craniotomy (including under the temporal or frontal lobe or in the interhemispheric fissure), epidural electrode grids can cover only the exposed area. In addition, cortical stimulation with epidural electrodes may cause pain because of stimulation of meningeal nerve fibers.

As electrodes become more invasive, they tend to provide more detailed and precisely localized information, at the expense of more limited sampling. The most invasive techniques, such as depth electrodes and epidural or subdural grids, are helpful in answering specific neurophysiological questions concerning a restricted cortical area, but they are less useful in exploring more widespread localization problems between large cortical areas. Therefore these techniques should be reserved for cases in which basic localization problems have already been resolved by scalp EEG and other diagnostic studies.

C. Surgical Procedures
1. Temporal Lobe Seizures
Temporal lobe seizures may arise from the anteromedial area or the lateral area (Table 10-4). Studies have shown that 60% of persons with refractory partial seizures of anteromedial origin are free of disabling seizures 1 year after surgery. The American Academy of Neurology recommends that such patients be offered surgery with an explanation of risks and benefits.

The evidence is not as complete or as compelling for surgical removal of lateral temporal foci. The risk–benefit analysis of surgery in this area requires further study.

2. Nontemporal Lobe Seizures
Temporal lobectomy is the most frequent type of epilepsy surgery among patients overall, but extratemporal resection is becoming more common. Locating a seizure focus in nontemporal lobe structures is more difficult than in the temporal lobe, unless the patient has a structural lesion. Locating the seizure focus is particularly difficult when the seizures are suspected to arise from the frontal lobe. The large surface of the frontal lobe, and anatomic structures like the mesial and orbital regions that are far removed from the recording electrodes, make it difficult to localize either interictal or ictal EEG abnormalities. Focal EEG seizures may also arise in a "silent" region of the frontal lobe, producing clinical symptoms only after a seizure spreads to neighboring frontal lobe structures or to the temporal lobe.

The task is made even more complicated by the existence of a functional network of pathways permitting spread of discharges within and outside the frontal lobes. The bidirectional spread of epileptic discharges through the uncinate fasciculus and the cingulate gyrus in seizures arising from the frontal lobe may be falsely localized to the temporal lobe and vice versa. Because of this difficulty in localizing abnormalities, electroclinical correlation of ictal events is poorer in the frontal lobe than elsewhere. Most patients with frontal lobe seizures who do not have structural lesions on MRI require invasive electrode monitoring.

The incidence of excellent outcome with patients seizure free or with a significant reduction in seizure frequency after extratemporal resection is only 50% to 60%. However, with improving anatomic and functional neuroimaging, the incidence is likely to increase. There remains a need to study the risk–benefit ratio of extratemporal resection.

Table 10-4. Summary of surgical procedures for patients with medically intractable seizures

Procedure	Seizure Type	Electroencephalogram (EEG)	Risks	Benefits
Temporal lobectomy	Partial[a] ± general[b]	*Interictal:* Temporal or frontal spikes, sharp waves. *Ictal:* Initially discharges (spikes, sharp waves, beta activity, or rhythmic slowing) from temporal lobe, may then spread	Quadrantanopic field deficit; cerebrovascular accident; third-nerve palsy	Seizure control or significant reduction of seizures
Nontemporal resections	Partial[a] ± general[b]	*Interictal:* Focal spikes/sharp waves, occasional generalized spike waves *Ictal:* Focal spikes, beta activity, rapid spikes, spike–wave, polyspike–wave	Dependent on surgical site; weakness; visual-field cut	Seizure control or significant reduction in seizures; improved development
Corpus callosotomy	Partial[a] ± general[b] seizure; tonic, atonic, drop attacks	*Interictal:* Multifocal spikes/sharp waves, generalized spike–wave, polyspike–wave *Ictal:* Rapid spikes, spike–wave, polyspike–wave	Disconnection syndrome; speech deficits; increased frequency or intensity of partial seizures	Reduction in drop and generalized seizures; rarely do seizures totally remit

Procedure	Seizure types	EEG findings	Side effects	Outcome
Hemispherectomy	Unilateral partial[a] ± general[b], hemiparesis	*Interictal:* Preponderance of lateralized EEG discharges over involved hemisphere; may have bilateral spikes. *Ictal:* Lateralized onset to seizure over involved hemisphere	Hemiparesis; homonymous; hemianopsia	Seizure control; improved behavioral and cognitive state
Subpial transection	Simple or complex partial ± general	*Interictal:* Focal spikes/sharp waves, occasional generalized spike–wave. *Ictal:* Focal spikes, beta-activity, rapid spikes, spike–wave, polyspike–wave	Dependent on surgical site; weakness; aphasia	Seizure control or significant reduction in seizures
Vagal nerve stimulation	All seizure types	All EEG abnormalities	Voice change, shortness of breath, nausea, ventricular asystole	Seizure control (rare) or significant reduction in seizures

[a]Simple or complex partial seizures.
[b]Secondarily generalized tonic–clonic seizures.

3. Hemispherectomy

The removal of all or most of one hemisphere is one of the most drastic yet effective means to treat seizures. The procedure is typically used in patients with severe unilateral motor seizures who already have a hemiparesis and nonfunctional hand. Patients with Rasmussen encephalitis and Sturge–Weber syndrome are frequently candidates for this type of surgery. In addition, patients with hemimeganencephaly and other disorders of cerebral dysgenesis, cerebral infarctions, and trauma may also benefit from the surgery.

The presurgical evaluation must establish that the patient is not a candidate for a more-restricted surgical resection. Bilateral interictal spikes are common in patients with unilateral hemisphere pathology, but determination that the seizures begin unilaterally is essential. This may be difficult to establish in patients with severe atrophy of the hemisphere, when only surface EEG monitoring is performed because the ictal discharges may not propagate well to the surface of the head. In these cases, the clinical features of the seizures and functional neuroimaging can be useful in lateralizing the epileptic focus.

The response to the procedure is gratifying; more than three fourths of patients have a favorable outcome after the procedure. Because of late complications, including superficial hemosiderosis with obstructive hydrocephalus, bleeding into the hemispherectomy cavity, and fatal brainstem shift, some surgeons have been performing modified hemispherectomies that isolate, but do not remove, the frontal and occipital poles, or hemicortectomies.

4. Corpus Callosotomy

In some patients, despite extensive evaluations, a focus cannot be identified. In others, presurgical evaluation detects more than one focus. These patients may benefit from a corpus callosotomy. In this procedure, epileptic tissue is not removed, but the spread of the seizures is altered.

No firm criteria are available that can be used to predict which patients will benefit from corpus callosotomy. Factors that have been associated with favorable outcomes by some, but not all, investigators have included normal intelligence; focal EEG abnormalities; focal abnormalities on CT scan or MRI; and the presence of generalized tonic–clonic, tonic, and atonic seizures and hemiparesis. The procedure is usually reserved for patients with very frequent seizures, particularly drop attacks (atonic and tonic seizures).

Although complications from corpus callosotomy are relatively few, the procedure is not without risk. Infection and infarction have occurred after the procedure, and, rarely, patients may die. A disconnection syndrome has been described after the callosotomy. Patients may have difficulties with speech and motor functioning for days to weeks after the surgery. A decrease in the spontaneity of speech may occur that may be as severe as complete mutism or as mild as a slowness in initiating speech. In addition, variable degrees of paresis of the nondominant leg, forced grasping of the nondominant hand, and incontinence are present. These deficits usually improve with speech and physical therapy. However, reports have been made of permanent language disturbances after isolated anterior, posterior, or complete callosotomy, but only in patients with mixed cerebral dominance. When the hemisphere with language dominance is not the hemisphere controlling handedness, language deficits are more likely to develop. In these patients, a prior injury to the dominant hemisphere may cause transfer of some expressive language to the contralateral hemisphere, without changing the preferred hand.

5. Multiple Subpial Transection

Multiple subpial transection (MST) is increasingly used in the treatment of patients in whom seizures arise from a vital area of cortex, such as the language or motor cortex. This procedure is based on the observation that seizures are transmitted through horizontally oriented neurons, whereas cortical function is transmitted by vertical pathways. By cutting these horizontal fibers, the propagation of seizures can be prevented without resulting neurologic deficits.

A meta-analysis of MST studies found more than 95% seizure reduction in 71% of generalized seizure cases, 62% of complex partial seizure cases, and 63% of simple partial cases. Slightly better results were obtained when MST was combined with cortical resection.

6. Vagus Nerve Stimulation

Vagus nerve stimulation (VNS) is approved for use as adjunctive treatment for medically refractory partial-onset seizures in adolescents and adults. Several antiepileptic drugs have usually failed, and the patients are not candidates for (or have failed) a cortical-resection procedure.

VNS requires implantation of a programmable signal generator subcutaneously in the chest. Electrodes carry electrical signals from the generator to the left vagus nerve. Testing of the device in the operating room is necessary because asystole with stimulation has been reported in a few patients.

The mechanism of suppression of seizures by stimulation of the vagus nerve is probably by alteration of vagal afferent activities. Activities are altered in the reticular activating system, central autonomic network, the limbic system, and the diffuse nonadrenergic projection system.

Three large trials of VNS reported similar results. Approximately one third of patients with refractory partial seizures had a 50% or greater reduction in partial seizure frequency. A growing body of evidence suggests that seizure reduction improves with continued use of VNS. Patients who predictably have auras may be particularly helped by VNS because the device can be turned on by the patient, possibly aborting a seizure.

The common side effects of VNS are voice alteration, cough, pharyngitis, dyspnea, hoarseness, throat pain, paresthesias, and muscle pain. Left vocal cord paralysis and lower facial muscle paresis are rare complications of the procedure. Evidence indicates that VNS may have positive effects on memory, mood, and drowsiness.

Table 10-4 summarizes the common epilepsy surgical procedures.

D. Special Considerations in Children

Although many of the principles applied to adult patients with epilepsy are relevant to children with medically intractable seizures, epilepsy surgery in children presents a number of unique challenges and differences from that in adults. Some seizure disorders in children are catastrophic. In disorders such as infantile spasms or Sturge–Weber syndrome, the clinician is often faced not only with frequent, medically intractable seizures but with a plateau or even decline in development. Children may have major neurologic impairment from recurrent seizures or from the effects of antiepileptic drugs during the crucial early years of learning. Removing the focal brain abnormality, theoretically, allows the remainder of the brain to develop free of the undesirable influences of the abnormal epileptic tissue and antiepileptic drug therapy.

However, many childhood seizure disorders remit spontaneously, and performing surgery on a child who has a reasonable likelihood of going into remission is inappropriate. Although knowing the natural course of the seizure disorder is not always possible, surgery should not be considered unless a high likelihood exists that remission is not going to occur. It should also be remembered that although epilepsy surgery offers hope to a number of children with severe epilepsy, it is not free of risk. The risk of creating a permanent deficit must be balanced against the likelihood that the surgery will eliminate or significantly reduce the frequency of the seizures.

XV. THE KETOGENIC DIET

The ketogenic diet consists of a high proportion of fats and small amounts of carbohydrate and protein. Typically, the diet consists of a fat-to-carbohydrate and protein ratio of 3:1 or 4:1. The basis of the therapeutic effectiveness of the ketogenic diet is thought to be the ketosis that develops when the brain is relatively deprived of glucose as an energy source and must shift to the use of ketone bodies as the primary fuel. This results in increased cerebral energy reserves and increased GABA shunt activity, which are possible mechanisms of action.

The ketogenic diet is first-line treatment for seizures in association with glucose transporter protein deficiency and pyruvate dehydrogenase deficiency. In both cases, the ketogenic diet effectively treats the seizures and provides fuel for cerebral activity.

The ketogenic diet is of proven efficacy for children with cryptogenic or symptomatic generalized seizures such as Lennox–Gastaut syndrome. The effectiveness for refractory partial seizures is uncertain.

Although the difficulties of initiating and maintaining the diet are substantial, parents and children readily adapt to the rigors of the diet if it is effective in reducing seizure frequency.

Significant problems are associated with the ketogenic diet. These include weight loss, lethargy, renal stones, hemolytic anemia, hypoproteinemia, renal tubular acidosis, and elevation of hepatic enzymes. The ketogenic diet requires hospitalization, involves risks, and requires complex protocols and monitoring. It is best administered by centers with expertise in the regimen.

A low-glycemic-index diet has also been shown to be effective in the treatment of difficult-to-control seizures. The diet allows more liberal use of carbohydrates but uses foods that produce low levels of glucose. However, the diet has yet to be widely used, and further information about efficacy and adverse effects is needed.

REFERENCES

1. American Academy of Neurology Quality Standards Subcommittee. Practice parameter: a guideline for discontinuing antiepileptic drugs in seizure-free patients: summary statement. *Neurology* 1996;46:600–602.
2. Bailey EE, Pfeifer HH, Thiele EA. The use of diet in the treatment of epilepsy. *Epilepsy Behav* 2005;6:4–8.
3. Berg AT, Shinnar S, Levy SR, et al. Two-year remission and subsequent relapse in children with newly diagnosed epilepsy. *Epilepsia* 2001;42:1553–1562.
4. Browne TR. Pharmacokinetics of antiepileptic drugs. *Neurology* 1998;51(suppl 4):2–7.
5. Bund OK. Antiepileptic drug withdrawal: a good idea? *Pharmacotherapy* 1998;18:235–241.
6. Camfield P, Camfield C. The office management of epilepsy. *Semin Pediatr Neurol* 2006;13:201–207.
7. Cascino GD. Advances in neuroimaging: surgical localization. *Epilepsia* 2001;42:3–12.
8. Chang BS, Lowenstein DH. Practice parameter: antiepileptic drug prophylaxis in severe traumatic brain injury: report of Quality Standards Committee of the American Academy of Neurology. *Neurology* 2003;60:1–16.
9. Commission on Neuroimaging of the International League Against Epilepsy. Guidelines for neuroimaging evaluation of patients with uncontrolled epilepsy considered for surgery. *Epilepsia* 1998;39:1375–1376.
10. Cornaggia CM, Schmitz B, Trimble MR. Psychotropic drugs and epilepsy. *Epilepsia* 2002;43:1–50.
11. Cramer JA, Fisher R, Ben-Mencehem E, et al. New antiepileptic drugs: comparison of key clinical trials. *Epilepsia* 1999;40: 598–680.
12. Cramer JA, Glassman M, Rienzi V. The relationship between poor medication compliance and seizures. *Epilepsy Behav* 2002; 3:338–342.
13. Devinsky O. Current concepts: patients with refractory seizures. *N Engl J Med* 1999;340:1565–1570.
14. Duchowny M, Jayakas P, Resnick T, et al. Epilepsy surgery in the first 3 years of life. *Epilepsy* 1998;39:737–743.
15. Engle J, Wiebe J, French J, et al. Practice parameter: temporal lobe and localized neocortical resections for epilepsy: report of the Quality Standards Subcommittee of American Academy of Neurology in association with the American Epilepsy Society and the American Society of Neurological Surgeons. *Neurology* 2003;60:538–548.

16. Farhat G, Yamout B, Mikati MA, et al. Effect of antiepileptic drugs on bone density in ambulatory patients. *Neurology* 2002; 58:1348–1353.

17. Glantz MJ, Cole BF, Forsyth PA, et al. Practice parameter: anticonvulsant prophylaxis in patients with newly diagnosed brain tumors: report of the Quality Standards Committee of the American Academy of Neurology. *Neurology* 2000;54: 1886–1893.

18. Hammen T, Kerling F, Schwarz M, et al. Identifying the affected hemisphere by (1)H-MR spectroscopy in patients with temporal lobe epilepsy and no pathological findings in high resolution MRI. *Eur J Neurol* 2006;13:482–490.

19. Hansten PD, Horn JR. *Drug interactions: analysis and management*. Vancouver: Applied Therapeutics, updated quarterly.

20. Hauser WA, Hesdorffer DC. Remission, intractability, mortality and comorbidity of seizures. In: Wyllie E, ed. *The treatment of epilepsy: principles and practice*. Philadelphia: Lippincott Williams & Wilkins, 2001:139–148.

21. Hernandez TD, Naritoku DK. Seizures, epilepsy, and functional recovery after brain surgery. *Neurology* 1997;48:1383–1388.

22. Hirtz D, Berg A, Bettis D, et al. Practice parameter: treatment of the child with a first unprovoked seizure: report of the Quality Standard Committee of the American Academy of Neurology and the Practice Committee of the Child Neurology Society. *Neurology* 2002:60:166–175.

23. Inpatient/outpatient EEG monitoring. *J Clin Neurophysiol* 1999; 16:91–140.

24. Kanner AM, Balabnov A. Depression and epilepsy: how closely related are they? *Neurology* 2002;58(suppl 5):S27–S39.

25. Kramer G. Epilepsy and EEG. *Epilepsia* 2000;41(suppl 3):1–74.

26. Krsek P, Hajek M, Dezortova M, et al. (1)H MR spectroscopic imaging in patients with MRI-negative extratemporal epilepsy: correlation with ictal onset zone and histopathology. *Eur Radiol* 2007;17:2126–2135.

27. Kuzniecky R. Magnetic resonance and epilepsy: III International Magnetic Resonance and Epilepsy Symposium. *Epilepsia* 2002; 43(suppl 1):1–77.

28. Lee SK, Lee SH, Kim SK, et al. The clinical usefulness of ictal SPECT in temporal lobe epilepsy: the lateralization of seizure focus and correlation with EEG. *Epilepsia* 2000;41:955–962.

29. McIntosh AM, Wilson JS, Bercovic SF. Seizure outcome after temporal lobectomy: current research, practice, and findings. *Epilepsia* 2001;42:1288–1307.

30. Neuroimaging Subcommittee of the International League Against Epilepsy, Commission on Diagnostic Strategies. Recommendations for functional neuroimaging of persons with epilepsy. *Epilepsia* 2000;42:1350–1356.

31. Nordil NR, DeVivo DC. The ketogenic diet. In: Wyllie E, ed. *The treatment of epilepsy: principles and practice*. Philadelphia: Lippincott Williams & Wilkins, 2001:1001–1006.

32. O'Dell C, Shinnar S. Initiation and discontinuation of antiepileptic drugs. *Neurol Clin* 2001;19:289–311.

33. Patsalos PN, Froscher W, Pisani F, et al. The importance of drug interactions in epilepsy surgery. *Epilepsia* 2002;43:365–385.

34. Pfeifer HH, Thiele EA. Low-glycemic-index treatment: a liberalized ketogenic diet for treatment of intractable epilepsy. *Neurology* 2005;65:1810–1812.
35. Potschka H, Loscher W. In vivo evidence for P-glycoprotein–mediated transport of phenytoin at the blood–brain barrier of rats. *Epilepsia* 2001;42:1231–1240.
36. Schachter SC, Wheless JW. Vagus nerve stimulation 5 years after approval: a comprehensive update. *Neurology* 2002;59(suppl 4): 1–61.
37. Shinnar S, Berg AT, Moshe SL, et al. Risk of seizure recurrence following a first unprovoked seizure in childhood: a prospective study. *Pediatrics* 1990;85:1076–1085.
38. Spencer S. Selection of candidates for temporal resection. In: Wyllie E, ed. *The treatment of epilepsy: principles and practice.* Philadelphia: Lippincott Williams & Wilkins, 2001:1077–1094.
39. Spencer SS, Schramm J, Wyler A, et al. Multiple subpial transection for intractable partial seizures: an international meta-analysis. *Epilepsia* 2002;43:141–145.
40. Vining EP, Freeman JM, Pillas DJ, et al. Why would you remove half a brain? The outcome of 58 children after hemispherectomy: the Johns Hopkins experience 1968–1996. *Pediatrics* 1997;100: 163–171.
41. Wheless JW, Castillo E, Maggio V, et al. Magnetoencephalography (MEG) and magnetic source imaging (MSI). *Neurologist* 2004;10: 138–153.
42. Wiebe S, Blume WT, Girvin JP, et al. A randomized, controlled trial of surgery for temporal lobe epilepsy. *N Engl J Med* 2001; 345:311–318.
43. Williamson PD, Jobst BC. Selection of candidates for extratemporal resection. In: Wyllie E, ed. *The treatment of epilepsy: principles and practice.* Philadelphia: Lippincott Williams & Wilkins, 2001:1031–1041.
44. Willmore LJ. Epilepsy emergencies: the first seizure and status epilepticus. *Neurology* 1998;51(suppl 4):34–48.
45. Wolf P. Behavioral therapy. In: Engel J, Pedley TA, eds. *Epilepsy: a comprehensive textbook.* Philadelphia: Lippincott-Raven, 1997: 1359–1364.

Antiepileptic Drugs

This chapter reviews the mechanisms of action, indications, pharmacokinetics, and clinical use of common antiepileptic drugs. Drugs are reviewed in alphabetic order. Principles of drug administration, drugs of choice for various seizure types, and discontinuing antiepileptic drug therapy are reviewed in Chapter 10.

I. MECHANISM OF ACTION

Marketed antiepileptic drugs work by varying combinations of mechanisms.

A. Sodium Currents

The firing of an action potential by an axon requires passage of sodium into the axon through sodium channels. Sodium channels exist in three states: (a) resting (able to allow passage of sodium), (b) active (allowing passage of sodium), and (c) inactive (not allowing passage of sodium). After activation, a percentage of sodium channels become inactivated for a period of time. With repetitive axonal firing, enough sodium channels become inactivated that the axon can no longer propagate an action potential. Some antiepileptic drugs stabilize the inactive form of sodium channels, preventing its return to the active state. This, in turn, prevents sustained repetitive firing of the axon. Drugs such as phenytoin and carbamazepine, felbamate, lamotrigine, topiramate, oxcarbazepine, valproate, and zonisamide have been demonstrated to attenuate voltage-gated Na^+ channels in a use-dependent fashion.

B. γ-Aminobutyric Acid (GABA)$_A$ Receptor Currents

Attachment of γ-aminobutyric acid (GABA) to GABA$_A$ receptors facilitates the passage of chloride ions through chloride channels into cells. Chloride ions are negatively charged. Their passage into the cell makes the resting membrane potential more negative inside the cell and makes it more difficult for the cell to depolarize. Some antiepileptic drugs are agonists of this type of GABA-mediated chloride conductance. The GABA$_A$ receptor has benzodiazepine and barbiturate receptor sites. Activation of the benzodiazepine receptor enhances the frequency of openings of the GABA$_A$ receptor. Activation of the barbiturate receptor increases the duration of openings of the GABA$_A$ receptor.

A large number of AEDs exert their effects through enhanced inhibition by augmenting the effect of GABA. This is accomplished by the drug acting directly at the GABA$_A$ site, allosterically influencing the chloride current (barbiturates, benzodiazepines, and felbamate), by antagonizing neuronal and glial reuptake of GABA (tiagabine), or by interfering with the metabolic breakdown of GABA (vigabatrin). Valproate and gabapentin increase GABA synthesis and turnover.

C. Reduction of Voltage-sensitive Calcium Currents

Calcium ions are positively charged. Their passage into a cell renders the cell membrane less polarized. T-calcium currents are low-voltage, rapidly inactivated currents that act as pacemakers for normal rhythmic brain activity, especially in the thalamus. T-calcium currents also appear to have an important role in pacing the three-per-second spike–wave activity of absence seizures (but not other seizure types). Drugs inhibiting T-calcium currents specifically inhibit absence seizures.

The L-, N-, P-, R-, and Q-calcium channels are high-voltage activated channels distinct from low-voltage T-calcium currents. Levetiracetam, lamotrigine, phenobarbital, felbamate, and topiramate target high-voltage calcium channels. Gabapentin and pregabalin bind to the $\alpha_2\delta$ subunit of the P/Q voltage-gated calcium channel. As a result, gabapentin and pregabalin reduce the calcium current at the terminal, reducing the release of glutamate, noradrenaline, and substance P.

D. Glutamate-receptor Antagonists

Excitation in the human nervous system is produced principally by binding of the excitatory amino acid glutamate to three types of ionotropic glutamate receptors: N-methyl-D-aspartate (NMDA), α-amino-3-hydroxy-5-methyl-4-isoxazole propionate (AMPA), and kainate. Binding of glutamate to these receptors facilitates passage of calcium and sodium into the cell and potassium out of the cell. The net effect is reduction of the negative resting-membrane potential, making the cell less electrically stable. Some antiepileptic drugs act by antagonism of one or more types of glutamate receptor. Felbamate has a dual action, blocking NMDA channels and enhancing the GABAergic effect. Topiramate has been shown to attenuate non-NMDA (AMPA) and kainate currents.

E. Other Mechanisms

Recently, another target of AEDs, the H (hyperpolarization induced, cyclic nucleotide gated) channel, has been characterized. The H-channel has a high permeability to potassium and tends to stabilize the membrane potential toward the resting potential against both hyperpolarizing and depolarizing inputs. Drugs such as lamotrigine and gabapentin target the H-channels by increasing the hyperpolarization-activated cation current.

The mechanism of action of levetiracetam is not entirely clear. However, the drug blocks N-type Ca^{2+} channels and reverses the inhibition by the negative allosteric modulators zinc and β-carbolines on neuronal GABA- and glycine-gated currents. In addition, the drug binds to a synaptic protein (SV2). How binding to a synaptic protein results in reduced excitability (or enhanced inhibition) is not clear.

Figures 11-1 and 11-2 depict the primary mechanisms of antiepileptic drug action at excitatory and inhibitory synapses.

III. BASIC PHARMACOKINETIC PRINCIPLES

An understanding of basic principles of pharmacokinetics and pharmacodynamics of antiepileptic drug therapy is necessary for the optimal management of patients with epilepsy.

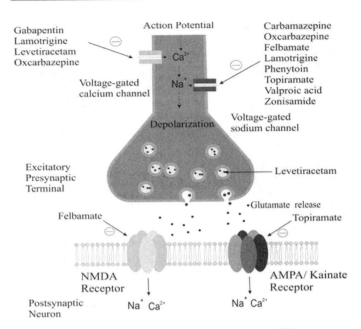

Fig. 11-1.   Excitatory pre- and postsynaptic neurons. AEDs may modify Na$^+$ or Ca^{2+} channels or work at the postsynaptic NMDA or non-NMDA receptor.

Pharmacokinetics is a measure of the action of drugs in the body over a period of time, including the processes of absorption, distribution, localization in tissues, biotransformation, and excretion. Pharmacodynamics is the study of the biochemical and physiological effects of drugs and the mechanisms of their actions, including the correlation of action and effects of drugs with their chemical structure. Whereas pharmacokinetic data are critical in determining dosage, frequency of administration, and time of steady state, pharmacodynamics provides information about efficacy and side effects of the administered drugs. In other words, pharmacokinetics is the study of what the body does to a drug, whereas pharmacodynamics is the study of what a drug does to the body.

The drug's bioavailability provides information about the degree to which a drug becomes available to the target tissue after administration. Bioavailability is dependent on absorption and first-pass hepatic metabolism, in the case of oral administration. In general, most antiepileptic drugs are well absorbed. The one exception is gabapentin, for which the rate of absorption is dose dependent. The drug is transported into the blood from the gut by a saturable transport mechanism, the L-amino-acid transport system. Because of this dose-dependent bioavailability, plasma concentrations of the drug are not directly propor-

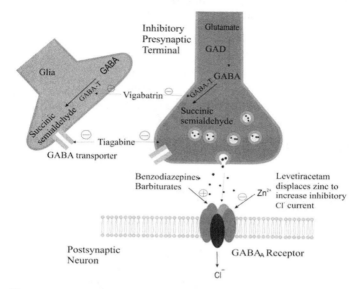

Fig. 11-2.   Inhibitory pre- and postsynaptic neurons. AEDs can enhance $GABA_A$ effect by increasing the frequency or duration of the channel opening. Levetiracetam can displace Zn^{2+}, which reduces Cl^- currents, from the $GABA_A$ channel. Vigabatrin inhibits GABA-transaminase, thereby increasing intracellular GABA. Tiagabine inhibits the uptake of GABA from the synaptic cleft, which increases extracellular GABA.

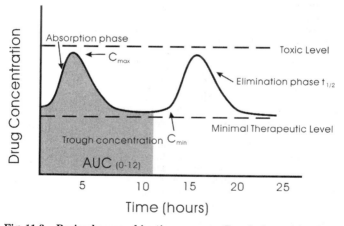

Fig. 11-3.   Basic pharmacokinetic measures. C_{max} is the maximum or peak concentration and is influenced by absorption as well as first-pass hepatic metabolism. The C_{min} is the minimal concentration. Toxicity is most likely to occur at C_{max}, whereas seizure recurrence is most likely to occur at C_{min}. The elimination half-life is the time required for the drug to decrease by one half of its concentration. The AUC is the area under the curve and indicates the amount of the drug to which the patient is exposed.

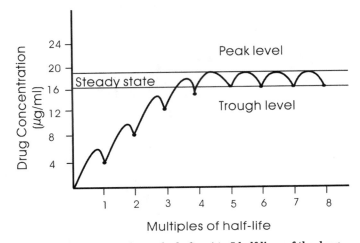

Fig. 11-4. Steady state is reached after 4 to 5 half-lives of the drug. Steady state is an equilibrium in which absorption of drug is balanced by clearance of the drug, and the serum concentration remains steady from day to day. During steady state, daily fluctuations occur between C_{min} and C_{max} .

tional to dose throughout the range of doses administered. With increasing dosages of gabapentin, no proportional increase in blood level occurs.

Compared with adults, drug absorption is compromised in newborns but is increased in children. Food does slow the rate of absorption (but not total amount absorbed), and rapid transit through the gut can reduce blood levels. In most cases, it is not important whether the drug is taken with or without food. However, it is recommended that the patients be consistent and take the drug either with or without food on a regular basis. Because rapid absorption of tiagabine can result in toxicity, it is recommended that tiagabine be taken with food.

The peak concentration of the antiepileptic drug, C_{max}, is related to the rapidity of absorption (Fig. 11-3). The C_{max} is often is the time when the drug should have its greatest effect and also is most likely to cause side effects. However, whether the peak efficacy and toxicity occur at C_{max} is dependent on the pharmacodynamics profile of the drug. For example, toxicity and efficacy of drugs such as vigabatrin, which inhibits GABA transaminase, may have a poor correlation with serum concentration of the drug.

One of the most important properties of a drug to know is clearance. Clearance represents the body's ability to eliminate drug completely from a particular volume of fluid (usually plasma) per unit of time. Clearance can be defined for particular organs, such as the liver or kidney. Total clearance represents the sum of the various organ clearances resulting in drug elimination (e.g., hepatic and renal clearance). Total clearance determines steady-state serum blood concentration:

Concentration = Bioavailability × Dose/Total clearance

Clearance represents a good parameter by which to evaluate age-related changes in drug elimination. Although half-life, the period over which the concentration of the drug decreases to half of its original concentration in serum, is an important pharmacokinetic feature, it is dependent on the volume of distribution (V_D), which is a measure of how the drug is distributed in the body (between blood and tissues, in particular). **V_D** is the amount of drug in the body divided by the concentration in the blood. Drugs that are highly lipid soluble have a very high volume of distribution, whereas drugs that are lipid insoluble remain in the blood and have a low V_D. Half-life is defined as

$$T_{1/2} = \frac{0.693 \; V_D}{\text{Total clearance Cls}}$$

Because V_D varies significantly as a function of age and body distribution of fat, it is not a good measure of longitudinal changes in clearance of the drug from the body. However, half-life is a valuable practical pharmacokinetic measure.

Steady state is the condition in which the drug is in a dynamic equilibrium in which the rate of clearance is equal to the rate of administration. Drugs will accumulate within the body if the drug has not been fully eliminated before the next dose. Steady-state concentration is reached after four to five half-lives (Fig. 11-4).

Antiepileptic drugs can be excreted unchanged in the urine or be metabolized in the liver through the cytochrome (Cyp) P450 system (CYP1A2, CYP2A6, CYP2C8, CYP2C9, CYP2C19, CYP2D6, CYP2E1, CYP3A) or via uridine 5'-diphosphate-glucuronosyltransferase. The majority of antiepileptic drugs that are metabolized in the liver go through the Cyp system. Lamotrigine is primarily metabolized via uridine 5'-diphosphate-glucuronosyltransferase. Table 11-1 lists the effects of antiepileptic drugs on the Cyp system, and Table 11-2 lists the antiepileptic drugs that are metabolized in the liver or excreted in the urine.

As a general rule, neonates and infants have slow hepatic metabolism, whereas hepatic metabolism is increased in children. Likewise, renal clearance of drugs is lower than that in adults, whereas renal clearance is greater in children than adults.

A constant fraction of the drug in the body is eliminated per unit time. The rate of elimination is proportional to the amount of drug in the body. The majority of drugs are eliminated in this way. When the rate of elimination is proportional to the amount of drug in the body, the drug has linear kinetics. For most antiepileptic drugs, the kinetics are linear. However, with phenytoin, when the enzymes responsible for its metabolism become saturated, the rate of elimination, in terms of the amount of the drug eliminated in a given period, does not increase in response to an increase in concentration. This is termed zero-order kinetics (Fig. 11-5).

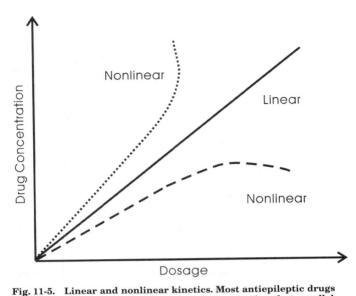

Fig. 11-5. Linear and nonlinear kinetics. Most antiepileptic drugs
have a proportional increase in serum concentration that parallels
the increase in dosage. In nonlinear kinetics, this proportional
increase in concentration with dosage does not occur. In the case of
phenytoin, enzyme saturation occurs, and the liver cannot increase
metabolism with increases in dosage. This results in marked
increases in serum concentration with modest increases in dosage.
This saturation may occur at serum levels in the therapeutic range.
In the case of gabapentin, dose-dependent absorption of the drug
occurs. With increasing doses of gabapentin, decreased absorption
of the drug results in a nonlinear relation between serum concentration and dosage.

Table 11-1. Effects of AEDs on cytochrome P450

Inducers	Inhibition or No Effect
Carbamazepine	Ethosuximide
Oxcarbazepine	Felbamate
Phenobarbital	Gabapentin
Phenytoin	Lamotrigine
Primidone	Levetiracetam
Topiramate	Tiagabine
	Valproate
	Vigabatrin

Table 11-2. Renal and hepatic excretion of antiepileptic drugs

Renal	Hepatic
Gabapentin	Carbamazepine
Levetiracetam	Clobazam
Pregabalin	Levetiracetam
Topiramate	Oxcarbazepine
Vigabatrin	Phenytoin
Zonisamide	Phenobarbital
	Tiagabine
	Topiramate
	Zonisamide
	Valproate

IV. DRUG INTERACTIONS

Drug interactions are common when antiepileptic drugs are given in combination with other antiepileptic drugs or with other classes of drug. Drug interactions can be pharmacodynamic or pharmacokinetic. Pharmacodynamic drug interactions occur when one drug affects the activity of another drug without altering the concentration of the other drug. For example, lamotrigine may enhance the toxicity of carbamazepine without altering plasma concentrations of carbamazepine or carbamazepine epoxide. Pharmacokinetic drug interactions occur when one drug affects the concentration on another drug at its site of action. The mechanism of the interaction may be an alteration in absorption, distribution (including protein binding), biotransformation (especially for drugs metabolized by the cytochrome P450), or excretion. Pharmacokinetic drug interactions can also be bidirectional. For example, phenytoin reduces carbamazepine plasma concentration by induction of CYP3A4, whereas carbamazepine increases plasma concentration of phenytoin, probably by inhibition of CYP2C9/19. One useful rule of thumb is that drugs eliminated by the kidney (e.g., pregabalin, gabapentin, levetiracetam, and topiramate) have a lower risk of drug interactions.

V. CARBAMAZEPINE (TEGRETOL)

A. Mechanism of Action
See section **I** and Table 11-3.

B. Indications, Advantages, and Disadvantages
Carbamazepine is indicated as initial or adjunctive therapy for complex partial and tonic–clonic seizures. It was found to be one of the two safest and most effective drugs for these seizure types in comparative studies of older drugs (phenytoin is the other.) It is relatively nonsedating (sedation is mild and similar to that of phenytoin) and does not have the cosmetic side effects of phenytoin.

Table 11-3.   Mechanism(s) of action and pharmacokinetics of antiepileptic drugs

Drug	Predominant Mechanism of Action[a]	Elimination Half-life in Children (hr)	Elimination Half-life in Adults (hr)	Time to Steady-state Plasma Concentration (d)	Protein Binding (%)
Carbamazepine (Tegretol)	A	14–27 (children), 8–28 (neonates)	9–27	3–4	85
Clobazam (Frezium)	B	10–20 (N-desmethylclobazam)	15–50 (N-desmethylclobazam)	3–5	85
Clonazepam (Klonopin)	B	20–40	10–40	—	95–98
Diazepam (Diastat)	B	17	36	—	40
Ethosuximide (Zarontin)	C	20–60	20–60	7–10	0
Gabapentin (Neurontin)	B, D	—	5–7	—	0
Lamotrigine (Lamictal)	A	—	See text	—	55
Levetiracetam	D, F	—	6–8	2	0
Oxcarbazepine (Trileptal)	A	5–8	7–11[b]	2–3	40
Phenobarbital	B	37–73	40–136	12–21	40–60
Phenytoin (Dilantin)	A	5–14 (children), 10–60 (neonates)	12–36	7–28	69–96

Pregabalin (Lyrica)	B, D	4–6	5–7	1–2	0
Primidone (Mysoline)	B	5–11	6–18	4–7	0
Tiagabine (Gabitril)	B	—	4–7	2	96
Topiramate (Topamax)	A, B, E	10–15, 6–8[c]	20–30, 12–15[c]	—	15
Valproic acid (Depakene, Depakote)	A, B	8–15	6–15	1–2	80–95
Vigabatrin (Sabril)	B	4–7	5–8	1–2	0
Zonisamide (Zonegran)	A, C	—	27–46	10–12	40

A, sodium currents; B, γ-aminobutyric acid-A receptor currents; C, T-calcium currents; D, voltage-gated calcium channel currents; E, glutamate receptor antagonist; F, synaptic vesicle protein.

[a]See section I of this chapter for discussion.

[b]Monohydroxy metabolite.

[c]In the presence of enzyme-inducing drugs such as carbamazepine, phenobarbital, or primidone.

A loading dose of carbamazepine cannot be administered by any route. The drug must be given in divided doses. Carbamazepine must be started at a low dose, and the dosage must be built up over time. Carbamazepine may exacerbate absence seizures in some patients. An increased risk exists of spina bifida in infants born to mothers taking carbamazepine during pregnancy.

C. Pharmacokinetics

Approximately 75% to 85% of an orally administered dose of brand-name Tegretol, 200-mg tablets, is slowly absorbed after oral administration. The bioavailability of generic carbamazepine is sometimes less than that of brand-name Tegretol. Carbamazepine is 70% to 80% protein-bound. Carbamazepine is metabolized by the liver into 32 or more metabolites, some of which (especially carbamazepine epoxide) possess antiepileptic activity. Carbamazepine biotransformation exhibits time-dependent pharmacokinetics (self-induction), which means that the plasma concentration may decrease unexpectedly during the first 2 months of administration when self-induction occurs.

D. Usual Pediatric and Adult Dosages

See Tables 11-4 and 11-5.

E. Formulations

Carbamazepine is marketed as standard 200-mg tablets (both brand-name Tegretol and generic), 100-mg chewable tablets (Tegretol), and suspension of 100 mg per 5 mL. These formulations are labeled for t.i.d. or q.i.d. administration.

Two sustained-release carbamazepine formulations (Carbatrol and Tegretol-XR) are available for b.i.d. administration. Although the two formulations use different technologies, they both perform well with b.i.d. administration. Sustained-release preparations may improve compliance, reduce toxicity associated with peak levels, and reduce breakthrough seizures at times of trough blood levels. Carbatrol is available as 200-mg and 300-mg capsules. Tegretol-XR is available as 100-mg, 200-mg, and 400-mg tablets. Sustained-release formulations of carbamazepine are the preferred mode of administration.

F. Toxicity

Local toxicity consists of gastric irritability that is usually managed if the patient takes the drug after meals. Common dose-related toxicity includes diplopia or blurred vision, dizziness, drowsiness, ataxia, and headache. At high plasma concentrations, the following may occur: tremor, dystonia, chorea, depression, irritability, psychosis, convulsions, water retention (inappropriate antidiuretic hormone–like syndrome), congestive heart failure, and cardiac arrhythmias.

Idiosyncratic toxicities are rash (common) and, more rarely, anemia, agranulocytosis, leukopenia, thrombocytopenia, hypersensitivity syndrome (dermatitis, eosinophilia, lymphadenopathy, splenomegaly), and cholestatic and hepatocellular jaundice. The rate of fatal idiosyncratic reactions with carbamazepine is estimated currently at 1 in 100,000 to 200,000 patients. Although this factor is a matter of concern, the risk is in a range similar to that of other commonly used drugs, such as penicillin.

The issue of reduced bone marrow density is discussed in Chapter 10.

G. Drug Interactions

Adding carbamazepine may increase the plasma concentration of fluoxetine, phenytoin, and tricyclic antidepressants. Adding carbamazepine may reduce the plasma concentrations of antiviral and anticancer drugs metabolized by CYP450, benzodiazepines, corticosteroids, cyclosporine, felbamate, griseofulvin, haloperidol, lamotrigine, oral contraceptives, oxcarbazepine, theophylline, tiagabine, topiramate, valproic acid, warfarin, and zonisamide. Propoxyphene, erythromycin, clarithromycin, chloramphenicol, isoniazid, verapamil, grapefruit juice, and cimetidine may increase the carbamazepine plasma concentration, whereas phenobarbital, phenytoin, felbamate, Saint John's wort, and primidone may reduce the carbamazepine plasma concentration. Adding valproic acid to carbamazepine may increase plasma carbamazepine epoxide concentration. Adding lamotrigine to carbamazepine may enhance the usual neurotoxic side effects of carbamazepine.

H. Disease States

Carbamazepine may precipitate or enhance congestive heart failure. Its use should be avoided in this setting or in cases in which major arrhythmias are a concern. Plasma concentrations and potential toxicity must be closely watched when the drug is used in patients with renal or hepatic disease.

I. Pregnancy

A 0.5% to 1% risk of spina bifida exists in infants born to mothers who took carbamazepine during the first trimester. Reports are found of increased risk of other congenital malformations in infants born to mothers taking antiepileptic drugs. The potential risks and benefits of using this drug in pregnancy must be carefully weighed for each patient. Because alternative antiepileptic drugs do not increase the risk of spina bifida, the authors generally prefer to use one of the alternative drugs (any other antiepileptic drug except valproic acid) in women of childbearing potential.

The drug is excreted in breast milk. The risks of exposure of the infant to the drug are unknown. The benefits of breast-feeding, the risk to the infant of drug exposure, and the risk to the mother of stopping the drug must be weighed in each case.

VI. CLOBAZAM (FREZIUM)

A. Mechanism of Action

See section I and Table 11-3.

B. Indications, Advantages, and Disadvantages

Clobazam currently is not available in the United States but is widely used throughout the world. Clobazam is a benzodiazepine

Table 11-4. Usual pediatric dosages of antiepileptic drugs

Drug	Starting Dose	Dosing Regimen	Dose-escalation Rate (in daily dose/ Time interval)	Maintenance Dose	Therapeutic Range of Plasma Concentration $(\mu g/mL)^a$
Carbamazepine (Carbatrol, Tegretol, Tegretol-XR)	<6 yr: 10–15 mg/kg/d 6–12 yr: 100 mg b.i.d.	Carbatol or Tegretol-XR b.i.d.; other forms, t.i.d.; b.i.d.	<6 yr: 5 mg/kg/1 wk >6 yr: 100–200 mg/1 wk	10–30 mg/kg/d	4–12
Clonazepam (Klonopin)	10 yr or <30 kg: 0.01–0.3 mg/kg/d >10 yr: 1–1.5 mg/d	t.i.d.–q.i.d.	<10 yr: 0.02 mg/kg/1 wk >10 yr: 0.5 mg/1 wk	0.1–0.3 mg/kg/d	0.02–0.08
Clobazam (Frezium)	<12 yr: 5 mg/d >12 yr: 10 mg/d	b.i.d.	5–10 mg/day/wk	0/25–1 mg/kg/d (maximum, 40 mg)	Not established
Diazepam (Diastat)	See text				
Ethosuximide (Zarontin)	<6 yr: 10–15 mg/kg, not to exceed 250 mg/d >6 yr: 250 mg/d	t.i.d–q.i.d.	125–250 mg/1 wk	15–40 mg/kg/d	120
Gabapentin (Neurontin)	10 mg/kg/d	t.i.d.	300 mg/1 d	30–100 mg/kg/d	Not established
Lamotrigine (Lamictal)	On enzyme inducers: 1 mg/kg/d On enzyme inducers and inhibitors	t.i.d.–b.i.d.	On enzyme inducers: 1 mg/kg/2 wk On enzyme inducers and inhibitors (valproate):	With enzyme inducers: 15 mg/kg/d With enzyme inducers and	Not established

Drug	Starting dose	Frequency	Titration	Maintenance dose	Therapeutic level
	0.3–0.5 mg/kg/d On enzyme inhibitor: 0.1–0.3 mg/kg/d Monotherapy: 0.5 mg/kg/d		On enzyme inhibitor: 0.1–0.3 mg/kg/2 wk Monotherapy: 0.5 mg/kg/2 wk	(valproate): 10 mg/kg/d With enzyme inhibitor: 5 mg/kg/d Monotherapy: 10 mg/kg/d	
Oxcarbazepine (Trileptal)	10 mg/kg/d	b.i.d.	10 mg/kg/2 wk	30 mg/kg/d	Not established
Phenobarbital	<1 yr: 3–5 mg/kg/d >1 yr: 2–4 mg/kg/d	b.i.d.–q.d.	1–2 mg/kg/2 wk	<1 yr: 3–5 mg/kg/d >1 yr: 2–4 mg/kg/d	10–40
Phenytoin (Dilantin)	5 mg/kg/d	b.i.d.	1–2 mg/kg/2 wk	5–8 mg/kg/d	10–25
Pregabalin (Lyrica)	1–2 mg/kg	b.i.d.	1–2 mg/kg/wk	5–20 mg/kg/d	Not established
Primidone (Mysoline)	<6 yr: 50 mg/d >12 yr: 100 mg/d	q.i.d.–t.i.d.	25–50 mg/2 wk	12–25 mg/kg/d	5–12
Tiagabine (Gabitril)	0.05–0.10 mg/kg/d (not to exceed 4 mg)	b.i.d.–q.i.d.	0.05–0.10 mg/kg/wk	1–2 mg/kg/d	Not established
Topiramate (Topamax)	1–3 mg/kg/d	b.i.d.	1–3 mg/kg/wk or 2 wk	5–9 mg/kg/d	Not established
Vigabatrin (Sabril)	50 mg/kg/d	b.i.d.	50 mg/kg/d	150–200 mg/kg/d	Not established
Valproic acid (Depakene)	15–20 mg/kg/d	q.i.d.–t.i.d.	5–10 mg/kg/d	30–80 mg/kg/d	50–150
Divalproex sodium (Depakote)	15–20 mg/kg/d	b.i.d.	5–10 mg/kg/d	30–80 mg/kg/d	50–150

[a]See Appendix I for conversion to molar units.

Table 11-5. Usual adult dosages of antiepileptic drugs (16 years and older)

Drug	Starting Dose (mg/d)	Dosing Regimen	Escalation Rate (in Daily Dose (mg/Time Interval)	Maintenance Dose (mg/d)	Maximum Dose (mg/d)	Therapeutic Range of Plasma Concentration ($\mu g/mL$)[a]
Carbamazepine (Tegretol)	200	Carbatrol or Tegretol-XR b.i.d.; other forms, t.i.d.	200/1 wk	600–1,200	1,600	4–12
Clobazam (Frezium)	10	b.i.d.	5/1 wk	20–40	80	Not established
Clonazepam (Klonopin)	1.5	t.i.d.	0.5/4 d	2–6	20	0.02–0.08
Diazepam (Diastat)	See text					
Ethosuximide (Zarontin)	500	t.i.d.	250/1 wk	1,000–2,000	—	40–120
Gabapentin (Neurontin)	300	t.i.d.	300/daily	900–3,600	—	Not established
Lamotrigine (Lamictal)	See text	b.i.d.	See text	See text	700	Not established
Levetiracetam (Keppra)	1,000[b]	b.i.d.	1,000/2 wk	1,000–3,000	3,000	Not established

Drug	Starting dose (mg/d)	Schedule	Titration	Usual dose (mg/d)	Maximum (mg/d)	Therapeutic level
Oxcarbazepine (Trileptal)	600 (monotherapy) 600 (adjunctive)	b.i.d.	300/3 d	1,200	2,400	Not established
Phenobarbital	90	b.i.d. q.d.[a]	300–600/3 d 30/4 wk	1,200 90–120	2,400 —	Not established 10–40
Phenytoin (Dilantin)	5 mg/kg/d	q.d.[c]	30–100[d]/4 wk	300–500	—	10–20
Primidone (Mysoline)	100–125	t.i.d.	50 mg/wk	750–1000	2000	5–12
Pregabalin (Lyrica)	75–150	b.i.d.	50/wk	150–600	600	Not established
Zonisamide (Zonegran)	100	b.i.d.	100/2 wk	100–400	400	Not established
Tiagabine (Gabitril)	4	b.i.d.–q.i.d.	4–8/1 wk	32–56	56	Not established
Topiramate (Topamax)	25–50	b.i.d.	See text	200–400	1,600	Not established
Valproic acid (Depakene) (Depakote)	1,000	Valproic acid t.i.d.; divalproex sodium b.i.d.	250/1 wk	1,000–3,000	4,000 (60 mg/kg/d)	50–150

[a]See Appendix I for conversion to molar units.
[b]Lower starting dose may reduce start-up toxicity. See text.
[c]Once-daily drugs are usually given at bedtime to avoid toxicity associated with peak plasma concentrations.
[d]Increments of 100 mg/d if plasma concentration <10 mg/mL; increments of 30 to 50 mg/d if plasma concentration is >10 mg/mL.

that has achieved popularity because it is highly effective as adjunctive therapy for partial and generalized seizures. It is far better tolerated than other benzodiazepines. The main disadvantage is the development of tolerance in many patients.

C. Pharmacokinetics

Clobazam is absorbed well by the alimentary tract. Clobazam is about 85% protein bound. Clobazam is extensively biotransformed. Eight metabolites are known, with N-desmethylclobazam, an active metabolite, being the most important. The elimination half-life of clobazam ranges from 10 to 30 hours, whereas N-desmethylclobazam is 36 to 46 hours.

D. Usual Pediatric and Adult Doses

See Tables 11-4 and 11-5.

E. Formulations

Clobazam in available in 10-mg tablets.

F. Toxicity

Dose-related toxicity includes drowsiness, ataxia, behavioral change (irritability, depression, psychosis), typically at a much lower rate than with other benzodiazepines, such as clonazepam. Idiosyncratic toxicity includes skin rash and, rarely, systemic lupus erythematosus.

G. Drug Interactions

Enzyme-inducing drugs, such as phenobarbital, phenytoin, and carbamazepine, can increase metabolism of clobazam and increase concentrations of the active N-desmethylclobazam. Although toxicity could ensue, this drug interaction is rarely of clinical significance.

H. Disease States

Hepatic disease may alter both protein binding and clobazam elimination, with potentially marked effects on clobazam levels.

I. Pregnancy

Little information is available on clobazam and pregnancy. Clobazam passes into breast milk and should be avoided by nursing mothers.

VII. CLONAZEPAM (KLONOPIN)

A. Mechanism of Action

See section I and Table 11-3.

B. Indications, Advantages, and Disadvantages

Clonazepam is the third-choice drug for absence seizures, because disabling side effects (drowsiness, ataxia, behavior disturbance) and development of tolerance to the antiepileptic effect of the drug are more common with clonazepam than with ethosuximide or valproic acid. Clonazepam also is indicated as initial or adjunctive therapy for atypical absence, atonic, and myoclonic seizures.

C. Pharmacokinetics

Clonazepam appears to be absorbed well by the alimentary tract. It is 47% protein bound. Extensive biotransformation takes place, and less than 0.5% is recovered from the urine as clonazepam.

D. Usual Pediatric and Adult Doses

See Tables 11-4 and 11-5.

E. Formulations

Tablet sizes include 0.5, 1.0, and 2.0 mg for both generic and brand0-name products. Clonazepam also is available in 0.125-, 0.25-, and 0.50-mg dissolvable tablets.

F. Toxicity

Dose-related toxicity includes drowsiness, ataxia, behavioral change (irritability, depression, psychosis), dysarthria, and diplopia. Idiosyncratic toxicity commonly includes skin rash and, rarely, hair loss, anemia, leukopenia, and thrombocytopenia.

G. Drug Interactions

Phenobarbital may reduce the clonazepam plasma concentration. Concurrent use of amphetamines and methylphenidate may cause central nervous system (CNS) depression and respiratory irregularities. Depressant effects may also be enhanced by alcohol, antianxiety and antipsychotic drugs, antidepressants, and other antiepileptic drugs.

H. Disease States

Renal disease is unlikely to affect the elimination of clonazepam, but liver disease may require a decrease in dosage.

I. Pregnancy

Because of experience with other members of the benzodiazepine class, clonazepam is assumed to be capable of causing an increased risk of congenital abnormalities when administered to a pregnant woman during the first trimester. Clonazepam is excreted in breast milk and can produce sedation in the neonate.

VIII. DIASTAT (DIAZEPAM RECTAL GEL)

A. Mechanism of Action

See section I and Table 11-3.

B. Indications, Advantages, and Disadvantages

Diastat is a gel formulation of diazepam intended for rectal administration in the management of selected patients with refractory epilepsy who are taking stable regimens of antiepileptic drugs but require intermittent use of diazepam to control bouts of increased seizure activity. Use of Diastat provides an opportunity for the caregiver to intervene immediately, reduce the likelihood of further seizures, and reduce the need for emergency-department care. Somnolence is the most commonly reported side effect.

C. Pharmacokinetics

Diastat is well absorbed after rectal administration. The minimum antiepileptic plasma concentration of diazepam (200 ng/mL) is reached within 15 minutes, and peak diazepam concentration is reached in 90 minutes. The absolute bioavailability of rectally administered Diastat relative to intravenously administered diazepam is 90%. The pharmacokinetics of diazepam derived from Diastat are similar to the pharmacokinetics of diazepam derived from other formulations. The major active metabolite of diazepam is desmethyl-diazepam. The demethylation involves cytochromes P450 (CYP) 2C19 and 3A4. The elimination half-life of diazepam is 46 hours, and the elimination half-life of desmethyl-diazepam is 71 hours. Both diazepam and desmethyl-diazepam bind extensively to plasma proteins (95% to 98%).

D. Usual and Adult Dosage

The recommended dose depends on age and weight: age 2 through 5 years, 0.5 mg/kg; age 6 through 11 years, 0.3 mg/kg; 12 years and older, 0.2 mg/kg. In elderly and debilitated patients, adjusting the dosage downward (because of reduced clearance) is recommended to reduce risks of sedation and ataxia. See package insert for details.

E. Formulations

Diastat (diazepam rectal gel) rectal delivery system is a nonsterile diazepam gel provided in a single-dose rectal delivery system. The system includes a plastic applicator with a flexible, molded tip available in two lengths (pediatric and adult). Applications are available starting at 2.5 mg and increasing in 2.5 mg up to 20 mg.

F. Toxicity

The most common adverse event reported with Diastat in clinical trials was somnolence (23%). Less frequent adverse events were dizziness, headache, pain, abdominal pain, nervousness, vasodilation, diarrhea, ataxia, euphoria, incoordination, asthma, rhinitis, and rash (which occurred in 2% to 5% of patients). In two of 573 patients, hypoventilation developed.

G. Drug Interactions

Other psychotropic agents may potentiate the actions (especially sedative actions) of diazepam. These agents include barbiturates, valproic acid, narcotics, phenothiazines, monoamine oxidase inhibitors, and other antidepressants. The clearance of diazepam can be delayed by cimetidine. Because *in vitro* studies suggest that diazepam is metabolized by CYP 2C19 and CYP 3A4, drugs metabolized by these isoforms could have an effect on diazepam clearance, and vice versa.

H. Disease States

Clearance of diazepam is reduced in patients with hepatic impairment. Diazepam clearance also is reduced in the elderly. The pharmacokinetics of diazepam have not been studied in renally impaired subjects.

I. Pregnancy

Some reports suggest an increased risk of congenital malformations in infants born to mothers taking long-term diazepam during the first trimester of the pregnancy. It is not known if a single dose of diazepam carries the same risk. The risks of status epilepticus to the mother and fetus are so great that it probably makes sense to use the drug when appropriate.

Because diazepam and its metabolites may be present in breast milk for prolonged periods after short-term use of Diastat, patients should be advised not to breast-feed for an appropriate period after receiving treatment with Diastat.

IX. ETHOSUXIMIDE (ZARONTIN)

A. Mechanism of Action

See section **I** and Table 11-3.

B. Indications, Advantages, and Disadvantages

Ethosuximide is typically used for the treatment of absence epilepsy. In general, the drug is effective and well tolerated. The common side effects of ethosuximide, gastrointestinal upset and drowsiness, tend to occur early in therapy and then diminish as tolerance develops. The drug seldom causes behavioral or cognitive disturbances. In approximately 1% to 7% of patients taking ethosuximide, leukopenia develops, which is reversible if detected early. Ethosuximide is ineffective against tonic–clonic and myoclonic seizures, which sometimes accompany absence seizures.

C. Pharmacokinetics

Ethosuximide is readily and almost completely absorbed in the alimentary tract. Little or no binding to serum proteins occurs. The drug is transformed in the liver to either a ketone or an alcohol metabolite, which is then excreted with or without glucuronide conjugation.

D. Usual Pediatric and Adult Dosages

See Tables 11-4 and 11-5.

E. Formulations

Ethosuximide is available as a 250-mg capsule or as a syrup (250 mg per 5 mL).

F. Toxicity

Local toxicity includes gastric irritation, anorexia, nausea, and vomiting. Dose-related toxicity includes drowsiness, dizziness, and headache. Idiosyncratic toxicity commonly includes rash and leukopenia and, very rarely, pancytopenia, agranulocytosis, aplastic anemia, psychosis, systemic lupus erythematosus (SLE), and parkinsonian changes.

G. Drug Interactions

No known drug interactions of clinical significance occur with ethosuximide.

H. Disease States
Renal and hepatic disorders do not appear to pose major problems for enhanced toxicity of ethosuximide.

I. Pregnancy
No adequate studies have been done of the drug in pregnancy. Some reports cite increased risk of congenital malformations in infants born to mothers taking antiepileptic drugs. The potential risks and benefits of using this drug in pregnancy must be carefully weighed for each patient. Ethosuximide freely enters the breast milk in concentrations similar to those in the maternal serum. No adverse effects on the nursing infant have been reported.

X. FELBAMATE (FELBATOL)
Felbamate is an antiepileptic drug introduced in 1993. Because of relatively high risk rates for aplastic anemia and hepatotoxicity, the drug must be used cautiously. The drug is reserved for adults and children with severe epilepsy refractory to other therapies, especially for patients with Lennox–Gastaut syndrome.

XI. GABAPENTIN (NEURONTIN)
A. Mechanism of Action
See section **I** and Table 11-3.

B. Indications, Advantages, and Disadvantages
Gabapentin is a structural but not functional analogue of γ-aminobutyric acid (GABA). GBP (Neurontin) has FDA approval for adjunctive therapy of partial seizures (with or without secondary generalization) in children 3 years of age or older. Gabapentin has no serious toxicity, minimal dose-dependent toxicity, and no drug interactions. No need exists to monitor laboratory values. Gabapentin appears to be a good drug in the elderly because of its low incidence of side effects and absence of drug interactions.

A t.i.d. dosing regimen is recommended. Parenteral administration is not possible.

C. Pharmacokinetics
Gabapentin has a bioavailability of approximately 60% at low doses. At higher doses, bioavailability decreases because gabapentin is absorbed through the saturable L-amino-acid transport system in the proximal small intestine. Gabapentin is less than 3% protein bound. The drug is eliminated by renal excretion as unchanged gabapentin. Gabapentin is not appreciably metabolized in humans. The gabapentin elimination half-life is 5 to 7 hours and is not affected by dose or other drugs. In the elderly and in patients with renal failure, the half-life is longer. A therapeutic range for gabapentin plasma concentration has not been established.

D. Usual Pediatric and Adult Dosages
Early experience indicated that daily doses of 900 to 1,800 mg are effective and well tolerated when gabapentin is used as add-

on therapy for refractory partial or tonic–clonic seizures in adults (Tables 11-4 and 11-5). More recent experience indicates that higher doses, up to 3,600 mg per day, are usually well tolerated and produce better seizure control in some patients. The initial dose is 900 mg per day with a t.i.d. regimen. Further increases may be made in increments of 300 to 900 mg per day as needed, with a t.i.d. regimen. The maximum time between doses should not exceed 12 hours.

E. Formulation
Gabapentin is formulated as 100-, 300-, and 400-mg capsules, as 400- and 800-mg tablets, and also a 250-mg/5 mL oral solution.

F. Toxicity
No unique side effects have been identified as presumably caused by gabapentin. A minority of patients experience one or more of the following CNS side effects: drowsiness, fatigue, dizziness, ataxia, diplopia, nonpitting leg edema, weight gain, and myoclonus. No idiosyncratic or long-term toxicity has been demonstrated. Gabapentin administered to children can occasionally precipitate emotional lability, hostility, thought disorder, or hyperkinesia.

G. Drug Interactions
No known drug interactions exist between gabapentin and other antiepileptic drugs. Naproxen increases gabapentin absorption. Maalox decreases gabapentin absorption. Gabapentin reduces hydrocodone levels.

H. Disease States
The clearance of gabpentin is reduced in patients with reduced renal function, including the elderly. Consult the package insert for dosage instructions when renal function is reduced.

I. Pregnancy
No adequate studies exist of the drug in pregnancy. Reports indicate increased risk of congenital malformations in infants born to mothers taking antiepileptic drugs. The potential risks and benefits of using this drug in pregnancy must be carefully weighed in each patient.

The drug is excreted in breast milk. The risks of exposure of the infant to the drug are unknown. The benefits of breast-feeding, the risk to the infant of drug exposure, and the risk to the mother of stopping the drug must be weighed in each case.

XII. LAMOTRIGINE (LAMICTAL)

A. Mechanism of Action
See sections **I.A** and **I.D** and Table 11-3.

B. Indications, Advantages, and Disadvantages
Lamotrigine is indicated as adjunctive therapy for adults with partial seizures that are not controlled with first-choice drugs, such as carbamazepine or phenytoin. Lamotrigine has minimal dose-dependent toxicity, and no need exists to monitor laboratory

values. Rash, occasionally with Stevens–Johnson syndrome, is a recognized side effect and a significant concern, especially when the drug is used in children. Lamotrigine cannot be given as a loading dose, and parenteral administration is not possible.

Lamotrigine also is indicated for conversion to monotherapy in adults receiving a single enzyme-inducing antiepileptic drug. Safety and effectiveness have not been established (a) as initial monotherapy; (b) for conversion to monotherapy from non–enzyme-inducing antiepileptic drugs (e.g., valproic acid, gabapentin); or (c) simultaneous conversion to monotherapy from two or more concomitant epileptic drugs.

Lamotrigine is one of the few drugs that are Food and Drug Administration (FDA) approved as adjunctive therapy for the Lennox–Gastaut syndrome in children and adults. The drug was found to have efficacy for major motor seizure types (atonic, tonic, myoclonic, and tonic–clonic). The drug is also approved as adjunctive treatment of primarily generalized tonic–clonic (PGTC) seizures in children and adults, aged 2 years and older. The risk of serious rash is higher in children (especially those taking valproic acid) than in adults.

C. Pharmacokinetics

Lamotrigine is rapidly and completely absorbed after oral administration. Protein binding is 55%. Lamotrigine undergoes hepatic metabolism and is excreted primarily as the 2-N-glucuronide metabolite. In adults, the elimination half-life of lamotrigine is 30 hours when it is taken alone, and this value does not change with prolonged administration. Coadministration with carbamazepine, phenytoin, or phenobarbital reduces the elimination half-life to 15 hours. Coadministration with valproic acid increases the elimination half-life of lamotrigine to 60 hours or more. In children, the elimination half-life of lamotrigine is 7 hours in patients taking enzyme-inducing antiepileptic drugs, 20 hours in patients taking drugs with no interaction with lamotrigine, and 45 to 65 hours in patients taking lamotrigine and valproic acid in combination.

A therapeutic range for lamotrigine plasma concentration has not been established. Preliminary data indicate that few patients have a good response with plasma concentrations less than 5 μg/mL; patients with good responses usually have plasma concentrations of 5 to 15 μg/mL; patients with concentrations greater than 15 μg/mL often have side effects.

D. Usual Pediatric and Adult Dosages

In adults taking enzyme-inducing antiepileptic drugs (carbamazepine, phenobarbital, phenytoin, primidone) and no valproic acid, the starting dosage of lamotrigine is 50 mg once daily for weeks 1 and 2 (Tables 11-4 and 11-5). The dosage is escalated to 50 mg b.i.d. for weeks 3 and 4. Further adjustments are made at the rate of 100 mg per day every week. The usual maintenance dose is 300 to 500 mg per day in two divided doses.

For patients taking an enzyme-inducing antiepileptic drug converting to lamotrigine monotherapy, lamotrigine is added by using the regimen just described. After attaining a maintenance dose of lamotrigine (usually 500 mg per day in two divided doses), the dosage of the concomitant enzyme-inducing antiepileptic drug is reduced by 20% decrements over a 4-week period.

In adults taking enzyme-inducing antiepileptic drugs and valproic acid, the starting dosage of lamotrigine is 25 mg every other day for weeks 1 and 2. The dosage is escalated to 25 mg once daily for weeks 3 and 4. Further adjustments are made at the rate of 25 to 50 mg per day every 1 or 2 weeks. The usual maintenance dosage is 100 to 150 mg per day in two divided doses.

The differences in doses are caused by metabolic drug interactions (see section **IX.G**). The slow initiation of therapy is to reduce risk of rash.

A large number of dosing regimens are used in children depending on age, weight, and concomitant drugs. See package insert for details.

Lamotrigine clearance increases by more than 50% during pregnancy. This change occurs early in pregnancy and reverts quickly after delivery. Lamotrigine plasma concentration should be monitored before, during, and after pregnancy.

E. Formulations

Lamotrigine is available as scored tablets in the following strengths: 25, 100, 150, and 200 mg. Lamotrigine also is available as chewable dispersible tablets in the following strengths: 2, 5, and 25 mg.

F. Toxicity

No unique side effects have been identified as presumably caused by lamotrigine. The following common side effects of antiepileptic drugs are increased in frequency or severity in some patients (especially those taking carbamazepine) when lamotrigine is added: drowsiness, dizziness, diplopia, headache, ataxia, tremor, and nausea. Rash is an idiosyncratic toxicity occurring in 10% of patients and progressing to Stevens–Johnson syndrome in some. The risk is 3 in 1,000 in most adults, 10 in 1,000 in adults taking valproic acid, and 10 to 20 in 1,000 in children. Most rashes occur during the first 6 weeks of therapy. The risk of rash is reduced by slow upward titration of dosage. Long-term toxicity has not been reported.

G. Drug Interactions

Carbamazepine, phenytoin, phenobarbital, and primidone reduce the plasma concentration of lamotrigine. Lamotrigine does not affect the plasma concentration of carbamazepine, phenobarbital, phenytoin, primidone, or valproic acid. Sertraline and valproic acid increase plasma concentrations of lamotrigine.

When lamotrigine is added to carbamazepine, symptoms of carbamazepine toxicity sometimes develop (drowsiness, dizziness, diplopia). The plasma concentration of carbamazepine is unchanged, and disagreement exists as to whether the plasma concentration of carbamazepine epoxide (active metabolite) is elevated. This incompletely understood drug interaction is managed by reduction in carbamazepine dosing rate (often a reduction of

200 mg per day is adequate), and it should not be mistaken for toxicity caused directly by recently added lamotrigine.

Oral contraceptives (OCPs) can increase metabolism of lamotrigine, and adjustments of the dosage may be required. Patients are at risk for seizures when they are taking the active component of the drug, and for toxicity when they transition to the inert component of the OCP.

H. Pregnancy

No adequate studies exist of the drug in pregnancy. Reports suggest increased risk of congenital malformations in infants born to mothers taking antiepileptic drugs. The potential risks and benefits of using this drug in pregnancy must be carefully weighed for each patient.

The drug is excreted in breast milk in significant quantities. In addition, infants do not metabolize lamotrigine well and subsequently may have blood levels higher than expected from the dose received in the breast milk. The risks of exposure of the infant to the drug are unknown. The benefits of breast-feeding, the risk to the infant of drug exposure, and the risk to the mother of stopping the drug must be weighed in each case.

XIII. LEVETIRACETAM (KEPPRA)

A. Mechanism of Action

The mechanism of action of levetiracetam is unknown. Levetiracetam has been tested for all of the known mechanisms of action of antiepileptic drugs and found to have no effect. Laboratory studies have found a number of possible mechanisms: reduction of high-voltage activated calcium currents, reduction of delayed-rectifier potassium currents, and reverse inhibition of GABA- and glycine-gated currents induced by negative allosteric modulators. The drug is highly bound to the synaptic vesicle protein SV2. It is likely that the primary mechanism of action is through this binding to vesicles. See Section I and Table 11-3.

B. Indications, Advantages, and Disadvantages

Levetiracetam is indicated as adjunctive therapy in the treatment of partial seizures in patients 4 years and older, adjunctive therapy in the treatment of myoclonic seizures in adults and adolescents 12 years and older with juvenile myoclonic epilepsy, and primarily generalized tonic–clonic seizures in adults and children 6 years of age and older with idiopathic generalized epilepsy.

Levetiracetam has a high responder rate for refractory partial seizures (relative to other antiepileptic drugs), a favorable pharmacokinetic profile, no serious toxicity, no drug interactions, and twice-daily administration. Levetiracetam causes drowsiness and dizziness in some patients. Levetiracetam can cause behavioral problems in a small percentage of patients.

C. Pharmacokinetics

Levetiracetam is rapidly and almost completely absorbed after oral administration. The absorption and elimination of levetiracetam are linear. Levetiracetam is less than 10% protein bound. Sixty-six percent of a dose of levetiracetam is excreted unchanged in the urine. The major metabolic pathway of levetiracetam (24% of dose) is enzymatic hydrolysis of the acetamide group. This does not involve cytochrome P450 enzymes. The metabolites have no known pharmacologic activity and are excreted in the urine. The elimination half-life is 6 to 8 hours in healthy adults. The half-life is longer in the elderly and in patients with impaired renal function.

D. Usual Adult Dosage

The recommended starting dose of levetiracetam is 500 mg, twice daily. The authors often use lower starting doses (250 or 500 mg at bedtime) to reduce start-up toxicity, especially in patients receiving polytherapy. The daily dose can be raised by 250 or 500 mg at weekly intervals to attain the target dose of 500 mg, twice daily. The dose can be increased by 500 mg, twice daily, at intervals of 2 weeks if necessary. The full benefit of the drug is realized after 2 weeks of administration. No evidence exists that doses greater than 3,000 mg per day confer any additional benefit. In children, the dose is usually started at 10 mg/kg; it can be increased weekly or every two weeks. Doses as high as 60 mg/kg/day are well tolerated in children.

E. Formulations

Levetiracetam comes in 250-, 500-, and 750-mg tablets, a liquid preparation of 100 mg/ml, and an intravenous preparation of 500 mg/ml.

F. Toxicity

No reports exist of serious toxicity with levetiracetam. The common side effects of levetiracetam are drowsiness and dizziness. These usually occur early in treatment and can be reduced by slow drug initiation or dose reduction or both. Levetiracetam can cause behavioral problems in a small percentage of patients.

G. Drug Interactions

Levetiracetam is excreted by the kidney. Levetiracetam produces no inhibition of cytochrome P450 isoforms, epoxide hydrolase, or uridine diphosphate (UDP)-glucuronide enzymes *in vitro*. To date, no reports are known of drug interactions between levetiracetam and antiepileptic drugs or other drugs, including oral contraceptive pills, warfarin, or digoxin.

H. Disease States

Levetiracetam clearance is reduced in patients with renal impairment. A table for the dose reduction of levetiracetam in renal impairment may be found in the package insert. No need exists to alter the levetiracetam dose in patients with hepatic impairment.

I. Pregnancy

No adequate studies have been made of the drug in pregnancy. Reports suggest increased risk of congenital malformations in infants born to mothers taking antiepileptic drugs. The potential risks and benefits of using this drug in pregnancy must be carefully evaluated in each patient.

The drug is excreted in breast milk. The risks of exposure of the infant to the drug are unknown. The benefits of breast-feeding, the risk to the infant of drug exposure, and the risk to the mother of stopping the drug must be weighed in each case.

XIV. OXCARBAZEPINE (TRILEPTAL)

A. Mechanism of Action

Oxcarbazepine is a 10,11-dihydro-10-oxo derivative of carbamazepine. The mechanism of action is similar to that of carbamazepine. See Section I and Table 11-3.

B. Indications, Advantages, and Disadvantages

Oxcarbazepine is indicated for use as monotherapy or adjunctive therapy in the treatment of partial seizures (simple, complex, secondarily generalized) in adults and children, including newly diagnosed patients. The drug is also indicated for adjunctive therapy for partial seizures in children aged 4 to 16 years.

When used as initial monotherapy, oxcarbazepine has efficacy similar to phenytoin, valproic acid, and (probably) carbamazepine. Fewer patients taking oxcarbazepine stop drug treatment because of side effects than do those taking phenytoin or valproic acid. The risk of rash is probably lower with oxcarbazepine than with carbamazepine or phenytoin.

When used as adjunctive therapy, oxcarbazepine has a favorable 50% responder rate (40% to 50%) when compared with alternative drugs. Thus risks of side effects and drug interactions may be less with oxcarbazepine than with carbamazepine, phenytoin, or valproic acid.

Oxcarbazepine has some of the same side effects as carbamazepine. The risks of teratogenesis, aplastic anemia, and hepatitis have not been firmly established for oxcarbazepine.

C. Pharmacokinetics

The antiepileptic activity of oxcarbazepine is exerted primarily by its 10-monohydroxy (MHD) metabolite. After oral administration oxcarbazepine is completely absorbed and extensively metabolized to its active MHD metabolite. Maximal plasma concentration of MHD occurs 4.5 hours after administration. Food has no effect on the rate or extent of absorption of oxcarbazepine. MHD is 40% protein bound (to albumin) and has an apparent volume of distribution of 0.7 L/kg. Cytosolic enzymes in the liver rapidly reduce oxcarbazepine to MHD. Oxcarbazepine has an elimination half-life of 1.3 to 2.3 hours, whereas MHD has an elimination half-life of 9.3 ± 1.8 hours in adults and children older than 8 years. Oxcarbazepine and MHD exhibit linear pharmacokinetics at usual therapeutic doses. Steady-state MHD plasma concentrations are reached within 2 to 3 days in patients taking oxcarbazepine twice daily. Only a small amount of the drug found in plasma is oxcarbazepine; most is MHD. MHD is further metabolized via glucuronide formation. Approximately 80% of an administered dose of oxcarbazepine is excreted as MHD or MHD glucuronide. Oxcarbazepine does not exhibit autoinduction of its own metabolism.

D. Dosage

For monotherapy or adjunctive therapy in adults, oxcarbazepine should be initiated with a dose of 600 mg per day (8 to 10 mg/kg per day), given in two divided doses. Good therapeutic effects are seen at doses between 600 and 2,400 mg per day. If clinically indicated, the dose may be increased by a maximum increment of 600 mg per day at approximately weekly intervals from the starting dose to achieve the desired clinical response. As the total antiepileptic drug load of the patient is increased, the dose of concomitant antiepileptic drugs may need to be reduced, the oxcarbazepine dose increased more slowly, or both.

For monotherapy or adjunctive therapy in children, oxcarbazepine should be initiated with a dose of 8 to 10 mg/kg per day, given in two divided doses. In adjunctive therapy, good therapeutic effects were seen at a median maintenance dose of approximately 30 mg/kg per day. This upward titration can be performed over a 2-week period.

Children younger than 2 years have not yet been studied in controlled clinical trials.

In patients with impaired renal function (creatinine clearance <30 mL per minute), oxcarbazepine therapy should be initiated at one-half the usual starting dose (300 mg per day) and increased slowly to achieve the desired clinical response.

E. Formulations

Oxcarbazepine is available as 150-, 300-, and 600-mg tablets and as 300 mg/mL oral suspension.

F. Toxicity

The most commonly observed adverse events associated with use of oxcarbazepine at dosing rates of 300 to 1,800 mg per day during initial monotherapy studies were headache, somnolence, dizziness, viral infection, and nausea. The most commonly observed adverse events associated with oxcarbazepine in trials as adjunctive therapy for partial seizures were headache, dizziness, somnolence, nausea, fatigue, and ataxia. In double-blind comparisons with phenytoin and valproic acid as initial monotherapy, fewer patients taking oxcarbazepine dropped out because of side effects. Weight gain is unusual with oxcarbazepine.

The reported rate of skin rash with oxcarbazepine is 4% to 7% versus 5% with placebo and 10% to 15% with carbamazepine, phenobarbital, and phenytoin. Approximately 25% to 30% of patients who have skin rash with carbamazepine will have skin rash with oxcarbazepine. A multiorgan hypersensitivity disorder characterized by rash, lymphadenopathy, abnormal liver functions, eosinophilia, and arthralgias has been reported. Cases of Stevens–Johnson syndrome and SLE have been reported. The risks of aplastic anemia and hepatitis with oxcarbazepine have not been established. Minor decreases in counts of red blood cells, granulocytes, leukocytes, or platelets may occur.

Oxcarbazepine is associated with hyponatremia (125 mM or less) in 3% of patients.

G. Drug Interactions

Carbamazepine, phenobarbital, phenytoin, and valproic acid may decrease MHD plasma concentration. Oxcarbazepine may increase plasma concentrations of phenytoin and phenobarbital and decrease plasma concentrations of carbamazepine and carbamazepine epoxide. Oxcarbazepine decreases plasma levels of the active components of oral contraceptive pills (ethynylestradiol and levonorgestrel) by 50%. This may render these contraceptives less effective. Oxcarbazepine may reduce plasma levels of felodipine. Verapamil may decrease plasma levels of oxcarbazepine. Oxcarbazepine does not appear to interact with cimetidine, erythromycin, or warfarin.

H. Age and Disease States

In children 8 years of age and younger, the clearance of MHD is greater, and the elimination half-life of MHD is shorter than in young adults. In the elderly, the reverse is true. These observations appear to correlate with age-related changes in creatinine clearance.

Mild to moderate hepatic impairment does not affect the pharmacokinetics of oxcarbazepine or MHD. Renal impairment reduces clearance of MHD.

I. Pregnancy

No adequate studies of oxcarbazepine have been performed in pregnant women. It is not known whether the risks of fetal epilepsy syndrome and spinal bifida for oxcarbazepine are greater or lesser than those for carbamazepine. Until more data are available, the teratogenicity of oxcarbazepine should be considered similar to that of carbamazepine, a known teratogen.

The drug is excreted in breast milk. The risks of exposure of the infant to the drug are unknown. The benefits of breast-feeding, the risk to the infant of drug exposure, and the risk to the mother of stopping the drug must be weighed in each case.

XV. PHENOBARBITAL

A. Mechanism of Action

See section I and Table 11-3.

B. Indications, Advantages, and Disadvantages

Phenobarbital is FDA approved as initial or adjunctive therapy for partial and tonic–clonic seizures. Parenteral phenobarbital is used for treatment of status epilepticus.

Serious toxicity is rare with phenobarbital. Parenteral administration is possible, and a loading dose may be given by the oral or intravenous route. Phenobarbital is inexpensive and need be taken only once a day by many adults. Phenobarbital is less effective than phenytoin or carbamazepine for partial seizures. Phenobarbital also causes sedation, irritability, hyperactivity (in children), and impairment of higher intellectual function in a higher percentage of patients.

C. Pharmacokinetics

Phenobarbital is absorbed slowly (over a 6- to 18-hour period) but completely from the small intestine. The drug is 40% to 60% protein bound. Approximately one third of an administered dose of phenobarbital is excreted unchanged in the urine, and two thirds is excreted as metabolites created by hepatic biotransformation. Phenobarbital exhibits linear (non–concentration-dependent) pharmacokinetics with an elimination half-life of approximately 4 days in adults. Phenobarbital steady-state plasma concentration is attained 14 to 20 days after initiating therapy or changing dosing rate.

D. Usual Pediatric and Adult Dosages

See Tables 11-4 and 11-5.

E. Formulations

Phenobarbital is available as tablets (15, 30, 60, and 100 mg), elixir (20 mg per 5 mL), and sodium phenobarbital for injection (65 mg per mL and 130 mg per mL).

F. Toxicity

Dose-related toxicity includes sedation, irritability, hyperactivity (in children), slowed mentation, and ataxia. Rash is a common idiosyncratic toxicity, and agranulocytosis, aplastic anemia, and hepatitis are very rare idiosyncratic reactions. Long-term toxicity includes folic acid, vitamin K, and vitamin D deficiency. The issue of decreased bone-marrow density is discussed in Chapter 10.

G. Drug Interactions

The phenobarbital plasma concentration is increased after the addition of tricyclic antidepressants or valproic acid. Phenobarbital may reduce the plasma concentrations of benzodiazepines, haloperidol, griseofulvin, antiviral and anticancer drugs metabolized by cytochrome P450, cyclosporine, carbamazepine, valproic acid, lamotrigine, oxcarbazepine, oral contraceptive pills, theophylline, corticosteroids, tiagabine, topiramate, zonisamide, warfarin, theophylline, and cimetidine.

H. Disease States

The risk of phenobarbital intoxication must be monitored carefully in patients with renal or hepatic disease.

I. Pregnancy

Available reports are conflicting as to whether phenobarbital is or is not teratogenic when it is taken alone, although newer data suggest that the drug is teratogenic. Phenobarbital in combination with other antiepileptic drugs appears to increase the risk of teratogenesis.

The drug is excreted in breast milk and can cause sedation and decreased feeding in infants. The benefits of breast-feeding, the risk to the infant of drug exposure, and the risk to the mother of stopping the drug must be weighed in each case. The authors generally recommend that breast-feeding not be done by mothers taking phenobarbital.

XVI. PHENYTOIN (DILANTIN)

A. Mechanism of Action
See section **I** and Table 11-3.

B. Indications, Advantages, and Disadvantages
Phenytoin is indicated for initial or adjunctive treatment of complex partial or tonic–clonic seizures. Phenytoin was found to be one of the two safest and most effective drugs for these seizure types in comparative studies of older drugs (carbamazepine is the other). Phenytoin also is effective for generalized-onset tonic–clonic seizures. Parenteral phenytoin is used for treatment of status epilepticus (see Chapter 12). Phenytoin is relatively nonsedating (sedation is mild and similar to that of carbamazepine), and serious toxicity is rare. Parenteral administration of phenytoin is possible, and a loading dose may be given by the oral, intramuscular, or intravenous route. Phenytoin need be taken only once a day by many adults and is inexpensive. Use of phenytoin may result in reversible gingival hyperplasia and other cosmetic side effects (hirsutism, acne, coarsening of facial features; these are not conclusively proven to be caused by phenytoin).

C. Pharmacokinetics
Approximately 85% of an orally administered dose of brand-name phenytoin (Dilantin, 100-mg extended-release Kapseals) is absorbed slowly over a period of 24 hours. Intramuscular sodium phenytoin for injection is slowly and erratically absorbed, whereas the fosphenytoin preparation (see section **XIII.D.2**) is rapidly and completely absorbed by the intramuscular route. Phenytoin is 69% to 96% protein bound and is biotransformed by the liver. Phenytoin has concentration-dependent (nonlinear) pharmacokinetics that have the following consequences: (a) plasma concentration increases (or decreases) faster than the dosing rate when the dosing rate is increased (or decreased), (b) the time to reach steady state after a change in the dosing rate may vary from 5 to 28 days, and (c) the plasma concentration at one dosing rate does not directly predict the plasma concentration at another dosing rate.

D. Formulations
1. Oral
Phenytoin is available in 30-mg capsules (prompt release), 100-mg capsules (extended release), and 50-mg tablets as brand name Dilantin. Phenytoin 100-mg, 200-mg, and 300-mg capsules (extended release) are also available in generic formulation. A syrup for oral dosage (125 mg per 5 mL) is available.

2. Parenteral
Parenteral preparations include injectable sodium phenytoin (injectable Dilantin and generic; 50 mg/mL) and fosphenytoin (Cerebyx; 50 mg phenytoin equivalent per mL).

Standard injectable sodium phenytoin is poorly soluble in water. When injected into muscle, it is slowly and unpredictably absorbed and may cause local tissue damage. Fosphenytoin is a water-soluble phosphate ester of phenytoin that is rapidly and predictably absorbed by the intramuscular route and causes minimal local tissue damage. Thus fosphenytoin is preferable to injectable sodium phenytoin for intramuscular administration. Once in the circulation, fosphenytoin is cleaved by alkaline phosphatase in red blood cells and liver to yield phenytoin. Fosphenytoin by the intramuscular route may be used in place of oral or intravenous phenytoin for short-term maintenance dosing or for administration of a loading dose.

Phenytoin may be administered by the intravenous route for maintenance dosing or for administration of a loading dose. Standard, injectable sodium phenytoin is insoluble in standard intravenous fluids (requiring undiluted direct administration) and may cause local irritation and phlebitis at the infusion site, as well as purple-glove syndrome (constriction of blood vessels of the hand with hand damage). Fosphenytoin is the preferred preparation because it is freely soluble in all standard intravenous fluids and causes less hypotension and local irritation.

Parenteral phenytoin, fosphenytoin, and loading-dose procedures are discussed in detail in Chapter 12.

E. Usual Pediatric and Adult Dosages

The usual adult starting dose of phenytoin is 300 mg once daily, by using an extended-release formulation (Tables 11-4 and 11-5). A better way to calculate starting dose is 5 mg/kg/day because of the dose-dependent pharmacokinetics of phenytoin. A dose of 300 mg per day is the correct dose only for 60-kg patients. Most 70-kg patients are underdosed on a dose of 300 mg per day. Some patients should receive extended-release phenytoin in two divided doses daily: (a) those who have unacceptable toxicity associated with peak plasma concentration with once-daily administration, (b) children (children have shorter phenytoin elimination half-lives than adults), and (c) those who do not obtain complete seizure control with once-daily administration. (Seizures may occur at the time of trough plasma concentration.) Patients receiving a prompt-release phenytoin preparation (i.e., a preparation that is not an extended-release preparation) should use a twice-daily regimen. Because of the concentration-dependent pharmacokinetics of phenytoin, the authors use two special rules for titrating dosage: (a) daily dosing rates should be changed by only 30 or 50 mg when the phenytoin plasma concentration is 10 µg/mL or higher; and (b) 28 days should be allowed for attainment of steady-state plasma concentration after a change in dosing rate.

F. Toxicity

Local toxicity includes gastric distress (can often be alleviated if the medication is taken with meals).

Common dose-related side effects are nystagmus, ataxia, dysarthria, and sedation. High plasma concentration may be associated with changes in mental state ranging from dysphoria and mild confusion to coma, choreiform movements, external ophthalmoplegia, and increased seizure frequency. Idiosyncratic toxicity commonly includes rash (usually morbilliform and appearing within the first 12 weeks of therapy). Rare side effects include agranulocytosis, thrombocytopenia, aplastic anemia, Stevens–Johnson syndrome, hepatitis, nephritis, lymphoma-like syndrome, thyroiditis, SLE, and hyperglycemia. Gingival hyperplasia occurs in approximately 20% of patients taking long-term phenytoin. The gingival hyperplasia can be treated with good oral hygiene or, rarely, gingivectomy. The gingival hyperplasia usually resolves within a few months if phenytoin is discontinued. Hirsutism, acne, and coarsening of facial features have all been attributed to phenytoin, but definitive scientific evidence for a cause-and-effect relation with phenytoin has never been published for any of these. The following laboratory abnormalities (usually asymptomatic) have been associated with long-term phenytoin administration: decreased levels of folic acid, vitamin K, vitamin D, and immunoglobulin A; decreased bone density; decreased motor nerve conduction velocity; and increased plasma alkaline phosphatase levels. The issue of decreased bone marrow density is discussed in Chapter 10.

G. Drug Interactions

Adding phenytoin may cause a short-term increase in the plasma concentration of warfarin with a resulting increase in prothrombin time. Adding phenytoin may decrease the plasma concentrations of benzodiazepines, haloperidol, griseofulvin, antiviral and anticancer drugs, cyclosporine, carbamazepine, valproic acid, felbamate, lamotrigine, tiagabine, topiramate, zonisamide, oxcarbazepine, oral contraceptive pills, corticosteroids, digoxin, tricyclic antidepressants, warfarin (with long-term administration), methadone, theophylline, and oral contraceptives. The following drugs may increase the plasma concentration of phenytoin: carbamazepine, felbamate, fluconazole, fluoxetine, cimetidine, warfarin, omeprazole, tricyclic antidepressants, chloramphenicol, isoniazid, and disulfiram. The following drugs may reduce the plasma concentration of phenytoin: Saint John's wort, rifampin, antacids, and valproic acid. (Free-phenytoin plasma concentration is unchanged.)

H. Disease States

Phenytoin intoxication is not likely in patients with renal disease, but relatively high plasma concentrations of unbound drug are present and may need to be specifically determined at times. Some risk of phenytoin intoxication exists in hepatic dysfunction.

I. Pregnancy

No adequate studies of the drug in pregnancy have been performed. Reports suggest increased risk of congenital malformations in infants born to mothers taking antiepileptic drugs. The potential risks and benefits of using this drug in pregnancy must be carefully weighed for each patient.

The drug is excreted in breast milk. The risks of exposure of the infant to the drug are unknown. The benefits of breast-feeding, the risk to the infant of drug exposure, and the risk to the mother of stopping the drug must be weighed in each case.

XVII. PREGABALIN (LYRICA)

A. Mechanism of Action

See section **I** and Table 11-3.

B. Indications, Advantages, and Disadvantages

Pregabalin (PGB; Lyrica) is approved for adjunctive therapy of partial seizures (with and without secondary generalization) in adults. Like gabapentin the drug is a structural but not functional analogue of GABA. The drug is well tolerated and has few side effects. It is a schedule IV drug because of some mild mood enhancement. In a study of recreational users ($n = 15$) of sedative/hypnotic drugs, including alcohol, pregabalin reported subjective ratings of "good drug effect," "high," and "liking," to a degree that was similar to a single dose of diazepam. Serious toxicity is rare with pregabalin. The drug is administered twice daily. In clinical studies with more than 5,500 patients, 4% of the pregabalin group and 1% of the placebo group reported euphoria as an adverse effect. Whether such side effects occur in children is not yet known.

C. Pharmacokinetics

Absorption is extensive, rapid, and proportional to dose. PGB absorption from the gastrointestinal tract is proportional to doses up to 150 mg/kg, which contrasts to the partially saturable absorption of gabapentin. Time to maximal plasma concentration is approximately 1 hour, and steady state is reached within 24 to 48 hours. Absorption with food has no clinically relevant effect on the amount of pregabalin absorbed.

Pregabalin does not bind to plasma proteins and is excreted virtually unchanged (<2% metabolism) by the kidneys. It is not subject to hepatic metabolism and does not induce or inhibit liver enzymes such as the cytochrome P450 system. Pregabalin has a clearance (mL/min) of 45 to 75 and has a half-life of 5 to 7 hours. Pregabalin demonstrates highly predictable and linear pharmacokinetics in adults.

Pregabalin has no substantial pharmacokinetic drug–drug interactions.

D. Usual Pediatric and Adult Dosages

In adults, pregabalin in doses of 150 to 600 mg/day have been shown to be effective as adjunctive therapy in the treatment of partial-onset seizures (Tables 11-4 and 11-5). No guidelines exist for dosing in children.

E. Formulations

Pregabalin comes in 25-, 50-, 75-, 100-, 150-, 200-, 225-, and 300-mg capsules. No liquid or intravenous preparation is available. No guidelines exist for dosing in children.

F. Toxicity

The drug was well tolerated, with most adverse side effects based in the central nervous system. In adult patients, the adverse effects are dose dependent and occur within the first

2 weeks of treatment. Up to 33% of patients receiving pregabalin and 10% of those receiving placebo withdrew from the
clinical trials because of adverse events. Common side effects
associated with pregabalin, occurring in >10% of patients in
epilepsy studies, include dizziness, somnolence, ataxia, asthenia,
and weight gain. More than 20% of patients will report dizziness
and somnolence.

G. Drug Interactions
Pregabalin has no substantial pharmacokinetic drug–drug
interactions.

H. Disease States
The risk of pregabalin toxicity is enhanced in instances of renal
disease. Because the drug is not metabolized in the liver, hepatic
disease does not typically affect pregabalin levels.

I. Pregnancy
The teratogenicity of pregabalin has not been determined in
humans.

XVIII. PRIMIDONE (MYSOLINE)

A. Mechanism of Action
See section I and Table 11-3.

B. Indications, Advantages, and Disadvantages
Primidone is indicated for use as initial or adjunctive therapy of
simple partial, complex partial, and tonic–clonic seizures. Serious
toxicity is rare with primidone. Primidone is less effective than
phenytoin or carbamazepine for these types of seizures. A high
incidence of toxicity is seen at the time of initiation of therapy
(nausea, dizziness, ataxia, somnolence). Primidone causes disabling sedation, irritability, impairment of high intellectual
function, or some combination of these during prolonged administration in a relatively high percentage of patients. Parenteral
administration of primidone is not possible, and a loading dose
cannot be administered by the oral or intravenous route. The drug
is administered in a thrice-daily regimen.

C. Pharmacokinetics
Primidone is rapidly absorbed from the gastrointestinal tract.
Protein binding is minimal. Biotransformation of primidone
leads to the formation of two metabolites, phenobarbital and
phenylethylmalonamide. Each has antiepileptic activity, as does
primidone *per se*. The rate of conversion to phenobarbital is
enhanced by concurrent use of enzyme-inducing drugs, such as
phenytoin. When primidone is given as monotherapy, the derived
phenobarbital concentration may be less than the serum concentration of primidone. Concurrent use of enzyme-inducing drugs
often produces plasma concentrations of primidone that are one
third those of the metabolically derived phenobarbital. Concurrent
use of primidone and phenobarbital should be avoided to prevent
phenobarbital toxicity.

D. Usual Pediatric and Adult Dosages

Special care is needed with the initiation of therapy (Tables 11-4 and 11-5). Patients must be forewarned about side effects such as dizziness, nausea, sedation, and ataxia. Patients 8 years of age and older may be started according to the following schedule: days 1 to 3, 100 to 150 mg at bedtime; days 4 to 6, 100 to 125 mg b.i.d.; days 7 to 9, 100 to 125 mg t.i.d.; and day 10, 250 mg t.i.d. A t.i.d. regimen typically is used to reduce side effects associated with peak plasma concentrations.

E. Formulations

Tablets of 50 and 250 mg and a suspension (250 mg per 5 mL) are available.

F. Toxicity

Common side effects are dysphoria, sedation, dizziness, and ataxia, especially when therapy is initiated. Idiosyncratic toxicity includes rash and, rarely, leukopenia and thrombocytopenia, agranulocytosis and aplastic anemia, lymphadenopathy, hepatitis, and SLE. Prolonged therapy may be associated with folic acid, vitamin D, and vitamin K deficiencies. The risks of decreased bone marrow density are discussed in Chapter 10.

G. Drug Interactions

Valproic acid and isoniazid may increase the plasma concentrations of primidone. Carbamazepine and phenytoin increase the plasma concentration of the phenobarbital derived from primidone. Primidone decreases the plasma concentration of carbamazepine, lamotrigine, oral contraceptive pills, theophylline, warfarin, corticosteroids, tricyclic antidepressants, benzodiazepines, haloperidol, griseofulvin, certain antiviral and anticancer drugs, cyclosporine, valproic acid, tiagabine, and zonisamide.

H. Disease States

The risk of primidone toxicity is enhanced in instances of renal disease. Its effect in patients with hepatic disease is less clear.

I. Pregnancy

The teratogenicity of primidone *per se* has not been determined in humans. Phenobarbital is a metabolite of primidone and may be teratogenic. Phenobarbital in combination with other antiepileptic drugs appears to increase the risk of teratogenesis.

Phenobarbital is excreted in breast milk and can cause sedation and decreased feeding in infants. The benefits of breast-feeding, the risk to the infant of drug exposure, and the risk to the mother of stopping the drug must be weighed in each case. The authors generally recommend breast-feeding not be done by mothers taking phenobarbital or primidone.

XIX. TIAGABINE HYDROCHLORIDE (GABITRIL)

A. Mechanism of Action

See section **I** and Table 11-3.

B. Indications, Advantages, and Disadvantages

Tiagabine is indicated as adjunctive therapy for persons 12 years and older with partial seizures that are not controlled by first-choice drugs. The drugs used as adjunctive therapy for partial seizures are compared in Table 10-2. In comparison with other drugs for this indication, tiagabine has a lower responder rate, a fairly high rate of troublesome side effects (dizziness, tremor, abnormal thinking, and depression); frequent drug interactions; and inconvenient dosing (2 to 4 times daily).

C. Pharmacokinetics

Tiagabine is absorbed well, with food altering the rate but not the extent of absorption. Tiagabine is 96% bound to human plasma proteins. The drug is metabolized by ring oxidation (probably by hepatic cytochrome P450 family 3A) to 5-oxotiagabine (inactive) and by glucuronidation. The elimination half-life of tiagabine is 7 to 9 hours in normal volunteers, but only 4 to 7 hours in patients receiving hepatic enzyme-inducing drugs (carbamazepine, phenytoin, primidone, and phenobarbital). After multiple dosing, steady-state plasma concentration is reached within 2 days. Tiagabine pharmacokinetics demonstrate a diurnal effect with lower plasma concentration in the evening. No clear relation exists between tiagabine plasma concentration and clinical efficacy.

D. Usual Pediatric and Adult Dosages

In adolescents 12 to 18 years old, tiagabine should be initiated at 4 mg once daily (Tables 11-4 and 11-5). Modification of concomitant antiepileptic drugs is not necessary unless clinically indicated. The total daily dose of tiagabine may be increased by 4 mg at the beginning of the second week of therapy. Thereafter, the total daily dose may be increased by 4 to 8 mg at weekly intervals until clinical response is achieved or up to 32 mg per day. The drug should be given with food in two to four divided doses.

In adults, tiagabine should be initiated at 4 mg once daily. Modification of concomitant antiepileptic drugs is not necessary unless clinically indicated. The total daily dose of tiagabine may be increased by 4 to 8 mg at weekly intervals until clinical response is achieved, or up to 50 mg per day. The drug should be given with food in two to four divided doses.

E. Formulations

Tiagabine is available as tablets in the following strengths: 2, 4, 12, 16, and 20 mg.

F. Toxicity

The most common CNS side effects seen with use of tiagabine in controlled studies were dizziness, asthenia, somnolence, nervousness, tremor, difficulty with concentration/attention, insomnia, ataxia, depression, and confusion. Rash occurred in 5% of patients taking tiagabine and 4% of patients taking placebo.

G. Drug Interactions

Carbamazepine, phenytoin, phenobarbital, and primidone decrease tiagabine plasma concentration. Valproate significantly reduces tiagabine protein binding *in vitro*.

Tiagabine has no effect on steady-state plasma concentrations of carbamazepine or phenytoin and probably has no effect on steady-state plasma concentrations of phenobarbital or primidone. Tiagabine causes about a 10% decrease in steady-state valproate plasma concentrations.

Tiagabine steady-state plasma concentration does not appear to be altered by the presence of cimetidine or triazolam. Tiagabine does not appear to alter the pharmacokinetics of theophylline, warfarin, digoxin, triazolam, oral contraceptives, or antipyrine.

H. Disease States

The pharmacokinetics of tiagabine do not appear to be altered in renal failure, including renal failure requiring hemodialysis. Clearance of tiagabine is reduced in patients with impaired liver function. Such patients may require reduced initial and maintenance doses.

I. Pregnancy

No adequate studies of the drug in pregnancy have been reported. Reports suggest increased risk of congenital malformations in infants born to mothers taking antiepileptics. The potential risks and benefits of using this drug in pregnancy must be carefully considered in each patient. The extent of excretion of tiagabine in breast milk is unknown.

XX. TOPIRAMATE (TOPAMAX)

A. Mechanisms of Action

See section I and Table 11-3.

B. Indications, Advantages, and Disadvantages

Topiramate is indicated as adjunctive therapy for partial seizures, primarily generalized tonic–clonic seizures, and seizures associated with Lennox–Gastaut syndrome in patients aged 2 years and older. The drug is approved as initial monotherapy in patients aged 10 years and older with partial onset or primarily generalized tonic–clonic seizures. Topiramate also has an indication for prophylaxis treatment of migraine. The drugs used for adjunctive therapy in partial seizures are compared in Table 10-2. Topiramate had the highest reported responder rate in controlled trials for refractory partial seizures. Topiramate has few drug interactions and may be given twice per day. Whereas some anticonvulsants can cause clinically significant weight gain, topiramate has been associated with weight loss. Chronic weight gain with anticonvulsant therapy (e.g., more than 5% increase in body weight) can decrease compliance and exacerbate weight-related illnesses such as diabetes and other cardio- and cerebrovascular diseases.

CNS side effects are not uncommon with topiramate. Renal stones occurred in 1.5% of study patients.

C. Pharmacokinetics

Topiramate is rapidly absorbed, with peak plasma concentrations occurring 1 to 4 hours after oral administration. Oral bioavailability is greater than 80% and unaffected by food or dosage size. Protein binding is approximately 15%. In the absence of enzyme-inducing drugs, 80% of a dose is excreted unchanged in the urine with an elimination half-life of 20 to 30 hours. In the presence of enzyme-inducing drugs, 50% to 80% of a dose is excreted unchanged in the urine, with an elimination half-life of 12 to 15 hours. The metabolic products of topiramate are formed in the liver and do not appear to be biologically active.

Pediatric patients have a 50% higher clearance and lower elimination half-life than adults. As in adults, hepatic enzyme–inducing antiepileptic drugs decrease the steady-state plasma concentration of topiramate.

D. Usual Pediatric and Adult Dosages

The recommended total dose as adjunctive therapy in adults is 200 to 400 mg per day in two divided doses (Tables 11-4 and 11-5). A daily dosage of 200 mg per day is effective and may be better tolerated than 400 mg per day. Also, doses of 200 mg per day and less do not reduce the effectiveness of oral contraceptive pills. It is recommended that therapy be initiated at 25 to 50 mg per day, followed by titration of 25 to 50 mg per day at weekly intervals to a total dose of 200 to 400 mg per day. Slower titration (25 mg per day in weekly increments) may reduce neurotoxicity in patients receiving polytherapy. Daily dosages higher than 1,600 mg have not been studied. For pediatric patients (ages 2 to 16 years), the recommended total daily dose of topiramate as adjunctive therapy is 5 to 9 mg/kg per day in two divided doses. Titration should begin at 25 mg (or less, based on a range of 1 to 3 mg/kg per day) nightly for the first week. The dose should then be increased at 1- or 2-week intervals by increments of 1 to 3 mg/kg per day (administered in two divided doses) to achieve optimal clinical response.

E. Formulations

Topiramate is available as 25-, 100-, and 200-mg tablets and as 15- and 25-mg sprinkle capsules.

F. Toxicity

The most common side effects with topiramate are CNS related. The side-effect profile differs when used as monotherapy versus polytherapy. Paresthesia is the most common complaint with monotherapy; drowsiness and fatigue are the most common side effects with adjunctive therapy. Cognitive effects such as decreased attention or impaired concentration, confusion, and impaired memory have been reported, particularly with rapid titration, high doses, and polytherapy. These side effects usually are mild to moderate, develop during the first weeks of therapy, and may decline over time. Weight loss occurs in most patients, but is only infrequently a cause for discontinuing the drug. The CNS side effects, including paresthesia, appear to be less in children when compared with adults. Weight loss in children is temporary and has not been associated with an adverse effect on overall growth.

Renal stones occurred in 1.5% of study patients. Renal-stone risk does not appear to be related to duration or dosage of therapy and may be related to individual patient susceptibility. A history or family history of renal stones increases the likelihood of renal stones in patients taking topiramate.

A rare idiosyncratic syndrome of acute myopia associated with secondary angle-closure glaucoma has been reported for persons taking topiramate. This may occur in children or adults and usually happens during the first month of topiramate therapy. Treatment is to withdraw topiramate as rapidly as possible.

Hepatotoxicity and bone marrow depression have not been observed. Monitoring tests of liver or bone marrow function is not necessary.

G. Drug Interactions

Enzyme-inducing drugs (phenytoin, carbamazepine, phenobarbital, primidone) may reduce topiramate plasma concentration. Valproic acid has no effect on topiramate plasma concentration. Topiramate may increase phenytoin plasma concentration, but it has no effect on carbamazepine or phenobarbital plasma concentration. Topiramate at doses of 200 mg per day or less does not significantly interact with oral contraceptives. Higher doses of topiramate may reduce their effectiveness.

H. Disease States

Topiramate dosing rate may have to be reduced in patients with renal impairment or hepatic impairment. Topiramate is cleared rapidly by hemodialysis; a supplemental dose of topiramate may be required during such treatment.

I. Pregnancy

No adequate studies of the drug in pregnancy have been performed. Reports suggest increased risk of congenital malformations in infants born to mothers taking antiepileptic drugs. The potential risks and benefits of using this drug in pregnancy must be carefully weighed for each patient.

The drug is excreted in breast milk. The risks of exposure of the infant to the drug are unknown. The benefits of breast-feeding, the risk to the infant of drug exposure, and the risk to the mother of stopping the drug must be weighed in each case.

XXI. VALPROIC ACID (DEPAKENE, DEPAKOTE)

A. Mechanism of Action
See section I and Table 11-3.

B. Indications, Advantages, and Disadvantages
Valproic acid is FDA approved as initial or adjunctive therapy of absence seizures and for adjunctive use in patients with multiple

seizure types (usually tonic–clonic, myoclonic, or both) that include absence seizures. Valproic acid also is FDA approved as monotherapy or adjunctive therapy for the treatment of complex partial seizures occurring alone or in association with other seizure types. The role of valproic acid in treating absence seizures and partial seizures is reviewed in Chapter 10.

C. Pharmacokinetics

Valproic acid is rapidly and completely absorbed after oral administration, with a slight delay in absorption when it is taken after meals. The valproic acid capsule, divalproex sodium capsule, and sprinkle forms deliver equivalent amounts of drug, although the time of maximal concentration and the maximal concentration may vary. The drug is approximately 90% protein bound. Protein binding varies with drug plasma concentration, and the free fraction increases with increasing plasma concentration (10% at 4 µg/mL, 18.5% at 130 µg/mL). Primary metabolism is by hepatic hydroxylation (mitochondrial beta oxidation) and conjugation with glucuronide. Eighty percent of an administered dose of valproic acid is metabolized via these two pathways and then excreted via the kidney. The remainder of a dose is excreted via other oxidized metabolites. Valproic acid clearance is reduced in neonates and the elderly.

D. Usual Pediatric and Adult Dosages

The package insert recommends starting at 10 to 15 mg/kg per day, but many experts start at a lower dosing rate to reduce start-up toxicity (Tables 11-4 and 11-5). Dosage is gradually increased by 5 to 10 mg/kg per day every week until therapeutic success is achieved, until a maximum dose of 60 mg/kg per day is reached, or until the plasma concentration exceeds 150 µg/mL.

E. Formulations

Valproic acid (Depakene and generics) is available in 250-mg capsules and as a syrup (250 mg per 5 mL). It is also available as enteric-coated divalproex sodium, a stable coordinate compound (Depakote), in 125-, 250-, and 500-mg tablets, and a sprinkle form (125 mg of divalproex sodium) that can be mixed with food. Valproic acid must be administered in three or more divided doses per day. Divalproex sodium can usually be administered twice daily and produces fewer gastrointestinal side effects than valproic acid in many patients, making it the preparation preferred by many experts.

An intravenous preparation (Depacon) is available for patients for whom oral drug administration is temporarily not possible. Depacon contains the equivalent of 100 mg of valproic acid per milliliter, must be diluted, must be infused slowly, and must be given in divided doses (see package insert for details).

F. Toxicity

Local toxicity includes anorexia, nausea, and indigestion. These symptoms may be reduced with the divalproex sodium preparations. Dose-related toxicities are action tremor (40% of adults, less frequent in children), elevated plasma transaminase (usually transient but may be a harbinger of serious hepatic disease), and hyperammonemia. Idiosyncratic toxicity includes hepatic necrosis (treatable with L-carnitine), thrombocytopenia, pancreatitis (0.5%, sometimes fatal), teratogenicity, stupor and coma, so-called worsened behaviors, and depression. The risk of hepatic fatality is greatest in children younger than 11 years and in persons taking valproic acid in combination with other antiepileptic drugs. Long-term toxicities are weight gain (20%), hair loss (4%), and platelet dysfunction.

Valproic acid may be associated with an increased risk of polycystic ovary syndrome in women. See Chapter 13 for discussion.

G. Drug Interactions
Valproic acid increases the plasma concentration of carbamazepine epoxide derived from carbamazepine, lamotrigine, and phenobarbital. Phenytoin, phenobarbital, primidone, and carbamazepine reduce the plasma concentration of valproic acid. Felbamate increases the plasma concentration of valproic acid. Valproic acid may reduce the total (but not free) plasma concentration of phenytoin.

H. Disease States
The use of valproic acid is best avoided in the presence of liver disease. Because of possible effects of valproic acid on hemostasis (thrombocytopenia, platelet dysfunction), persons taking valproic acid who are about to undergo surgery should have a thorough hemostasis evaluation.

I. Pregnancy
As with several other antiepileptic drugs, valproic acid may increase the risk of congenital abnormality. In addition, a 2% risk of spina bifida exists in infants born to mothers taking valproic acid (vs. 1 in 1,500 in the normal population). The risks and benefits of valproic acid therapy must be carefully weighed in women of childbearing potential. Because alternative antiepileptic drugs do not have an increased risk of spina bifida, the authors usually prefer to use one of these alternative drugs (any antiepileptic drug except carbamazepine) in women of childbearing potential.

Valproate is highly protein bound, and the amount of drug excreted in breast milk is quite small. The low serum concentrations in infants appear to have a negligible effect on the infant.

XXII. VIGABATRIN (SABRIL)

A. Mechanisms of Action
See section I and Table 11-3.

B. Indications, Advantages, and Disadvantages
Vigabatrin is a structural analogue of GABA with a vinyl appendage, designed as an enzyme-activated, irreversible, specific inhibitor of GABA transaminase. The drug increases intracellular GABA and is effective as for partial seizures as well as other specific seizure types. It is particularly useful in the treatment of

infantile spasms, particularly those associated with tuberous sclerosis. Unfortunately, because of retinal toxicity, the drug is not frequently used, except in patients with intractable partial epilepsy and infantile spasms. The drug is not approved for use in the United States.

C. Pharmacokinetics
Peak vigabatrin concentration is reached within 2 hours. Approximately 60% to 80% of vigabatrin is excreted in unchanged in urine, with the remainder presumably binding to GABA transaminase. No metabolites of vigabatrin are known. The elimination half-life is 5 to 8 hours.

D. Usual Adult Dosage
The initial dose of vigabatrin is 500 mg/day. The dose is increased weekly until a total daily dose of 2 to 3 grams is reached. In children, the drug is typically started at 50 mg/kg with escalation weekly by 50 mg/kg until the child is taking 150 to 200 mg/kg/day.

E. Formulations
Vigabatrin is available as 500-mg capsules.

F. Toxicity
The most common side effects of vigabatrin are sedation, fatigue, and weight gain. Rarely can vigabatrin be associated with psychosis and depression. The most serious side effect has been the development of concentric visual field defects. These defects occur in 20% to 40% of patients exposed to vigabatrin and appear to be a direct effect of high GABA concentrations in the retina. In some patients, the defects persist after the vigabatrin is discontinued. If patients are given vigabatrin, it is important that they be monitored closely by an ophthalmologist familiar with vigabatrin retinal pathology. If the patient does not respond well to the drug, it is recommended that it be discontinued quickly.

G. Drug Interactions
Because vigabatrin is not metabolized and is excreted unchanged in the urine, it neither induces nor inhibits hepatic enzymes. The drug has few interactions. Phenytoin levels have been reported to decrease with vigabatrin. Although the mechanism for this decrease is unclear, the changes in phenytoin concentration are rarely of clinical significance.

H. Disease States
Vigabatrin clearance is reduced in patients with renal insufficiency. The daily dose of vigabatrin may have to be reduced in patients with renal failure.

I. Pregnancy
No adequate studies of vigabatrin in pregnant women are available. No adequate studies have been performed to determine infant risk when the mother is breastfeeding with this drug.

XXIII. ZONISAMIDE (ZONEGRAN)

A. Mechanisms of Action
See section I and Table 11-3.

B. Indications, Advantages, and Disadvantages
Zonisamide is indicated for adjunctive therapy of partial seizures in adults that are not controlled with first-line drugs. Zonisamide has no effect on the plasma concentration of other antiepileptic drugs and may be given twice per day.

CNS side effects are not uncommon with zonisamide, especially during titration. Among 991 patients treated during the development of zonisamide, in 40 patients (4.0%) with epilepsy receiving zonisamide, possible or confirmed kidney stones developed. Zonisamide can cause a syndrome of oligohidrosis and hyperthermia in children and is not approved for use in this age group.

C. Pharmacokinetics
Peak zonisamide plasma concentration occurs 2 to 6 hours after oral administration. Food delays the time of absorption, but not the extent of absorption. Zonisamide is highly bound to red blood cells and has modest binding to plasma proteins (40% protein bound). Dose-to-plasma concentration relations are linear at doses of 100 to 400 mg. At higher doses, a nonlinear increase in plasma concentration occurs, possibly because of saturable red blood cell binding. Approximately 35% of a dose of zonisamide is excreted as unchanged drug. Most of the remainder is excreted via a pathway using hepatic CYP3A4 followed by glucuronidation. The elimination half-life of zonisamide is 60 hours in monotherapy and 27 to 46 hours when it is taken in combination with enzyme-inducing antiepileptic drugs. The time to steady-state plasma concentration after changing zonisamide dosing rate is 14 days. The metabolic products of zonisamide do not appear to be biologically active. Median steady-state plasma zonisamide concentration in controlled studies was 18 μg/mL (range, 1.9 to 55.3). Some evidence of increasing efficacy was seen with increasing plasma concentrations.

D. Usual Dosages
The initial dose of zonisamide is 100 mg per day (Tables 11-4 and 11-5). The fastest rate of upward titration is 100 mg per day at 2-week intervals, up to a dose of 400 mg per day. Doses higher than 100 mg per day are given in two divided doses. No evidence exists that doses higher than 400 mg per day produce better results. Children are typically started on a dose of 2 to 3 mg/kg/day. The dose is increased by 2 to 3 mg/kg/week until a dose of 8 to 10 mg/kg/day is reached.

E. Formulations
Zonisamide is available as 25-, 50-, and 100-mg capsules.

F. Toxicity
The most common side effects of zonisamide are dizziness, anorexia, tiredness, headache, nausea, diplopia, ataxia, confusion, memory difficulty, depression, irritability, insomnia, speech

abnormalities, tremor, mental slowing, and emotional lability. These side effects usually are mild to moderate, develop during the first few weeks of therapy, and may decline over time. Weight gain was reported in 5% of study patients.

Renal stones occurred with a frequency of 6 per 1,000 person-years in study patients. A history of renal stones may be a relative contraindication to zonisamide. Rash developed in 5% of study patients taking zonisamide. Serious rash developed in 0.3%. Zonisamide is a sulfonamide drug and is contraindicated in persons with a history of allergy to sulfonamides.

G. Drug Interactions
Phenytoin, carbamazepine, phenobarbital, primidone, and valproic acid decrease zonisamide plasma concentration. Other drugs that induce or inhibit CYP3A4 may induce or inhibit zonisamide metabolism, although this has not been reported to date. Zonisamide has no effect on the steady-state plasma concentrations of phenytoin, carbamazepine, or valproic acid.

H. Disease States
Zonisamide clearance is reduced in patients with renal insufficiency. The pharmacokinetics of zonisamide in patients with impaired liver function have not been studied.

I. Pregnancy
No adequate studies of zonisamide in pregnant women are available. In animal studies, zonisamide at plasma concentrations similar to human therapeutic concentrations produced teratogenicity and reproductive toxicity (decrease in corpora lutea, implantation, and live fetuses). Some reports have been made of abortions and congenital anomalies in human fetuses exposed to zonisamide. The risks and benefits of zonisamide should be carefully weighed in women with the potential to bear children.

It is not known whether zonisamide is excreted in breast milk.

XXIV. LESS COMMONLY USED ANTIEPILEPTIC DRUGS
The following drugs are occasionally used in treating partial (localization-related) and tonic–clonic seizures: acetazolamide (Diamox), clorazepate (Tranxene), diazepam (Valium), ethotoin (Peganone), mephenytoin (Mesantoin), mephobarbital (Mebaral), and phenacemide (Phenurone). The following drugs are occasionally used in treating absence seizures: acetazolamide (Diamox), diazepam (Valium), methsuximide (Celontin), paramethadione (Paradione), phensuximide (Milontin), and trimethadione (Tridione). In general, the less commonly used drugs are less safe, less effective, or less convenient than commonly used drugs.

REFERENCES
1. Beavis J, Kerr M, Marson AG. Pharmacological interventions for epilepsy in people with intellectual disabilities. *Cochrane Database Syst Rev* 2007;18:CD005399.
2. Ben-Menachem E. Vigabatrin. In: Levy RH, Mattson RH, Meldrum BS, et al., eds. *Antiepileptic drugs*, 5th ed. Philadelphia: Lippincott Williams & Wilkins, 2002:855–864.

3. Bohan TP, Helton E, McDonald I, et al. Effect of L-carnitine treatment for valproate-induced hepatotoxicity. *Neurology* 2001;56:1405–1409.
4. Canadian Study Group for Childhood Epilepsy. Clobazam has equivalent efficacy to carbamazepine and phenytoin as monotherapy for childhood epilepsy. *Epilepsia* 1998;39: 952–959.
5. Chapman SA, Wacksman GP, Patterson BD. Pancreatitis associated with valproic acid: a review of the literature. *Pharmacotherapy* 2001;21:1549–1560.
6. Cramer JA, Fisher R, Ben-Menachem E, et al. New antiepileptic drugs: comparison of key clinical trials. *Epilepsia* 1999;40: 590–600.
7. Dreifuss FE, Rosman NP, Cloyd JC, et al. A comparison of rectal diazepam gel and placebo for acute repetitive seizures. *N Engl J Med* 1998;338:1869–1875.
8. Dulac O. Use of antiepileptic drugs in children. In: Levy RH, Mattson RH, Meldrum BS, et al., eds. *Antiepileptic drugs*. 5th ed. Philadelphia: Lippincott Williams & Wilkins, 2002:119–130.
9. Elterman RD, Shields WD, Mansfield KA, et al. Randomized trial of vigabatrin in patients with infantile spasms. *Neurology* 2001;57:1416–1421.
10. French JA, Kanner AM, Bautista J, et al. Efficacy and tolerability of the new antiepileptic drugs, I: treatment of new onset epilepsy: report of the Therapeutics and Technology Assessment Subcommittee and Quality Standards Subcommittee of the American Academy of Neurology and the American Epilepsy Society. *Neurology* 2004; 62:1252–1260.
11. French JA, Kanner AM, Bautista B, et al. Efficacy and tolerability of the new antiepileptic drugs, II: treatment of refractory epilepsy: report of the Therapeutics and Technology Assessment Subcommittee and Quality Standards Subcommittee of the American Academy of Neurology and the American Epilepsy Society. *Neurology* 2004;62:1261–1273.
12. Gilman JT, Duchowny M. Antiepileptic drug hypersensitivity in children. *Epilepsia* 1998;39(suppl 7):1–32.
13. Isojarvi JT, Raltya J, Myllyia W, et al. Valproate, lamotrigine, and insulin related risks in women with epilepsy. *Ann Neurol* 1988;43:446–451.
14. Kalviainen R, Nousiainen I. Visual field defects with vigabatrin: epidemiology and therapeutic implications. *CNS Drugs* 2001;15:217–230.
15. Kohling R. Voltage-gated sodium channels. *Epilepsia* 2002;43: 1278–1295.
16. Leppik IE. Pharmacologic treatment of epilepsy: current tradeoffs and the role of levetiracetam. *Epilepsia* 2001;42(suppl 4):1–45.
17. Lesser RP, Krauss G. Buy some today: can generics be safely substituted for brand name drugs. *Neurology* 2001;57:571–573.
18. Levy RH, Mattson RH, Meldrum BS, et al. *Antiepileptic drugs*. 5th ed. Philadelphia: Lippincott Williams & Wilkins, 2002.
19. Mattson RH. Antiepileptic drug monotherapy in adults: selection and use in new onset epilepsy. In: Levy RH, Mattson RH, Meldrum BS, et al., eds. *Antiepileptic drugs*. 5th ed. Philadelphia: Lippincott Williams & Wilkins, 2002:72–95.

20. Mattson RH and the Department of Veterans Affairs Epilepsy Cooperative Study No. 118 Group. A comparison of carbamazepine, phenobarbital, phenytoin and primidone in partial and secondarily generalized tonic-clonic seizures. *N Engl J Med* 1985;313:145–151.

21. Mattson RH and the Department of Veterans Affairs Epilepsy Cooperative Study No. 264 Group. A comparison of valproate with carbamazepine for the treatment of complex partial seizures and secondarily generalized tonic-clonic seizures in adults. *N Engl J Med* 1992;327:765–771.

22. Moshé SL. Mechanisms of action of anticonvulsant drugs. *Neurology* 2000;55(suppl 1):32–40.

23. Nuwer M, Browne TR, Dodson WE, et al. American Academy of Neurology Position Statement: generic substitution for antiepileptic medication. *Neurology* 1990;40:1641–1643.

24. Patsalos PN, Frocher W, Pisani F, et al. The importance of drug interactions in epilepsy therapy. *Epilepsia* 2002;43:365–385.

25. Perucca E, Kupferberg H. Drugs in early clinical development. In: Levy RH, Mattson RH, Meldrum BS, et al., eds. *Antiepileptic drugs*. 5th ed. Philadelphia: Lippincott Williams & Wilkins, 2002:913–927.

26. Quality Standards Subcommittee. Practice advisory: the use of felbamate in the treatment of patients with intractable epilepsy: report of the Quality Standards Subcommittee of the American Academy of Neurology and the American Epilepsy Society. *Neurology* 1999;52:1540–1545.

27. Rogawski MA, Loscher W. The neurobiology of antiepileptic drugs. *Nat Rev Neurosci* 2004;5:553–564.

28. Schachter SC, Vazquez B, Fisher RS, et al. Oxcarbamazepine: double blind, randomized placebo-control monotherapy trial for partial seizures. *Neurology* 1999;52:732–737.

29. Schmidt D. Benzodiazepines: clinical efficacy and use in epilepsy. In: Levy RH, Mattson RH, Meldrum BS, et al., eds. *Antiepileptic drugs*. 5th ed. Philadelphia: Lippincott Williams & Wilkins, 2002:206–214.

30. Stevens RE, Limsakan TL, Evans E, et al. Controlled, multidose, pharmacokinetic evaluation of two extended release carbamazepine formulations (Carbatrol and Tegretol-XR). *J Pharm Sci* 1998;87:1531–1534.

31. Tran TA, Leppik IE, Blesi K, et al. Lamotrigine clearance during pregnancy. *Neurology* 2002;59:251–255.

32. Uthman BM, Beydoun A. Less commonly used antiepileptic drugs. In: Wyllie E, ed. *The treatment of epilepsy: principles and practice*. Philadelphia: Lippincott Williams & Wilkins, 2001: 985–1000.

33. White HS, Privetera M. Topiramate in epilepsy: a compendium of basic science and clinical work. *Epilepsia* 2000;41(suppl 1):1–94.

34. Wyllie E, ed. *The treatment of epilepsy: principles and practice*. Philadelphia: Lippincott Williams & Wilkins, 2001.

35. Poolos NP, Migliore M, Johnston D. Pharmacological upregulation of h-channels reduces the excitability of pyramidal neuron dendrites. *Nat Neurosci* 2002;5:767–774.

Status Epilepticus

I. OVERVIEW

A. Definitions

Status epilepticus is defined as a condition in which seizures occur so frequently that the patient does not fully recover from one seizure before having another. Status epilepticus is also defined as a single prolonged seizure. A seizure lasting more than 5 minutes (especially a tonic–clonic seizure in an older child or adult) should be considered status epilepticus. Several types of status epilepticus exist, depending on seizure type: tonic–clonic (grand mal); simple partial (focal); complex partial (psychomotor, temporal lobe); and absence (petit mal). Tonic–clonic status epilepticus is the most common and most life-threatening type.

B. Epidemiology

The frequency of status epilepticus occurrences (all types) is 50 per 100,000 population per year or 125,000 occurrences per year in the United States. Frequency is highest in children and in adults older than 60 years. In both children and adults, approximately 80% of cases are of the tonic–clonic type. Approximately one third of cases fall into each of three groups: (a) first unprovoked seizure, (b) patients with well-established epilepsy, (c) acute new neurologic disease. Approximately 12% of all patients with newly diagnosed epilepsy are first seen with status epilepticus. The lifetime incidence of status epilepticus among patients with known seizure disorders is 1% to 4% and is highest in patients with symptomatic focal epilepsy.

Children have a high incidence of status epilepticus cases, with infants during the first year of life having the highest incidence. Up to 70% of children whose epilepsy begins before age 1 year will have an episode of status epilepticus after the diagnosis.

Four risk factors for status epilepticus in children have been identified: focal background electroencephalographic (EEG) abnormalities, partial seizures with secondary generalization, first seizure as status epilepticus, and generalized abnormalities on neuroimaging.

II. TONIC–CLONIC STATUS EPILEPTICUS

A. Clinical Presentation

Tonic–clonic status epilepticus generally follows a predictable sequence of events that can be described in three categories: motor, EEG, and systemic. In both human and animal studies, the phenomenology of these phases differs between early tonic–clonic status epilepticus (phase I) and late tonic–clonic status epilepticus (phase II). The transition from phase I to phase II usually occurs after 30 to 60 minutes.

1. Motor Events, Phase I

Phase I motor events consist of a tonic phase (muscles continuously contracted) followed by a clonic phase (alternate contraction and relaxation of muscles). The seizures are bilaterally synchronous at onset in 45% of patients; in the remainder, they are aversive (head, eyes, or both turned to one side) or focal at onset.

2. Motor Events, Phase II

As tonic–clonic status epilepticus continues, seizures often become shorter in duration and more restricted in distribution. Focal or lateralized motor activity may occur and does not necessarily imply focal pathology. Later, the motor activity may be reduced to brief muscle jerks (myoclonus) of the face, hands, or feet or nystagmoid jerking of the eyes. Finally, no motor activity may be seen at times when prominent paroxysmal activity is present on the EEG (electromechanical dissociation).

3. EEG Events

A progressive succession of five EEG patterns occurs in patients with tonic–clonic status epilepticus: (a) discrete clinical and EEG seizures with interictal slowing, (b) waxing and waning of ictal discharges, (c) continuous ictal discharge, (d) continuous ictal discharges punctuated by flat periods, and (e) periodic epileptiform discharges on a flat background. In later stages, electromechanical dissociation may be present. Considerable variability exists in the duration of each of these stages, and not all patients will progress through each stage.

4. Systemic Events

During the early phase of status epilepticus, an increase in blood pressure and glucose and lactate levels occurs. As the status continues, the blood pressure returns to normal or decreases, glucose decreases, hyperthermia may occur, and the patient is at risk for respiratory compromise. Additional events may include oral trauma, head trauma, aspiration pneumonia, orthopedic injuries (especially compression fractures of thoracic or lumbar vertebrae), myoglobinuria (caused by muscle breakdown during seizures), pulmonary edema, cardiac arrhythmias, myocardial infarction, dehydration, disseminated intravascular coagulation, leukocytosis, and cerebrospinal fluid (CSF) pleocytosis. These last two events, combined with fever, may spuriously suggest a central nervous system (CNS) infection.

5. Clinical Significance of Phase II Tonic–Clonic Status Epilepticus

Phase II status epilepticus has five clinically significant aspects. First, the initial presentation (to the treating physician) of tonic–clonic status epilepticus can be a comatose patient with or without myoclonic jerks if the patient has had preceding tonic–clonic seizures, or has had only a few tonic–clonic seizures after a severe cerebral insult. Second, brain damage during experimental models of tonic–clonic status epilepticus occurs only during phase II, and not during phase I. Third, phase II tonic–clonic status epilepticus is more difficult to control with drugs than is phase I. Fourth, phase II tonic–clonic status epilepticus (periodic epileptiform discharges or continuous ictal discharge) is correlated with poor outcome. Fifth, these observations argue for aggressive therapy during phase I of tonic–clonic status epilepticus.

B. Pathophysiology

Several factors appear to account for the prolongation of the epileptic state in tonic–clonic and partial status epilepticus: (a) changes in extracellular environment (e.g., increased potassium); (b) increase in excitatory α-amino-3-hydroxy-5-methyl-4-isoxazolepropionic acid and N-methyl-D-aspartate neurotransmission; (c) decrease in inhibitory (γ-aminobutyric acid) neurotransmission; (d) activation of voltage-gated calcium channels; and (e) reverberating seizure activity between, for example, hippocampal and parahippocampal structures. The longer the status persists, the harder it is to treat. A change in neuroreceptor function is found with a decreased response to benzodiazepines as the seizure progresses.

C. Prognosis
1. Mortality

The mortalities of status epilepticus in the pediatric, adult, and elderly populations are 2.5%, 14%, and 38%, respectively, with an overall rate of 22%. Death may result from the basic disease process causing status epilepticus, medical complications, or overmedication. The mortality related to prolonged seizures *per se* is 2% to 5%.

2. Causes of Status Epilepticus

Status epilepticus due to acute processes (metabolic disturbances, CNS infection, head trauma, stroke, hypoxia) is often difficult to control and is associated with higher mortality. Status epilepticus due to chronic processes (breakthrough seizures or discontinuing medication in patients with chronic epilepsy, old tumor, old stroke) often responds well to treatment. Table 12-1 lists causes of status epilepticus as a function of age.

3. Future Seizures

Patients who have a first episode of status epilepticus are at a substantial risk for future episodes of status epilepticus and the development of chronic epilepsy.

4. Brain Damage

Status epilepticus lasting 30 to 45 minutes can cause cerebral damage, especially to the hippocampus, in animals and humans. Other brain areas may be damaged as well. The damage appears to be caused more by glutamate-mediated excitotoxicity than by excessive metabolic demands of repetitive neuronal firing. Systemic stresses such as hypertension, hypoxia, and hyperpyrexia exacerbate the extent of neuronal injury in

Table 12-1. Causes of status epilepticus

Newborns	Children (2 mo–12 yr)	Adults
Hypoxia–ischemia	Fever	Infection
Intracranial	Infection	Meningitis
hemmorrhage	Meningitis	Encephalitis
Intracerebral	Encephalitis	Trauma
Intraventricular	Trauma	Toxins
Subdural	Toxins	Neoplasms
Subarachnoid	Neoplasms	Degenerative
Hypocalcemia	Degenerative	disorders
Hypomagnesemia	disorders	Drug
Hypoglycemia	Drug withdrawal	withdrawal
Hyponatremia/		
hypernatremia		
Infection		
Congenital		
(intrauterine, e.g.,		
toxoplasmosis,		
rubella)		
Postnatal		
CNS malformation		
Inborn errors of		
metabolism		
Drug withdrawal		

animal models of status epilepticus and may have similar effects in humans.

Virtually no studies systemically evaluated neuropsychological function before and after status epilepticus in an unselected human population. However, a substantial number of studies in both children and adults suggest that tonic–clonic or partial status epilepticus may be accompanied by permanent neurologic and cognitive sequelae in humans. On the basis of these studies and animal work, it is believed that prolonged tonic–clonic or complex partial seizures may cause brain damage or cognitive dysfunction in humans and should be prevented with vigorous therapy.

D. Treatment of Tonic–Clonic Status Epilepticus

The treatment plan for tonic–clonic status epilepticus given here is based on the plan of the Working Group on Status Epilepticus of the Epilepsy Foundation of America, published in 1993; it is summarized in Table 12-2. The only modifications are the inclusion of fosphenytoin and results from a Veterans Administration Cooperative study (23), which were not available when the plan was formulated.

1. Immediate Treatment

As with that in any unresponsive patient, initial management of status epilepticus includes the ABCs of life support (maintaining

Table 12-2. A suggested timetable for the treatment of status epilepticus

Time (min)	Action
0–5	Diagnose status epilepticus by observing continued seizure activity or one additional seizure
	Give oxygen by nasal cannula or mask; position patient's head for optimal airway patency; consider intubation if respiratory assistance is needed
	Obtain and record vital signs at onset and periodically thereafter; control any abnormalities as necessary; initiate electrocardiographic monitoring
	Establish an i.v. line; draw venous blood samples for glucose level, serum chemistries, hematology studies, toxicology screens, and determinations of antiepileptic drug levels
	Assess oxygenation with oximetry or periodic arterial blood gas determinations
6–9	If hypoglycemia is established or a blood glucose is unavailable, administer glucose; in adults, give 100 mg of thiamine first, followed by 50 mL of 50% glucose by direct push into the i.v.; in children, the dose of glucose is 2 mL/kg of 25% glucose
10–60	Administer either 0.1 mg/kg of lorazepam at 2 mg/min (maximum dose of 8 mg) or 0.2 mg/kg of diazepam at 5 mg/min by i.v.; if diazepam is given, it can be repeated if seizures do not stop after 5 min
	For all patients given diazepam and for patients who continue to seize after lorazepam, administer 15–20 mg/kg phenytoin equivalent of fosphenytoin, no faster than 150 mg of phenytoin equivalent per minute in adults and 3 mg of phenytoin equivalent per kg per min in children by i.v.; monitor electrocardiogram and blood pressure during the infusion. For patients who stop seizing after lorazepam, administer 15–20 mg/kg of phenytoin equivalent of fosphenytoin at a slower infusion rate (e.g., 50 mg of phenytoin equivalent per min)
>60	If status does not stop after 20 mg/kg phenytoin equivalent of fosphenytoin, give additional doses of 5 mg of phenytoin equivalent per kg to a maximum dose of 30 mg of phenytoin equivalent per kg
	If status persists, give 20 mg/kg of phenobarbital by i.v. at 100 mg/min; when phenobarbital is given after a benzodiazepine, the risk of apnea or hypopnea is great, and assisted ventilation is usually required
	If status persists, give anesthetic doses of drugs such as pentobarbital; ventilatory assistance and vasopressors are virtually always necessary

From Epilepsy Foundation of America's Working Group on Status Epilepticus. Treatment of convulsive status epilepticus: recommendations of the Epilepsy Foundation of America's Working Group on Status Epilepticus. *JAMA* 1993;270:854–859, modified with permission.

an *a*irway, supporting *b*reathing, maintaining *c*irculation), gaining access to circulation, and when possible, identifying and treating the probable cause. Body temperature, blood pressure, the electrocardiogram, and respiratory function should be monitored closely as soon as status epilepticus is recognized. Status epilepticus should be managed in an emergency department or in an environment in which continuous skilled nursing care is available.

A. AIRWAY AND OXYGENATION. The head and mandible of the patient should be positioned to promote drainage of secretions, and if necessary, the airway should be suctioned to ensure patency. If it is feasible without undue force, an oral airway should be inserted. Oxygen should be administered by nasal cannula or mask and bag-valve-mask ventilator. If the need for respiratory assistance persists after the patient has been ventilated by bag-valve-mask, endotracheal intubation should be considered. If neuromuscular blockade is needed to facilitate intubation, use of a short-acting drug (e.g., vecuronium) enables the treating physician promptly to regain the ability to determine whether seizures are present clinically. Administering an antiepileptic drug is a top priority because managing the airway and assisting respiration are much easier after the convulsion is stopped.

B. GLUCOSE. Although hypoglycemia is a rare cause of status epilepticus, it may complicate other predisposing conditions, such as alcoholism. In most cases of status epilepticus, several factors result in early hyperglycemia. This, in turn, promotes insulin secretion. Late in status epilepticus (usually after 2 hours), secondary hypoglycemia can occur. Consequently, all patients should have a prompt determination of blood glucose level. If hypoglycemia is documented or if obtaining a measurement of blood glucose is impossible, intravenous (i.v.) glucose should be administered through an indwelling venous catheter. In adults, an initial bolus injection of 50 mL of 50% glucose is used. In children, 25% glucose, 2 mL/kg, is administered. Thiamine, 100 mg i.v., should precede glucose administration in adults.

C. BLOOD PRESSURE. During the first 30 to 45 minutes, status epilepticus usually produces hypertension; thereafter, blood pressure returns to normal or decreases below baseline values. Systolic blood pressure should be maintained at normal or high-normal levels during prolonged status, by using vasopressors if necessary.

D. INTRAVENOUS FLUIDS. Overhydration should be avoided because it can exacerbate the cerebral edema usually present in tonic–clonic status epilepticus.

E. BLOOD WORK. Blood should be drawn for a complete blood cell count; serum chemistry studies (including glucose, sodium, calcium, magnesium, and blood urea nitrogen determinations); and antiepileptic drug levels. Urine and blood samples should be obtained for toxicologic screening. In children, consideration should be given to metabolic testing if no other cause is determined. Adequate oxygenation should be confirmed by oximetry or periodic arterial blood gas determinations. In many patients in status epilepticus, acidosis develops, but this usually resolves promptly when status epilepticus terminates. Bicarbonate therapy is usually unnecessary, but it should be considered when a patient has severe acidosis.

F. BODY TEMPERATURE. Increased body temperature—sometimes to a striking degree—occurs in many patients with status epilepticus, primarily as a result of increased motor activity. Rectal temperature should be monitored frequently throughout treatment. Hyperthermia should be treated promptly with passive cooling because it may contribute to brain damage.

G. IDENTIFICATION AND TREATMENT OF PRECIPITATING FACTORS. The majority of cases of tonic–clonic status epilepticus do not occur randomly or as a result of a massive new cerebral lesion. Rather, a specific precipitating factor causes status epilepticus to develop in a patient with a known seizure disorder at a specific time. The most frequent causes of tonic–clonic status epilepticus are withdrawal from antiepileptic drugs and fever. Other precipitating factors include (a) withdrawal from alcohol or sedative drugs; (b) metabolic disorder (hypocalcemia, hyponatremia, hypoglycemia, hepatic or renal failure); (c) sleep deprivation; (d) acute new brain insult (meningitis, encephalitis, cerebrovascular accident, or trauma); and (e) drug intoxication (e.g., cocaine, amphetamines, phencyclidine, tricyclics, or isoniazid). The precipitating factors in a case of status epilepticus must always be vigorously sought and treated to facilitate seizure control and to ensure that any reversible cause of cerebral dysfunction is treated before it results in irreversible cerebral damage.

H. ROLE OF ELECTROENCEPHALOGRAPHY. When it is available, electroencephalograph (EEG) monitoring confirms the diagnosis of status epilepticus and the presence or absence of paroxysmal activity after treatment. This is useful information. Treatment should not be delayed because of EEG procedures, however, unless the EEG is needed to establish the diagnosis of status epilepticus.

That nonconvulsive status epilepticus (phase II tonic–clonic status epilepticus or partial status epilepticus) may persist after overt tonic–clonic seizures have been stopped has increasingly been recognized. The EEG is necessary to diagnose these conditions, and it should be performed on patients who do not quickly recover consciousness after tonic–clonic or partial status epilepticus is treated.

2. Pharmaceutical Treatment

A. PHARMACOLOGIC PRINCIPLES. The ideal therapeutic agent for status epilepticus should (a) enter the brain rapidly; (b) have an immediate onset of antiepileptic action; (c) not significantly depress consciousness or respiratory function; (d) have a long duration of antiepileptic action so that seizures do not recur; and (e) effectively block the motor, cerebral (EEG), and systemic effects of status epilepticus. The rate of brain entry of a drug is directly proportional to non–protein-bound drug plasma concentration, lipid solubility, and cerebral blood flow. Therefore status epilepticus is treated with i.v. infusion (to obtain high plasma concentration) of lipid-soluble antiepileptic drugs.

Drug volume of distribution increases with lipid solubility, and lipid-soluble drugs tend to redistribute out of the brain and plasma into body fat. Rapidly to attain and then maintain a therapeutic plasma and brain concentration of drug, a loading dose must be administered sufficient to attain the desired concentration throughout the volume of distribution.

The loading dose of a drug can be computed by using this simple equation:

Loading dose (mg/kg) = desired concentration (mg/L)
$$\div \text{ volume of distribution (L/kg)}$$

Thus a dose of 20 mg/kg of phenytoin (volume of distribution, 0.7 L/kg) produces a plasma concentration of 28.6 mg/L (1 mg/L = 1 μg/mL). This equation can also be used to determine the dose needed to elevate plasma concentration to a higher value by substituting the desired increase in plasma concentration for plasma concentration. Thus a dose of 5 mg/kg of phenytoin elevates plasma concentration by 7 mg/L.

B. AVAILABLE DRUGS. Diazepam, lorazepam, phenytoin, and phenobarbital are the four drugs commonly used to treat tonic–clonic status epilepticus (Table 12-3). Diazepam and lorazepam are the most lipid soluble of the group, enter the brain most rapidly, and stop status epilepticus most rapidly. Therefore diazepam or lorazepam usually is the first drug administered to a patient in active status epilepticus. Phenytoin and phenobarbital have longer durations of action and are used for long-acting seizure control.

C. BENZODIAZEPINES: DIAZEPAM AND LORAZEPAM. Diazepam and lorazepam rapidly enter the brain and stop status epilepticus. This makes them initial drugs of choice in patients who are actively seizing. However, use of these agents in status epilepticus is associated with a risk of cardiorespiratory depression (3% to 10%), hypotension (less than 2%), or impaired consciousness (20% to 60%). Therefore in patients not actively seizing, benzodiazepines are omitted, and therapy is usually initiated with phenytoin or phenobarbital.

Diazepam is highly lipid soluble and is rapidly taken up by fatty tissues. This results in a rapid decrease of plasma and brain levels and recurrence of seizures within less than 1 hour. Therefore administration of diazepam should be followed immediately by a loading dose of a long-lasting drug, usually phenytoin.

Lorazepam has a longer duration of action than diazepam (12 to 24 hours), but it is not a long-term therapy for tonic–clonic seizures. In patients thought to be at risk for recurring tonic–clonic seizures (or patients whose status epilepticus is not controlled with lorazepam), a loading dose of i.v. phenytoin usually is given in addition to lorazepam. The longer duration of action of lorazepam (in comparison to diazepam) permits more time for completion of diagnostic studies and slow infusion of phenytoin.

Diazepam is approved by the U.S. Food and Drug Administration (FDA) for treatment of status epilepticus;

Table 12-3. The major drugs used to treat status epilepticus: intravenous doses, pharmacokinetics, and major toxicities

	Diazepam	Lorazepam	Fosphenytoin[a] or phenytoin	Phenobarbital
Adult i.v. dose, mg/kg range (total dose)	0.15–0.25	0.1 (4–8 mg)	15–20	20
Pediatric i.v. dose, mg/kg range (total dose)	0.1–1.0	0.05–0.5 (1–4 mg)	20	20
Maximum administration rate (mg/min)	5	2	150 (fosphenytoin) 50 (phenytoin)	100
Time to stop status (min)	1–3	6–10	10–30	20–30
Effective duration of action (hr)	0.25–0.5	>12–24	24	>48
Elimination half-life (hr)	30	14	24	100
Volume of distribution (L/kg)	1–2	0.7–1.0	0.5–0.8	0.7
Potential side effects				
Depression of consciousness	10–30 min	Several hours	None	Several days
Respiratory depression	Rarely	Rarely	Infrequent	Occasional
Hypotension	Infrequent	Infrequent	Occasional	Infrequent
Cardiac arrhythmias	None	None	Rarely in patients with heart disease	None

[a]Fosphenytoin doses are in phenytoin equivalent units.

lorazepam is not. Nevertheless, many experts prefer lorazepam because of its longer duration of action.

The pharmacokinetics, dosing, timing of administration, and side effects of diazepam and lorazepam are shown in Tables 12-2 and 12-3.

D. PHENYTOIN AND FOSPHENYTOIN. Phenytoin and phenobarbital are the only long-acting antiepileptic drugs for tonic–clonic and partial seizures that can be given as an i.v. loading dose. Phenytoin is the usual first-choice drug over phenobarbital in older children and adults, because less sedation occurs after treatment of status epilepticus with phenytoin, and because phenytoin is preferred to phenobarbital for long-term treatment of seizures in this age group.

An i.v. loading dose of phenytoin can be administered by using either of two preparations: injectable sodium phenytoin or fosphenytoin. Injectable sodium phenytoin is poorly water soluble and is formulated in a vehicle containing concentrated sodium hydroxide (pH 11 to 12) and propylene glycol. This formulation is irritating to veins and does not dissolve in standard i.v. solutions. Sodium phenytoin i.v. should be injected undiluted into a large vein and flushed with normal saline to prevent phlebitis. Extravasated drug may cause local tissue damage.

Fosphenytoin is a phosphate-ester prodrug of phenytoin, developed as a replacement for standard injectable sodium phenytoin. Fosphenytoin is a simple aqueous solution with a pH of 8.8. After absorption, phenytoin is cleaved from fosphenytoin by alkaline phosphatase in red blood cells and other tissues. Advantages of fosphenytoin are that (a) it dissolves readily in any standard i.v. solution (allowing continuous infusion with less staff time and greater convenience); (b) fosphenytoin produces less local toxicity (pain, burning, itching) than injectable sodium phenytoin; (c) fosphenytoin produces less hypotension with rapid i.v. infusion than injectable sodium phenytoin; and (d) fosphenytoin has not been reported to cause the purple-glove syndrome of hand damage associated with i.v. use of phenytoin. For these reasons, fosphenytoin is now the preferred formulation. Fosphenytoin is labeled in "phenytoin equivalent" units. Such units describe the amount of phenytoin liberated from fosphenytoin. Injectable sodium phenytoin and fosphenytoin both deliver 50 mg of phenytoin per milliliter of solution, and fosphenytoin is labeled as "50-mg phenytoin equivalent per mL."

The loading dose of phenytoin is 20 mg/kg in adults; the reduced dose for elderly patients or patients with cardiac disease is 15 mg/kg. The maximum infusion rate in adults is 150 mg per minute (phenytoin equivalent) of fosphenytoin or 50 mg per minute of injectable sodium phenytoin (i.e., the maximum infusion rate is 3 times faster with fosphenytoin). Lower rates should be used in children (Table 12-2).

Phenytoin may cause hypotension, especially in older patients with preexisting cardiac disease or in severely ill patients with marginal baseline blood pressure. Phenytoin should be administered cautiously to patients with known cardiac-conduction abnormalities. Human and animal work indicates that risk of hypotension varies directly with phenytoin plasma concentration. Peak plasma phenytoin concentration occurs approximately 30 minutes after initiation of a loading dose with either sodium phenytoin for injection (infused at 50 mg per minute) or fosphenytoin (infused at 150 mg per minute, phenytoin equivalent). Blood pressure should be monitored for at least 30 minutes after administering a loading dose with either preparation. If significant hypotension develops, the infusion should be slowed or stopped. In any patient, the rate of administration should be slowed to reduce the risk of complications if seizures stop before the entire phenytoin loading dose is given. If feasible, the electrocardiogram should be observed during administration, and the rate of infusion should be slowed if the QT interval widens or if arrhythmias develop. Occasionally, phenytoin is associated with respiratory depression, although this is less common than with benzodiazepines or barbiturates. Phenytoin is also less likely than sedative drugs to impair consciousness.

The pharmacokinetics, dosing, timing of administration, and side effects of phenytoin and fosphenytoin are shown in Tables 12-2 and 12-3.

Fosphenytoin and phenytoin are absorbed too slowly by the intramuscular (i.m.) route for treatment of status epilepticus. However, a loading dose of phenytoin can be administered by using fosphenytoin i.m. for chronic administration. A loading dose of 9 to 12 mg/kg of fosphenytoin i.m. produces a maximum phenytoin plasma concentration of 12 μg/mL in 4 hours.

E. PHENOBARBITAL. Phenobarbital is often used as the first-choice long-acting drug for tonic–clonic status epilepticus in children younger than 6 years because of the perception (unproved in controlled trials) that phenobarbital may be more effective than phenytoin in this age group. Phenobarbital is used in patients of all ages whose seizures fail to be controlled with phenytoin or who are allergic to phenytoin.

The recommended dosage of phenobarbital is 20 mg/kg, but additional increments may be necessary to stop the convulsions. If the convulsion subsides before the entire dose is given, the rate of administration can be slowed, but the full dose should be given to reduce the risk of seizure recurrence. Doses of this magnitude administered to patients without previous exposure to sedative drugs usually produce substantial sedation and, occasionally, apnea or hypopnea. Hypotension is a potential side effect of phenobarbital, especially if it is given in combination with a benzodiazepine. Phenobarbital administration should be slowed if blood pressure begins to decrease.

The pharmacokinetics, dosing, timing of administration, and side effects of phenobarbital are shown in Tables 12-2 and 12-3.

F. COMPARATIVE TRIALS OF DRUGS FOR TONIC–CLONIC STATUS EPILEPTICUS. Only two comparative trials of drugs for tonic–clonic status epilepticus have been performed. In the first trial, patients received an unspecified loading dose of phenytoin. In addition, patients were randomly assigned to receive either lorazepam (4 to 8 mg) or diazepam (10 to 20 mg). Results were similar for the diazepam and lorazepam groups: seizure control,

83% versus 76% of patients; median latency of action, 2 versus 3 minutes; respiratory distress, hypotension, and sedation, 12% versus 13% of patients.

The second trial compared phenytoin, 18 mg/kg; diazepam, 0.15 mg/kg followed by phenytoin, 18 mg/kg; phenobarbital, 15 mg/kg; and lorazepam, 0.1 mg/kg, as initial therapy for phase I and phase II tonic–clonic status epilepticus. Success was defined as no clinical or electrical seizure activity from 20 to 60 minutes after the start of the i.v. infusion. Success rates for phase I were similar for diazepam plus phenytoin (68%), phenobarbital (76%), and lorazepam (73%). Success rates were lower for phenytoin (40%). Success rates for phase II were low for all drugs: diazepam plus phenytoin (11.1%), phenobarbital (28.0%), lorazepam (28.6%), and phenytoin (0%). Long-term success rates were not reported.

These data do not completely establish the regimen of choice for the initial treatment of tonic–clonic status epilepticus. A considerable delay in initiation of treatment occurred in the patients, with a mean duration of 2.5 hours before therapy was begun. However, the data do indicate that lorazepam alone is effective for at least 60 minutes, and phenytoin alone does not stop seizures within 20 to 60 minutes in many patients. For active tonic–clonic status epilepticus, many experts now advocate a regimen of immediate administration of lorazepam followed by slow infusion of phenytoin if lorazepam is successful in stopping seizures, or rapid infusion of phenytoin if lorazepam is unsuccessful in stopping seizures (Table 12-2).

G. **REFRACTORY TONIC–CLONIC STATUS EPILEPTICUS.** In general, a consultant neurologist should be called when the patient does not wake up, convulsions continue after the administration of a benzodiazepine and phenytoin, or diagnostic confusion exists during evaluation and treatment. EEG monitoring is also helpful under these conditions.

If status epilepticus does not respond to recommended initial doses of a benzodiazepine, phenytoin, and phenobarbital, consideration should be given to anesthetizing the patient to suppress the cerebral ictal discharge, by using midazolam, propofol, pentobarbital, or thiopental. Additional doses of phenytoin, greater than 30 mg/kg, are contraindicated, because high doses may exacerbate seizures. A sample protocol for treatment of refractory status epilepticus with midazolam is given in Table 12-4.

H. **OUT-OF-HOSPITAL TREATMENT.** Intravenous, intramuscular, subbuccal, or intranasal benzodiazepines can be effective in stopping status epilepticus before patients reach the hospital. In a randomized, double-blind trial to evaluate intravenous benzodiazepines administered by paramedics for the treatment of out-of-hospital status epilepticus, adults with prolonged (lasting 5 minutes or longer) or repetitive generalized convulsive seizures received diazepam (5 mg i.v.), lorazepam (2 mg i.v.), or placebo. Status epilepticus was terminated on arrival at the emergency department in more patients treated with lorazepam (59%) or diazepam (43%) than in patients given placebo (21%). Diazepam rectal gel (Diastat) may also be useful for this purpose and may

Table 12-4. Protocol for the treatment of refractory status epilepticus with either midazolam, pentobarbital, or propofol

1. Intubate and ventilate patient; admit to intensive care unit
2. Place electroencephalographic monitor
3. Place arterial catheter and central catheters, if indicated
4. Administer either midazolam at a loading dose of 0.2 mg per kg (slow i.v. bolus), then at a dose of 0.75 to 10 μg/kg/min; pentobarbital at a loading dose of 5–10 mg/kg (slow i.v. bolus), then at a dose of 0.5–3 mg/kg/h, or propofol at a dose of 1 to 2 mg/kg i.v., followed by a dose of 2 to 10 mg/kg/hr. Adjust maintenance dose on the basis of electroencephalographic monitoring results. Continue electroencephalographic monitoring throughout therapy (check hourly once patient achieves a stable response to the selected drug). Primary end point for therapy is suppression of electroencephalographic spikes. If blood pressure is adequate, secondary end point is burst-suppression pattern
5. Continue maintenance doses of phenytoin, phenobarbital, or levetiracetam; track concentrations to determine optimal doses
6. Use i.v. fluids and low-dose dopamine to treat hypotension. If necessary, add low-dose dobutamine. Decrease dosage of midazolam or propofol if any signs of cardiovascular compromise are seen
7. Taper infusion at 12 hr to observe for further seizure activity. If seizures recur, reinstate infusion in intervals of at least 12 hr

be given by relatives or by emergency medical technicians. However, rectal administration of medications can be difficult in adults, and alternative routes are generally preferable.

Intranasal midazolam is now routinely used to abort status epilepticus or to treat serial seizures. In a recent study, intranasal midazolam, 0.2 mg/kg, and intravenous diazepam, 0.2 mg/kg, were compared in treatment of acute seizures. Intranasal midazolam and intravenous diazepam were equally effective. The mean time to control of seizures was approximately 3.6 minutes in the midazolam group and 2.9 minutes in the diazepam group, not counting the time required to insert the intravenous line.

i. Lumbar Puncture. CNS infection is a major consideration in any patient with fever and status, especially a young child. In most of these situations, a lumbar puncture (LP) should be performed unless a contraindication, such as severe intracranial hypertension, suspected cerebral mass lesion, or obstructed CSF flow (e.g., hydrocephalus), is present. Unless the suspicion of CNS infection is high, brain imaging [usually a computed tomographic (CT) scan] should be performed before an LP is performed in adults. Performing a CT scan before the LP is not a "must"; however, if meningitis is not suspected and the LP is done electively with other diagnoses in mind, the CT scan is recommended first. If meningitis is suspected but an LP cannot be performed expediently, antibiotics should be administered immediately, rather than delayed until an imaging test and LP can be arranged. Notably, whereas some patients have CSF pleocytosis after status epilepticus (so-called benign postictal pleocytosis), meningitis is rare in patients with status epilepticus.

Although the presence of leukocytes in CSF samples usually does not indicate that the patient has a CNS infection, patients with CSF pleocytosis should be treated for suspected meningitis until the diagnosis is excluded by culture or other means.

ii. Emergency Neuroimaging Studies. In persons with status epilepticus of unknown origin after routine testing is performed, neuroimaging studies [magnetic resonance imaging (MRI) or CT scan with contrast] are recommended to be certain a treatable lesion is not being overlooked. Life support, seizure treatment, and routine tests should be accomplished before neuroimaging. Notably, old static lesions (e.g., posttraumatic, congenital, cerebrovascular) causing partial status epilepticus (simple, complex, or secondarily generalized) may exhibit edematous changes suggesting a new lesion (tumor, stroke, abscess). This edema resolves on follow-up neuroimaging.

3. Long-term Antiepileptic Drug Therapy after Tonic–Clonic or Partial Status Epilepticus

Patients whose seizures were previously well controlled on a tolerable regimen should be restarted on the same medications after status epilepticus. If an episode of status epilepticus was caused by an identifiable precipitating factor (e.g., fever, drug withdrawal, drug interaction), the patient should be counseled on how to avoid the precipitating factor. If no precipitating factor was identified, higher doses of medication or new medications should be considered.

Whereas efficacy of the second-generation antiepileptic drugs is similar to that of the first generation of antiepileptic drugs, tolerability of the new drugs is generally better. For that reason, it is recommended that long-term use of phenytoin, phenobarbital, and primidone be avoided. If phenytoin or phenobarbital was required to stop the status, the drugs can be maintained until patients have a therapeutic level of one of the newer antiepileptic drugs and then be discontinued. If phenytoin or phenobarbital was not used to stop the status epilepticus, patients can be given initial doses of valproate (20 mg/kg) or levetiracetam (1,000 mg in adults; 10 mg/kg in children) intravenously. Although topiramate and zonisamide do not have intravenous preparations, they typically demonstrate efficacy at low doses. Because of the slow titration rate of lamotrigine due to a risk of rash, most patients started on lamotrigine after status epilepticus will require another drug, such as clonazepam, to prevent seizures until the lamotrigine dosage is high enough to demonstrate efficacy.

Persons not subject to spontaneous, recurring seizures (e.g., drug withdrawal, drug intoxication, intercurrent illness) should be tapered off antiepileptic drugs.

4. Brain Imaging

All patients who have status epilepticus should have brain imaging performed at some point. Most patients with established epilepsy that has already been thoroughly evaluated do not need another brain-imaging procedure after a bout of status epilepticus. However, each patient should be considered individually. In some patients with known epilepsy, new problems develop, and brain imaging sometimes reveals a new cause for the seizures. Among the various imaging techniques, CT of the brain is the most widely available and can usually be obtained rapidly in an emergency. In most patients, CT scanning is sufficient. However, when the need for imaging is not urgent or when the patient has had previous imaging, MRI is preferred because it provides more-detailed images and occasionally reveals abnormalities that cannot be visualized on CT scans.

III. SIMPLE PARTIAL (FOCAL MOTOR) STATUS EPILEPTICUS

A. Clinical Presentation

Simple partial status epilepticus may occur in patients with chronic seizure disorders or as a presenting symptom of an acute neurologic event. Focal motor status epilepticus in patients with chronic seizure disorders tends to be localized to the face and eyes or to the face and upper limbs. Facial seizures tend to be more clonic, whereas seizures affecting the limbs are apt to be tonic–clonic. Even though the motor seizure activity remains localized, some impairment of consciousness or autonomic disturbances may occur.

B. Management

In managing focal motor status epilepticus, the relative risks and benefits of therapies must be weighed. Intravenous diazepam or lorazepam usually temporarily halts focal motor status epilepticus, and an i.v. loading dose of fosphenytoin often completely ends the attack. However, some risk is associated with i.v. administration of diazepam, lorazepam, or fosphenytoin, as mentioned earlier, in section **II.D.2**. If the focal motor seizures can be temporarily tolerated, administering an i.m. loading dose of fosphenytoin is less dangerous. Directions for using i.v. diazepam, i.v. lorazepam, and i.m. or i.v. fosphenytoin are given earlier, in sections **II.D.2.C** and **D**.

IV. COMPLEX PARTIAL (PSYCHOMOTOR, TEMPORAL LOBE) STATUS EPILEPTICUS

A. Clinical Presentation

Complex partial (psychomotor, temporal lobe) status epilepticus may take two forms in patients at all ages: (a) a prolonged twilight state with partial responsiveness, impaired speech, and quasipurposeful automatisms; or (b) a series of complex partial seizures with staring, total unresponsiveness, speech arrest, and stereotyped automatisms, with a twilight state between seizures.

A third type of prolonged partial complex status epilepticus has been described in children. Symptoms include repeated partial complex, simple partial, and secondarily generalized seizures with intervening, at times prolonged, interictal periods of psychotic behavior, hallucinations, delusions, aphasia, and neurovegetative symptoms. Resistance or tachyphylaxis to antiepileptic medication is a prominent feature of this syndrome.

Electroencephalograms recorded during complex partial status epilepticus may show intermittent EEG seizures (most common finding), merging EEG seizures, continuous ictal discharges, or periodic epileptiform discharges that may be lateralized (PLEDS) or bilateral (BLEDS).

B. Management

Therapy for complex partial status epilepticus consists of administering an i.v. loading dose of fosphenytoin or phenobarbital. Intravenous diazepam (FDA approved) or lorazepam (not FDA approved) may rapidly end an attack but carries some risk. Intravenous diazepam or lorazepam is indicated when the ongoing complex partial seizure activity represents an immediate serious threat or makes administration of fosphenytoin or phenobarbital impossible. Lorazepam is preferred by many experts because of its longer duration of action.

Animal studies indicate that nonconvulsive status epilepticus in animals can cause brain damage, and although controversial, some evidence exists that prolonged complex partial status epilepticus may result in permanent cognitive disability in humans. This type of status epilepticus, therefore, should be treated rapidly by using a protocol similar to that described earlier, in section **II.D**, for treatment of tonic–clonic status epilepticus.

V. ABSENCE (PETIT MAL) STATUS EPILEPTICUS

A. Clinical Presentation

The clinical presentation of absence status epilepticus is altered consciousness, often accompanied by mild clonic movements of the eyelids and hands and automatisms of the face and hands. The alteration of consciousness may range from a vague feeling, which can be recognized only subjectively, to stupor. Attacks may last 30 minutes to 12 hours or longer. Although absence seizures occur chiefly in children, a considerable percentage of cases of absence status epilepticus occur in adults. Adults who have failed to outgrow absence seizures seem particularly prone to absence status epilepticus developing, and some adults with previously undiagnosed absence seizures may first be seen in absence status epilepticus without a history of a seizure disorder. The differential diagnosis of absence status epilepticus includes drug intoxication, psychosis, metabolic encephalopathy, structural brain lesion, late (phase II) tonic–clonic status epilepticus, complex partial status epilepticus, and psychogenic seizures. The diagnosis of absence status epilepticus is definitively established by an EEG that shows spike–wave activity. The spike–wave activity may be continuous or discontinuous and may consist of regular three-per-second spike–wave or (more commonly) irregular two- to three-per-second spike–wave and polyspike–wave activity.

B. Management

Intravenous diazepam (FDA approved) or lorazepam (not FDA approved) at doses shown in Table 12-3 usually stops absence status epilepticus for a period. Lorazepam is preferred by many experts because of its longer duration of action. Therapy then continues with high-dose oral treatment with an antiabsence medication (e.g., ethosuximide, 250 mg q8h) and further intermittent doses of an i.v. benzodiazepine, if needed.

REFERENCES

1. Alldredge BK, Gelb AM, Isaacs SM, et al. A comparison of lorazepam, diazepam, and placebo for the treatment of out-of-hospital status epilepticus. *N Engl J Med* 2001;345:631–637.
2. Browne TR. The pharmacokinetics of antiepileptic drugs. *Neurology* 1998;51(suppl 4):2–7.
3. Burneo JG, Anandan JV, Barkley GL. A prospective study of the incidence of purple glove syndrome. *Epilepsia* 2001;42:1156–1159.
4. Classen J, Hirsch LJ, Emerson RG, et al. Treatment of refractory status epilepticus with pentobarbital, propofol, or midazolam: a systematic review. *Epilepsia* 2002;43:146–153.
5. DeLorenzo RJ, Pellock JM, Towne AR, et al. Epidemiology of status epilepticus. *J Clin Neurophysiol* 1995;12:310–325.
6. DeLorenzo RJ, Waterhouse EJ, Towne AR, et al. Persistent nonconvulsive status epilepticus after control of convulsive status epilepticus. *Epilepsia* 1998;39:833–840.
7. Dreifuss FE, Rosman NP, Cloyd JC, et al. A comparison of rectal diazepam gel and placebo for acute repetitive seizures. *N Engl J Med* 1998;338:1869–1875.
8. Drislane FW, Evidence against permanent neurologic damage from nonconvulsive status epilepticus. *J Clin Neurophysiol* 1999;16:323–331.
9. Drislane FW. Presentation, evaluation, and treatment of nonconvulsive status epilepticus. *Epilepsy Behav* 2000;1:301–314.
10. Garzon E, Fernandez RMF, Sakamoto C. Serial EEGs during human status epilepticus: evidence for PLED as an ictal pattern. *Neurology* 2001;57:1175–1183.
11. Hesdorffer DC, Logroscino G, Cascino G, et al. Incidence of status epilepticus in Rochester, Minnesota, 1965-1984. *Neurology* 1998;50:735–741.
12. Lansberg MG, O'Brien MW, Norbask AM, et al. MRI abnormalities associated with partial status epilepticus. *Neurology* 1999;52:1021–1027.
13. Leppik IE, Derivan AT, Homan RW, et al. Double blind study of lorazepam and diazepam in status epilepticus. *JAMA* 1983;249:1452–1454.
14. Lowenstein DH, Alldredge BK. Status epilepticus. *N Engl J Med* 1998;338:970–976.
15. Lowenstein DH, Bleck T, MacDonald RL. It's time to revise the definition of status epilepticus. *Epilepsia* 1999;40:120–122.

16. Lowenstein DH. Status epilepticus: an overview of the clinical problem. *Epilepsia* 1999;40(suppl 1):S3–S8.
17. Mahmoudian T, Zadeh MM. Comparison of intranasal midazolam with intravenous diazepam for treating acute seizures in children. *Epilepsy Behav* 2004;5:253–255.
18. Nei M, Lee JM, Shanker VL, et al. The EEG and prognosis in status epilepticus. *Epilepsia* 1999;40:157–163.
19. Noval G. Risk factors for status epilepticus in children with symptomatic epilepsy. *Neurology* 1997;49:532–537.
20. Pellock JM. Management of acute seizures in children. *J Child Neurol* 1998;13(suppl 1):1–33.
21. Riviello JJ Jr, Ashwal S, Hirtz D, et al. Practice parameter: diagnostic assessment of the child with status epilepticus (an evidence-based review): report of the Quality Standards Subcommittee of the American Academy of Neurology and the Practice Committee of the Child Neurology Society. *Neurology* 2006;67:1542–1550.
22. Epilepsy Foundation of America's Working Group on Status Epilepticus. Treatment of convulsive status epilepticus: recommendations of the Epilepsy Foundation of America's Working Group on Status Epilepticus. *JAMA* 1993;270:854–859.
23. Treiman DM, Meyers PD, Walton NY, et al. A comparison of four treatments for generalized status epilepticus. *N Engl J Med* 1998;339:742–798.
24. Treiman DM. Status epilepticus. In: Wyllie E, ed. *The treatment of epilepsy: principles and practice*. Philadelphia: Lippincott Williams & Wilkins, 2001:681–698.
25. Wu YW, Shek BA, Garcia PA, et al. Incidence and mortality of generalized convulsive status epilepticus in California. *Neurology* 2002;58:1070–1076.

Special Considerations in Women and the Elderly

Thomas R. Browne, Gregory L. Holmes, and Georgia D. Montouris

I. SPECIAL CONSIDERATIONS IN WOMEN

A. Hormonal Effects on the Brain

Predictable changes in seizure frequency over the course of the menstrual cycle (catamenial epilepsy) have been reported for many years. Seizure frequency often increases during phases of the menstrual cycle that are characterized by a high ratio of estrogen to progesterone (just before and during menstruation and at the time of ovulation). Estrogen induces structural and functional changes in hippocampal neurons that increase seizure susceptibility. Progesterone decreases seizure susceptibility in animal models of epilepsy.

Menarche is a risk factor for new onset of seizures and for exacerbation of existing seizures. This may be due to relatively high levels of estrogens and the neuroexcitatory steroids dehydroepiandrosterone and pregnenolone at the time of menarche.

B. Ovarian Dysfunction

Polycystic ovaries are common, occurring in 20% of the female population. Polycystic ovary syndrome (hirsutism, acne, obesity, hypofertility, hyperandrogenemia, and menstrual disorders) is less common. Some data suggest that the incidence of polycystic ovaries and polycystic ovary disease may be increased in women with epilepsy, and the incidence may be even greater in women taking valproic acid. Evidence also indicates that valproic acid may increase the risk of anovulatory cycles. It is the authors' practice to avoid use of valproic acid in women of childbearing potential because of issues of birth defects (spina bifida), polycystic ovary syndrome, anovulatory cycles, and weight gain.

C. Pregnancy

1. Seizure Frequency

Epilepsy is the most frequently encountered neurologic disorder during pregnancy. Approximately one third of women with epilepsy have an increase in seizure frequency during pregnancy. Some women have seizures only during pregnancy. Seizure exacerbation may occur at any time, but it is most frequently encountered at the end of the first and at the beginning of the second trimester. The likelihood of a change in seizure frequency appears to be independent of seizure type and frequency before pregnancy.

2. Pharmacologic Changes

Although some pregnant women have an exacerbation of their seizures because of noncompliance or sleep deprivation, in the majority of these women, a number of physiologic changes are responsible for the increase in seizure frequency. During pregnancy, hepatic metabolism of antiepileptic drugs is increased, presumably because of the stimulating effect of progesterone on the liver. During pregnancy, glomerular filtration and renal excretion increase. Antiepileptic drugs cleared by the renal route (gabapentin, lamotrigine, levetiracetam) often have an increase in clearance beginning early in pregnancy and ending abruptly soon after delivery. Body weight, total body water, and intravascular volume gradually increase throughout pregnancy. An increase in the volume into which the drug is distributed (volume of distribution) results in a lower plasma concentration, even if the rate of drug metabolism or renal excretion is not altered. Lower plasma concentrations of antiepileptic drugs during pregnancy, therefore, appear to be related to the combined effects of enhanced hepatic metabolism, increased renal clearance, and an increased volume of distribution. The greatest changes in plasma concentration occur during the first trimester with lamotrigine, phenobarbital, and phenytoin, and during the third trimester with carbamazepine.

Another important physiologic change occurring during pregnancy is the change in protein binding of antiepileptic drugs. Plasma albumin concentration tends to decline during pregnancy, which leads to a proportional reduction in the protein binding of drugs. Although the total plasma concentration of a drug may decrease during pregnancy, the free (non–protein-bound) fraction of highly bound drugs such as phenytoin and valproate may increase, so that the concentration of free drug, which is the pharmacologically active portion, may change very little. To monitor effective drug concentration, measuring concentrations of the free drug is sometimes necessary, especially for phenytoin and valproate.

After delivery, drug pharmacokinetic values often return to prepregnancy values within a few days for renally excreted drugs and a few weeks for drugs metabolized by the liver. Returning antiepileptic dosing rates to their prepregnancy values is usually necessary after delivery.

3. Eclampsia

See Chapter 8.

4. Birth Defects and Teratogenesis of Antiepileptic Drugs

An association between fetal malformations, maternal epilepsy, and antiepileptic drugs has long been noted. In the late 1960s, phenytoin was claimed to be associated with a number of birth anomalies, and the term *fetal hydantoin syndrome* was coined. However, many of the birth anomalies associated with phenytoin were observed in infants of mothers with epilepsy who were taking antiepileptic drugs other than phenytoin or who were not taking antiepileptic drugs. Although antiepileptic drugs increase the risk for congenital anomalies, the risk of malformations is increased in mothers with epilepsy, regardless of whether they are taking antiepileptic drugs.

Major malformations include cleft lip and palate, cardiac defects (ventricular septal defects), neural tube defects, and urogenital defects. Whereas congenital malformations in the general population range from 2% to 3%, the risk for malformations in infants of mothers with epilepsy is significantly higher. The risk if the mother is taking antiepileptic drugs is even higher. The risk of malformations in any individual pregnancy in a woman with epilepsy taking a single antiepileptic drug is estimated to be between 4% and 6% for the older antiepileptic drugs.

This risk of major malformations is also increased in mothers receiving polytherapy taking toxic levels of antiepileptic drugs. All of the antiepileptic drugs have been associated with congenital malformations, although the incidence and type of the malformations may vary with the drug. Trimethadione, which should never be used during pregnancy, results in major malformations or fetal loss in 87% of pregnancies. This figure is far higher than that for any other antiepileptic drug. The risk of spina bifida appears to be significantly greater in infants exposed to valproate or carbamazepine, but not other antiepileptic drugs.

In addition to major malformations, infants born to mothers taking antiepileptic drugs are at increased risk for minor anomalies, including epicanthal folds, hypertelorism, broad or flat nasal bridges, an upturned nasal tip, prominent lips, and fingernail hypoplasia. These minor anomalies, although more common than in the general population, do not influence general health.

5. Other Complications of Pregnancy

Infants of mothers with epilepsy are approximately twice as likely to have an adverse pregnancy outcome. Stillbirths and neonatal death rates of infants of mothers with epilepsy are approximately twice as high as in the general population. Premature births are more common, and birth weights are also lower. Infants of mothers with epilepsy also have a higher risk of mental retardation, learning disabilities, and epilepsy than the general population. Finally, infants born to mothers with idiopathic generalized epilepsy are at increased risk for developing epilepsy.

6. Developmental Delay

Limited available studies indicate a risk for impaired cognitive development in the offspring of women with epilepsy. The relative contributions of heredity, maternal epilepsy, antiepileptic drugs, and socioeconomic factors are not clear.

7. Breast-feeding

The concentration of a drug in breast milk is determined by the plasma concentration and the protein binding of the medication. Because antiepileptic drugs do not bind to protein in milk, the concentration of drug in milk is approximately the same as the free plasma concentration. The greater the plasma-protein binding, the lower the amount of drug excreted in the milk. Phenytoin is very poorly absorbed from the infant gastrointestinal tract and tightly bound to plasma proteins; consequently, no detectable amounts of phenytoin are usually found in the plasma of breast-fed infants whose mothers take phenytoin. The amount of phenobarbital and primidone obtained in breast milk can be significant, and some infants nursing from mothers taking phenobarbital have significant plasma concentrations of phenobarbital. Clinical symptoms such as poor suck, lethargy, and irritability may ensue. Lamotrigine is metabolized slowly in neonates, and blood levels may be higher than anticipated from the breast-milk concentration. Measurements of lamotrigine levels in the newborn may be beneficial if the infant becomes lethargic.

The specifics of breast-feeding for each antiepileptic drug are reviewed in Chapter 11. No absolute contraindications exist to breastfeeding while taking antiepileptic medications. The benefits of breast-feeding, such as reduced risk of infection, must be weighed against the immediate and long-term (unknown) risks of exposure to antiepileptic drugs. Women should make individual, informed choices.

8. Management

All women of childbearing potential should be told the risks associated with pregnancy. Decisions regarding antiepileptic drug therapy should be made before the woman becomes pregnant. If the woman is receiving polytherapy, attempts should be made to convert to monotherapy before she becomes pregnant. Monotherapy should be reduced to the lowest effective dose. All women contemplating pregnancy should be taking folic acid, 1 to 4 mg per day.

All of the commonly used antiepileptic drugs are associated with both minor and major malformations. The drug of choice, therefore, is whichever antiepileptic drug controls a woman's seizures without causing side effects. However, women with a family history of neural tube defects should probably avoid valproic acid and carbamazepine. During the pregnancy, toxic and subtherapeutic concentrations must be avoided. Monthly monitoring of antiepileptic drug levels during pregnancy is recommended. Because of the increased clearance of antiepileptic drugs during pregnancy, the dosages of antiepileptic drugs often must be increased. If the patient experiences signs of toxicity in the face of apparent therapeutic drug levels, a free phenytoin or valproate plasma concentration determination may be useful.

An ultrasonographic evaluation should be performed to rule out spina bifida, cardiac anomalies, or a limb defect at 16 to 18 weeks. If ultrasound examination is not conclusive, amniocentesis could be performed, and α-fetoprotein levels obtained.

Good nutrition and adequate sleep are essential. The patient must avoid use of other medications, except as directed by a physician. Smoking and the consumption of alcohol should be avoided, because they have been associated with fetal anomalies. Alcohol may also stimulate hepatic pathways, altering the metabolism of antiepileptic drugs, and, thus altering the risk that malformations may occur.

To prevent hemorrhagic disease of the newborn (possibly due to induction of enzymes degrading vitamin K), vitamin K oral supplementation at 10 mg per day should be carried out from the 36th week of gestation until delivery. This practice does not supplant the recommendation of the American Academy of Pediatrics and the American College of Obstetrics and Gynecology that all infants receive vitamin K at birth.

Although the risks to the mother with epilepsy and her offspring are greater than those of the normal population, it is important to remember that approximately 90% of women with epilepsy have an uneventful pregnancy and normal infant.

9. Pregnancy Registries

Large numbers of mothers and infants are needed to determine the teratogenic risks of pregnancy and of antiepileptic drugs. Several registries have been formed to collect these data, with two large international registries. One covers North America, and the other covers Europe, Australia, and India. Three registries exist for specific drugs: lamotrigine, gabapentin, and levetiracetam.

D. Reproductive Dysfunction

Reproductive dysfunctions are common in women with epilepsy. Menstrual cycle disruption; anovulatory cycles; disturbances of hypothalamic hormones, pituitary hormones, or both; and disturbances of gonadal steroids are increased in frequency among women with epilepsy. Fertility may be as low as two thirds of that expected in the general population. Sexual dysfunction can occur as disorders of either desire or physiologic arousal. The most common dysfunction appears to be an inadequate initial physiologic arousal response. Reproductive dysfunctions may be due to psychological, pharmacologic, or physiologic factors.

E. Contraception

The enzyme-inducing antiepileptic drugs carbamazepine, oxcarbazepine, phenytoin, phenobarbital, primidone, and topiramate (at doses greater than 200 mg/day) increase steroid hormone-binding globulins with a reduction in free hormone levels. This leads to a reduction in exogenous estradiol and progesterone levels in women using hormonal contraception and to failure of hormonal contraception. Progesterone levels are not affected by topiramate at any dose. Birth-control formulations containing at least 50 mg of estradiol or mestranol are recommended for women taking enzyme-inducing antiepileptic drugs. Enzyme induction does not appear to be a problem with valproic acid, felbamate, gabapentin, lamotrigine, levetiracetam, tiagabine, or zonisamide. Only lamotrigine is affected by oral contraceptives, reducing lamotrigine concentration by up to 52%.

F. Menopause

At the time of menopause, seizure frequency worsens in one third of patients, remains the same in one third, and improves in one third. Seizures begin for the first time during or after menopause in some women. Little is known about the effect of hormonal replacement for postmenopausal women with epilepsy.

II. SPECIAL CONSIDERATIONS IN THE ELDERLY

A. Epidemiology

The prevalence and cumulative incidence of epilepsy and the incidence of partial seizures increase dramatically in the elderly. The prevalence rate of active epilepsy (usually symptomatic focal) is approximately 1.5% among persons 65 years and older. Risk of recurrent seizures in this age group is 90% without treatment. A significant increase also occurs in the incidence of status epilepticus in the elderly. Approximately 10% of elderly nursing-home residents receive an antiepileptic drug.

B. Etiology

Most seizures with onset after age 65 are due to symptomatic focal epilepsies. Cerebrovascular disease is the etiology in approximately 75% of seizures in the elderly. Seizures may occur at the time of stroke onset (2% to 6% of cases), or later as recurring seizures (5% to 20% of cases). Seizures may be particularly common after subarachnoid hemorrhages, in patients with seizures immediately after a cerebral infarction, and in patients with recurrent cerebral infarction. The risk of seizures in patients with Alzheimer disease is 5 to 10 times that of the general population.

Early-onset (within 7 days) seizures occur in 2% to 6% of strokes and are a predictor of future seizures. Early-onset seizures are initially seen as status epilepticus 25% of the time. Early seizures are particularly common after lobar intracerebral hemorrhage (14%) and subarachnoid hemorrhage (8%).

C. Seizure Morphology

Most new-onset partial seizures in the younger population have a temporal lobe origin. In the elderly, a higher proportion of new-onset partial seizures arise from the frontal and parietal lobes, because of differences in etiology between the two age groups. In particular, this is reflective of the increased incidence of vascular disease in the elderly.

Younger patients tend to have symptoms referable to the temporal lobe (nausea, olfactory hallucinations, déjà vu, etc.). In the elderly, seizures appear as altered mentation, staring and unresponsiveness, and blackout spells with nonspecific prodromes. Because of more-subtle manifestations, seizures in the elderly are often underdiagnosed or misdiagnosed. The postictal period is often longer in the elderly than in younger patients and may go on for days.

D. Diagnosis: Electroencephalography

A number of normal patterns in the elderly can be mistaken for abnormalities suggesting epilepsy. These include benign temporal delta transients of the elderly, frontally dominant rhythmic activity at onset of drowsiness, and electrocardiograph artifact caused by ventricular premature contractions (may appear to be temporal spikes). Medications and disease states also may alter the electroencephalograph in the elderly.

Approximately 40% of EEGs on elderly patients with new-onset seizures show paroxysmal activity. Focal or generalized slowing are also common findings. Use of prolonged EEG recordings increases the yield of paroxysmal activity.

E. Differential Diagnosis
Epilepsy frequently must be distinguished from syncope, transient ischemic attacks, and transient global amnesia in the elderly. These differential diagnoses are discussed in Chapter 9.

F. Management: Clinical Pharmacology
The absorption, distribution, biotransformation, excretion, drug interactions, and toxicology of antiepileptic drugs are all affected by age.

1. Absorption
Gastrointestinal motility, absorptive surface area, and splanchnic blood flow decrease with age, and gastric pH increases with age. However, other factors, such as concomitant food intake, concomitant therapy, and underlying disease, have even greater importance in determining absorption. Overall, no consistent rules exist regarding how drug absorption varies with age.

2. Distribution: Volume of Distribution
With increasing age, total body water and lean body mass decrease, whereas fat mass increases. This results in a decreased volume of distribution and increased plasma concentration of water-soluble drugs such as ethanol and caffeine. Conversely, volume of distribution increases (and plasma concentration decreases) of lipid-soluble drugs such as valproic acid and clonazepam.

3. Distribution: Protein Binding
Plasma albumin (principal drug-binding protein) concentration decreases by 5% to 10% in the elderly. This results in less protein binding and a higher free (unbound) fraction for drugs that are tightly bound to albumin. This, in turn, results in greater efficacy and toxicity for a given total plasma concentration of drug in the elderly. Phenytoin and valproic acid demonstrate this phenomenon.

4. Biotransformation
Hepatic mass and volume decrease by 15% to 20% between young and old adults. Decreases in clearance through cytochrome oxidase (cytochrome P450) enzymes roughly correlate with decreased hepatic mass and volume for many (but not all) drugs metabolized by these enzymes. Carbamazepine, phenytoin, phenobarbital, and valproic acid exhibit this phenomenon. The extent of slowed metabolism varies greatly among individuals and is difficult to predict.

5. Excretion
A 10% to 20% decrease in renal mass, blood flow, size and number of nephrons, and glomerular surface area occurs between young and old adults. This is accompanied by a corresponding decrease in measures of renal function, such as creatinine clearance and

Table 13-1.   Antiepileptic drug dosages and pharmacokinetics in the elderly[a,b]

Drug	Starting Dose	Protein Binding	Half-life	Metabolism Route of Elimination	Comments
Carbamazepine	4–6 mg/kg/d	75%–85%	NA	Hepatic	Protein binding decreased with reduced serum albumin. Estimated dosage requirements were 40% less than for younger patients
Gabapentin	600 mg/d	<10%	NA	Renal	Elimination correlates with creatinine clearance. Dosage may need to be reduced by 30% to 50%
Lamotrigine	25–50 mg/d (if not taking valproate)	55%	31 hr	Hepatic: glucuronide conjugation	Dosage adjustment may not be necessary because conjugation reactions only slightly diminish with advancing age
Levetiracetam	750 mg/d	<10%	9	Renal	Elimination correlates with creatinine clearance. Dosage may need to be reduced by 30%–50%
Phenobarbital	2 mg/kg/d	50%	NA	Hepatic/renal	Half-life and clearance similar to younger adults
Pregabalin	150 mg/d	<10%	NA	Renal	Elimination correlates with creatinine clearance. Dosage may need to be reduced by 30%–50%
Phenytoin	3 mg/kg/d	80%–93%	$t_{1/2}$ Varies with concentration (e.g., at 15 µg/ml, $t_{1/2}$ = 40–60 hr)	Hepatic	Protein binding decreased with reduced serum albumin. Subsequent increases should be small (<10% of dose)

Primidone	50 mg/d	Primidone, 70%; Phenobarbital, 50%	12.1 ± 4.6 hr	Hepatic	Half-life and clearance similar to younger adults.
Tiagabine	2–4 mg/d	96%	7–10 hr	Hepatic	Pharmacokinetic information based on small number of patients
Topiramate	25 mg/d	9%–17%	NA	Hepatic/renal	Dosage may need to be reduced in elderly patients with diminished renal function
Valproic acid	5–10 mg/kg/d	80%–95%	11–17 hr	Hepatic	Protein binding decreased with reduced serum albumin. Dosage reduction of 30% to 40% may be needed
Zonisamide	100 mg/d	40%	63 hr	Hepatic/renal	Pharmacokinetics similar in young adults and elderly

NA, not available for elderly patients; $t_{1/2}$, half-life.

[a]Considerable variation may be seen among the elderly (young-old, old, and old-old). Data on which this table is based are limited. Clinical judgment and observation of responses are needed.

[b]Estimated doses based on clinical experience and adjustment for slower metabolism or renal clearance.

tubular excretory capacity, and a decrease in clearance of drugs cleared by direct renal excretion, such as gabapentin, pregabalin, topiramate, and zonisamide. Unlike hepatic biotransformation, renal excretion decreases consistently and predictably with age.

6. Drug Interactions

The elderly often take multiple types of drugs, putting them at risk for drug–drug interactions. Such interactions are particularly common when antiepileptic drugs metabolized by the hepatic cytochrome P450 system (carbamazepine, phenobarbital, phenytoin, primidone) are administered with each other or with other types of drugs also metabolized by the cytochrome P450. Physicians are advised to consult the package insert or an appropriate pharmacy reference or database before adding another drug to an antiepileptic drug or vice versa.

7. Toxicity

Certain toxicities of antiepileptic drugs appear to be more severe at a given free or total plasma concentration of certain drugs in the elderly than in younger patients. These toxicities and drugs include sedation and behavioral changes (clonazepam, phenobarbital, primidone), tremor (valproic acid), and hyponatremia (carbamazepine).

8. Consequences of Polypharmacy

The elderly often take multiple drugs; they constitute 12% of the population and consume 25% of prescription drugs. The average elderly resident in a long-term facility is taking five to six prescription drugs. This polypharmacy puts the elderly at risk for drug toxicity and drug–drug interactions. Side effects and interactions of prescription drugs account for 17% of hospitalizations in the elderly, versus 3% of hospitalizations in the overall population.

G. Management

1. Drug Selection

No rigorous trials of antiepileptic drugs in the elderly are available. What follows is based on extrapolation from findings in young and middle-aged patients.

Most seizures in the elderly are of the symptomatic focal type. Carbamazepine and phenytoin have been the drugs of choice for localization-related seizures, based on comparative studies of older antiepileptic drugs performed with nonelderly adults. Furthermore, phenobarbital, primidone, and valproic acid all have toxicity problems in the elderly.

The ideal antiepileptic drug for the elderly would have minimal protein binding, minimal oxidative metabolism, and minimal neurotoxicity. Carbamazepine and phenytoin fail all three of these criteria; the newer drugs gabapentin, pregabalin, levetiracetam, and lamotrigine pass. Gabapentin, pregabalin, and levetiracetam have the added advantages of no drug interactions and no serious toxicity. Gabapentin, pregabalin, lamotrigine, and levetiracetam are the drugs of choice for use as adjuncts to carbamazepine and phenytoin therapy in the elderly. Gabapentin, pregabalin, lamotrigine, or levetiracetam may become the initial drugs of choice for partial seizures in the elderly (not yet an indication approved by the U.S. Food and Drug Administration). Because gabapentin, pregabalin, and levetiracetam are excreted by the kidney, their dosage in elderly patients with reduced creatinine clearance should be reduced by following guidelines contained in the package insert.

Based on neurotoxicity profiles in younger patients, tiagabine, topiramate, and zonisamide may not be ideal agents for adjunctive therapy of partial seizures in the elderly. Topiramate has been found to have much less neurotoxicity when taken as monotherapy than when taken as part of combination therapy.

2. Drug Dosage

Table 13-1 contains a summary of pharmacokinetic and dosing information on each of the antiepileptic drugs commonly used in the elderly.

REFERENCES

1. Abbasi F, Krumholtz A, Kittner SJ, et al. Effects of menopause on seizures in women with epilepsy. *Epilepsia* 1999;40:205–210.
2. Beghi E, Annegers JF for the Collaborative Group for the Pregnancy Registries in Epilepsy. Pregnancy registries in epilepsy. *Epilepsia* 2001;42:422–425.
3. Controversies in Epilepsy. The association between valproate and polycystic ovary syndrome. *Epilepsia* 2001;41:295–315.
4. Foldvary N. Treatment of epilepsy during pregnancy. In: Wyllie E, ed. *The treatment of epilepsy: principles and practice.* Philadelphia: Lippincott Williams & Wilkins, 2001:775–786.
5. Harden CL. Pregnancy and epilepsy. *Semin Neurol* 2007;27: 453–459.
6. Harden CL, Leppik I. Optimizing therapy of seizures in women who use oral contraceptives. *Neurology* 2006;67(suppl 4): S56–S58.
7. Hernandez-Diaz S, Werler MM, Walker AM, et al. Folic acid antagonists during pregnancy and the risk of birth defects. *N Engl J Med* 2000;343:1608–1614.
8. Hesdorffer AC, Logroscino G, Cascino G, et al. Incidence of status epilepticus in Rochester, Minnesota, 1965–1984. *Neurology* 1998;50:735–741.
9. Holmes LB, Harvey LA, Coull SA, at al. Teratogenicity of anticonvulsant drugs. *N Engl J Med* 2001;344:1132–1138.
10. Klass DW, Brenner RP. Electroencephalography of the elderly. *J Clin Neurophysiol* 1995;12:116–131.
11. Klein P, van Passel-Clark LMA, Pezzullo JC. Onset of epilepsy at time of menarche. *Neurology* 2003;60:495–497.
12. Labovitz DL, Hauser WA, Sacco R. Prevalence and predictors of seizure and status epilepticus after first stroke. *Neurology* 2001;57:200–206.
13. Lackler TE, Cloyd J, Thomas LW, et al. Antiepileptic drug use in nursing home residents: effect of age, gender, and comedication on patterns of use. *Epilepsia* 1998;39:1083–1087.
14. Lackner TE. Strategies for optimizing antiepileptic drug therapy in elderly people. *Pharmacotherapy* 2002;22:329–364.

15. Leppik IE. Epilepsy in the elderly. *Epilepsia*. 2006;47(suppl 1): 65–70.
16. Leppik IE, Epilepsy Foundation of America. Choosing an antiepileptic: selecting drugs for older patients with epilepsy. *Geriatrics* 2005;60:42–77.
17. Morrell MJ, Flynn KL, Done S, et al. Sexual dysfunction, sex steroid hormone abnormalities, and depression in women with epilepsy treated with antiepileptic drugs. *Epilepsy Behav* 2005;6:360–365.
18. Morrell MJ. Antiepileptic drug use in women. In: Levy RH, Mattson RH, Meldrum BS, et al., eds. *Antiepileptic drugs*. 5th ed. Philadelphia: Lippincott Williams & Wilkins, 2002:132–148.
19. Ramsay RE, Pryor F. Epilepsy in the elderly. *Neurology* 2000;55(suppl 1):S9–S14.
20. Report of the Quality Standards Subcommittee of the American Academy of Neurology. Practice parameter: management issues for women with epilepsy (summary statement). *Neurology* 1998;51:944–948.
21. So EL, Annegers JF, Hanser WA, et al. Population-based study of seizure disorders after cerebral infarction. *Neurology* 1996;46: 350–355.
22. The North American Pregnancy and Epilepsy Registry. A North American registry for epilepsy and pregnancy: a unique public/private partnership of health surveillance. *Epilepsia* 1998;39:793–798.
23. Woolley CS, Schwartzkroin PA. Hormonal effects on the brain. *Epilepsia* 1998;39(suppl 8):2–8.

Comorbidities

Although a major goal in the treatment of epilepsy is stopping the seizures, it is not the only treatment goal. Patients with epilepsy are a risk for a number of comorbidities. Comorbidity refers to the cooccurrence of two supposedly separate conditions that occur together more than by chance. For example, depression occurs more frequently in patients with epilepsy than in the normal population, so that epilepsy and depression are comorbidities. Comorbidities are not necessarily causal. For example, because epilepsy and depression are comorbidities does not mean that epilepsy caused the depression or depression caused the epilepsy. Rather, it is possible that both conditions have a common biologic substrate or that another independent variable triggers one of the comorbidities. For example, epilepsy often leads to drug therapy, which could cause depression independent of the epilepsy. Although some overlap occurs, children and adults are considered separately.

I. CHILDREN

Children with epilepsy are far more likely to have a psychiatric disorder than are children without epilepsy or with other chronic disorders. In a large British survey, it was found that rates of psychiatric disorder in children with epilepsy was 37% compared with 11% in diabetes and 9% in control children. Emotional disorders, conduct disorders, attention disorder/hyperactive disorder (ADHD), anxiety, and autism-spectrum disorder are over-represented in children with epilepsy. Emotional, behavioral, and relationship difficulties are common in children with epilepsy and constitute a significant burden to the children and their families, indicating the need for effective mental health services for these children.

A. Attention Deficit/Hyperactivity Disorder
1. Definitions
Children with epilepsy are at substantial risk for ADHD. Clinical studies suggest a prevalence of 30% to 40%, several fold higher than that of the normal population. Children with epilepsy and ADHD differ from children with ADHD who do not have epilepsy by having a higher incidence of the inattentive form of the disorder. In addition, in the general population, ADHD is more common in boys than in girls, whereas in children with epilepsy, an equal female/male ratio is found.

2. Treatment
Educational and psychological evaluations are helpful in identifying ADHD and distinguishing the condition from depression and learning disabilities. Psychoeducational interventions can be quite useful. Children with ADHD typically work better if they are taught in a quiet and structured environment. A

personal aide can help redirect the child's attention. A consistent
educational program at home as well as in school is important,
and the parents should be engaged in the education plan.
Antiepileptic drugs, such as barbiturates and benzodiazepines
that may exacerbate the ADHD, should be avoided.

Although stimulant medications have been a mainstay in the
treatment of ADHD in children with epilepsy, concerns exist
that these drugs could lower the seizure threshold. Seizures
associated with stimulant medications are unusual, and drugs
such as dexedrine, methylphenidate, and atomoxetine can be
quite useful. Bupropion, an atypical antidepressant, should be
avoided because it can lower the seizure threshold.

B. Depression
1. Definitions
A higher-than-expected incidence of depression is found in children with epilepsy. In a study of adolescents with epilepsy, 23%
had symptoms of depression. It has been found that adolescents'
attitudes, attributions, and satisfaction with family relationships are related to depression and should be assessed in the
clinical setting. Children with epilepsy are at risk for suicide.

Children may not have the vocabulary to talk about such feelings and so may express their feelings through behavior.
Younger individuals with depression are more likely to show
phobias, separation anxiety disorder, somatic complaints, and
behavior problems, such as anger and aggression. The adolescent
may demonstrate academic decline, disruptive behavior, loss of
interest in activities, and problems with friends. Sometimes one
can also see aggressive behavior, irritability, and suicidal
ideation. The parent may say that the child hates himself or her-
self and everything else.

2. Treatment
All children with suspected depression should have a psychological evaluation with testing. Once diagnosed, patients may benefit from counseling. Antiepileptic drugs that could be contributing
to the problem should be discontinued and substituted with
drugs that might improve mood. For example, eliminating barbiturates and benzodiazepines and substituting lamotrigine, carbamazepine, or valproate, when appropriate for the child's seizure
disorder, can be very useful.

Selective serotonin reuptake inhibitors (SSRIs) have
improved the outlook for the medication treatment of child and
adolescent depression. The side effects are not as annoying as
those of the older medications. These medications are somewhat
less toxic in overdose. Fluoxetine has been shown to be effective
in depression and does not increase the risk of suicide.

C. Cognition
1. Definitions
Apart from control of the seizures, one of the most important factors in determining how well a child with epilepsy progresses
toward independence is cognition. Mental retardation is higher
in children with epilepsy than in the normal population. The

majority of the mental retardation in children with epilepsy is a result of the insult leading to the epilepsy. For example, children with hypoxic–ischemic insults, head trauma, or genetic causes of their epilepsy are retarded because of these insults. Most children with epilepsy have stable intelligence. In the small percentage of children that have a progressive decline in intelligence over time, the seizures are usually intractable.

2. Treatment

Recognizing that the child is retarded is critical. Inappropriate placement in a grade in which he or she is incapable of succeeding can result in considerable anxiety, frustration, and may result in a conduct disorder. All children with epilepsy who are not progressing in school should have psychological testing. Once identified, the child can be placed in the correct educational program. Antiepileptic drugs that could impair attention or learning, such as barbiturates or benzodiazepines, should be avoided.

D. Learning Disabilities
1. Definitions

A learning disability is a disorder in basic psychological processes involved in understanding or using language, spoken or written, that may manifest itself in an imperfect ability to listen, think, speak, read, write, spell, or use mathematical calculations. The term includes conditions such as perceptual disability, brain injury, minimal brain dysfunction, dyslexia, and developmental aphasia. In learning disabilities, the ability to learn is below what is expected for the child's IQ.

2. Treatment

Any child with epilepsy not doing well in school should undergo psychological testing. This can typically be done through the school. Children with specific learning difficulties and memory problems can benefit greatly from appropriate management. Benzodiazepines and barbiturates can contribute to learning difficulties and should be avoided when possible. Topiramate may rarely be associated with cognitive impairment. If appearance of the learning disabilities coincides with initiation of topiramate treatment, consideration should be given to discontinuing the medication.

E. Conduct Disorders
1. Definitions

A conduct disorder is a behavioral and emotional disorder of childhood and adolescence. Children with conduct disorder act inappropriately and irritate or upset parents, teachers, and other students. Children with conduct disorder act out aggressively and express anger inappropriately. They engage in a variety of antisocial and destructive acts, including violence toward people and animals, destruction of property, lying, stealing, truancy, and running away from home. Irritability, temper tantrums, and low self-esteem are common personality traits of children with conduct disorders. They often participate in risk-taking behaviors such as early sex and abuse of drugs and alcohol. Although a conduct disorder occurs in approximately 9% of boys and 2% to 9% of girls younger than 18 years, it is substantially increased with children with epilepsy.

Causes of conduct disorders include the epilepsy itself, the associated brain damage or dysfunction responsible for the epilepsy, the antiepileptic drug treatment, or the reactions to the epilepsy. The risk for developing a conduct disorder increases if the home environment is dysfunctional.

2. Treatment

The child with a conduct disorder should undergo psychological testing. For children with coexisting ADHD, substance abuse, depression, or learning disorders, treating these conditions first is preferred and may result in a significant improvement to the conduct disorder. Mental retardation and depression may be seen with a conduct disorder. Once a conduct disorder is identified, the child can be enrolled in a behavioral therapy program, which can work both with the family and school system to address and modify the child's behavior. Parents should be counseled on how to set appropriate limits with their child and be consistent and realistic when disciplining. Antiepileptic drugs that could be contributing to the problem should be discontinued and substituted with drugs that might improve mood. For example, eliminating barbiturates and benzodiazepines and substituting lamotrigine, carbamazepine, or valproate, when appropriate for the child's seizure disorder, can be very useful.

When aggressive behavior is severe, mood-stabilizing medication, including lithium buspirone or propranolol, may be an appropriate option for treating the aggressive symptoms. In some children, placing the child into a structured setting or treatment program such as a psychiatric hospital may be beneficial.

F. Anxiety Disorders

1. Definitions

Anxiety is overrepresented in children with epilepsy. Compared with normal children without epilepsy, significantly more patients have affective and anxiety disorder diagnoses (33%) as well as suicidal ideation (20%). Unfortunately, many children with anxiety disorders go underdiagnosed and poorly treated. Physical symptoms, such as a rapid heart beat, stomach or chest pain, or feeling short of breath may accompany anxiety. It is common to have more than one type of anxiety disorder or anxiety plus a mood disorder, such as depression.

2. Treatment

Children with suspected anxiety disorders should undergo a psychological evaluation. Supportive psychotherapy may help some children vent their feelings, Cognitive behavioral therapies improve self-confidence and coping by reducing tension and avoidance.

Antianxiety medications that enhance serotonin activity (e.g., SSRIs) are usually effective and well tolerated. Buspirone, propranolol, and benzodiazepines such as chlorazepate or diazepam may be useful. It is important to keep in mind that a dangerous cycle can develop when a benzodiazepine is used for the long-term treatment of anxiety or insomnia. Initially, the drug works well, but tolerance often develops, and the dose must be increased. The cycle can repeat until a high dose is reached, with cognitive and behavioral toxicity, but the role of the benzodiazepine may be overlooked because other factors also contribute.

G. Migraine
1. Definitions
A higher-than-expected incidence of migraine is found in children with epilepsy. Differentiating seizures from migraines may be a challenge.

An acute confusional state, which is considered to a rare form of a migraine, consists of a period of confusion that can last for minutes to hours. It may resemble complex partial status epilepticus and often requires an EEG to distinguish between the two. Benign paroxysmal vertigo occurs in children from 1 to 5 years of age and is characterized by episodes of vertigo, nystagmus, and anxiety. The child often vomits during the attack and is diaphoretic and pale. Benign paroxysmal vertigo is considered to be a form of migraine. As discussed in Chapter 10, abdominal migraine is a condition consisting of intermittent abdominal pain and vomiting occurring in school-age children.

2. Treatment
Fortunately, many of the antiepileptic drugs used to treat epilepsy are effective in migraine. For example, topiramate and valproate are excellent antimigraine drugs and have received approval for their use in migraine by the United States Food and Drug Administration. The other antiepileptic drugs are sometimes used in the treatment of migraine.

II. ADULTS
Many of the conditions described in the prior section on children may persist into adulthood. ADHD, cognitive impairment, conduct disorders, and learning disabilities can extend into adulthood. The strategies discussed for the children would generally be appropriate as well for the adults.

A. Depression
1. Definitions
Mood disorders are conditions that negatively affect an individual's emotional state. For people with epilepsy, the most common mood disorders are major depression and dysthymia. Adults with epilepsy often have sadness associated with a lack of pleasure in performing activities; problems with weight and sleep; tiredness; difficulty concentrating and making decisions; feelings of worthlessness or guilt; and frequent thoughts of suicide and death. A dysthymic disorder is similar to major depressive disorder, but it is less intense and includes depression for most days for at least 2 years. During this interval, two or more of the following symptoms must be present: change in appetite, lack of sleep, decreased energy, low self-esteem, poor concentration,

difficulty making decisions, and feelings of hopelessness. Another common mood disorder in people with epilepsy is bipolar affective disorder, also known as manic–depressive disease. It is characterized by two types of symptoms: depression and mania. Manic symptoms are characterized by excessive energy (agitation), excessive feelings of self-importance (grandiosity), excessive interest in sex (hypersexuality), and inability to sleep (insomnia), as well as distractibility and high-risk behavior.

The risk for suicide is higher in patients with epilepsy than in the normal population. Whereas depression often develops after the diagnosis of epilepsy is made, evidence suggests that depression is a risk factor for developing epilepsy, suggesting that a common pathologic substrate may exist for both conditions.

2. Treatment

The most common treatment of depression includes psychotherapy and medication. These forms may be used separately or together, but the overriding goal is eventually to eliminate symptoms of depression. Counseling for the adult or child also may help, and family therapy may be useful, as well, particularly if anyone else in the family has a mood disorder. The most frequently prescribed antidepressants for adults with epilepsy and depression are the SSRIs such as fluoxetine.

Antiepileptic drugs that could be contributing to the depression should be discontinued and substituted with drugs that might improve mood. For example, eliminating barbiturates and benzodiazepines and substituting lamotrigine or valproate, when appropriate for the seizure type and syndrome, can be very useful.

B. Anxiety

1. Definitions

The presence of anxiety in adults with epilepsy was recently found to be 20.5%. Epilepsy was associated with a history of depression, perceived side effects of antiepileptic medication, lower educational attainment, chronic ill health, female gender, and unemployment. Excessive anxiety can have significant effects of person's education, job performance, and interpersonal relationships. Although anxiety is best quantified and diagnosed through anxiety questionnaires, the diagnosis can often be suspected based on the patient's interview.

2. Treatment

Adults with suspected anxiety disorders should undergo a psychological evaluation, because the anxiety may coexist with depression. Supportive psychotherapy is often very useful in identifying anxiety-provoking issues and providing the patients with strategies to cope with these issues.

Antianxiety medications that enhance serotonin activity (e.g., SSRIs) are usually effective and well tolerated. Buspirone, propranolol, and benzodiazepines such as clorazepate or diazepam may be useful.

REFERENCES

1. Davies S, Heyman I, Goodman R. A population survey of mental health problems in children with epilepsy. *Dev Med Child Neurol* 2003;45:292–295.
2. Dunn DW, Austin JK, Harezlak J, et al. ADHD and epilepsy in childhood. *Dev Med Child Neurol* 2003;45:50–54.
3. Dunn DW, Kronenberger WG. Childhood epilepsy, attention problems, and ADHD: review and practical considerations. *Semin Pediatr Neurol* 2005;12:222–228.
4. Dunn DW, Austin JK, Huster GA. Symptoms of depression in adolescents with epilepsy. *J Am Acad Child Adolesc Psychiatry* 1999;38:1132–1138.
5. Caplan R, Siddarth P, Gurbani S, et al. Depression and anxiety disorders in pediatric epilepsy. *Epilepsia* 2005;46:720–730.
6. Bridge JA, Iyengar S, Salary CB, et al. Clinical response and risk for reported suicidal ideation and suicide attempts in pediatric antidepressant treatment: a meta-analysis of randomized controlled trials. *JAMA* 2007;297:1683–1696.
7. Austin JK, Dunn DW, Caffrey HM, et al. Recurrent seizures and behavior problems in children with first recognized seizures: a prospective study. *Epilepsia* 2002;43:1564–1573.
8. Rogawski MA, Loscher W. The neurobiology of antiepileptic drugs for the treatment of nonepileptic conditions. *Nat Med* 2004;10:685–692.
9. Hesdorffer DC, Hauser WA, Olafsson E, et al. Depression and suicide attempt as risk factors for incident unprovoked seizures. *Ann Neurol* 2006;59:35–41.
10. Hesdorffer DC, Hauser WA, Annegers JF, et al. Major depression is a risk factor for seizures in older adults. *Ann Neurol* 2000;47:246–249.
11. Mensah SA, Beavis JM, Thapar AK, et al. A community study of the presence of anxiety disorder in people with epilepsy. *Epilepsy Behav* 2007;11:118–124.

Counseling

I. COUNSELING ISSUES FOR CHILDREN

A. Activities

Although children with epilepsy are at increased risk for injury, limitations on activities should be relatively few. When restrictions are excessive, they may lead to significant psychological difficulties with impaired self-esteem.

Childhood is filled with inherent risks, and the child with epilepsy is at only a minimally greater risk than before the seizures began. Making guidelines that can be applied to all children with epilepsy is impossible because seizure type, duration, and frequency all may affect the number of restrictions.

Restrictions may also vary over the course of the disorder. Restrictions should be more stringent during the first 2 to 3 months after onset of the disorder, until the physician and family are in agreement that further seizures are unlikely, and for 2 to 3 months after discontinuing antiepileptic medication. In children with persistent, recurrent seizures, restrictions usually remain the same.

Parents must be particularly careful around water. Children with epilepsy are at higher risk for drowning than are children without epilepsy, whether in a bathtub or during recreational swimming. Recreational swimming should occur only with close supervision and in clear water. Swimming in lakes, rivers, and the ocean is very risky. Young children should never be left alone in the bathtub, even for a few seconds. Older children should be encouraged to use a shower and reminded not to lock the bathroom door when showering. Unsupervised swimming should never occur.

All children should avoid open fires, hot stoves and ovens, and dangerous machinery. Parents must assume that a seizure could occur at any time and should avoid allowing a child to be in a situation where a seizure could be deadly. For example, children should not stand near the edge of platforms of subway or train stations.

Very few restrictions should be placed on recreational activities. Activities in which the child is high off the ground, such as rock or rope climbing, should be discouraged. Although bike riding can be pursued safely by most children, it should be avoided by children with frequent seizures in whom impairment of consciousness occurs. Skating, roller-blading, and skateboarding should be restricted only in children with frequent seizures. Even in children with well-controlled epilepsy, these activities should not occur on busy streets. Skydiving and scuba diving should be prohibited.

The child with epilepsy should be encouraged to participate in organized sports. Although some physicians restrict contact sports in the belief that head trauma can precipitate seizures, no evidence exists that patients with epilepsy are at higher risk for seizures after minor head injury. Children who have a regular exercise program may actually have fewer seizures and side effects than do children who are sedentary.

Parents of young children are often terrified that the child will have an undetected seizure and die during sleep. Having the child sleep in the same room as the parents may be appropriate for the first few months after diagnosis. The parents should also be instructed to purchase an intercom that can be turned on and placed in the child's room, so they can be alerted by any crying or an abnormal breathing pattern. Soft or restricting sleeping surfaces should be avoided with infants and young children.

Caregivers other than the parents should be told that the child has epilepsy and be given a description of the seizure, along with first-aid measures. Because seizures can be extremely frightening, baby-sitters should be chosen with care. Local epilepsy support groups often have a list of experienced baby-sitters.

Children who are at risk for prolonged seizures present additional problems when the family travels or visits remote areas in which medical care may not be readily available. Before traveling, parents should inquire about the closest medical facility that can deal with a child with epilepsy. It is recommended that the parents be given instruction in administering rectal diazepam or other rescue medications, in case a prolonged seizure ensues.

B. Television and Video Games

Rarely, children have a seizure while watching television, playing an electronic screen game, or using a computer. Most of these children have a photoconvulsive response on electroencephalography. Television, computers, and video games should be restricted only when a consistent relation is seen between watching television or playing video games and seizures. Parents often erroneously blame video-game playing or television watching for a seizure, even when the seizure occurs some time after play. The parents must be informed that if television or the video game is responsible for the seizure, the seizure will occur during the activity.

C. School

Children with epilepsy are at significant risk for a variety of problems involving cognition and behavior. The distribution of IQ scores among children with epilepsy is skewed toward lower values, and the number of children requiring special education services varies from 10% to 33%. Behavioral and psychiatric disorders in children with epilepsy are also higher than in the normal population, with surveys demonstrating that the prevalence of psychiatric disease is 2 to 4 times greater among children with epilepsy than in control subjects. Although the cognitive and behavioral abnormalities may often be explained by the etiologic factors responsible for the epilepsy, evidence exists that some children with poorly controlled epilepsy have progressive declines of IQ on serial intelligence tests, and behavioral and psychiatric deterioration over time. Whether this decline is secondary to antiepileptic medications, to progression of the underlying encephalopathy responsible for the seizures, or to the seizures *per se* is not certain.

A number of factors place the child at increased risk for cognitive impairment: an early age at seizure onset, intractable seizures, and polytherapy. The etiology of the epilepsy is also important. Children with symptomatic epilepsy are at higher risk for cognitive impairment than are children with idiopathic epilepsy.

It is important that the physician and the child's teachers be aware of these potential difficulties, and the difficulties should be addressed as soon as they are identified. The child may benefit from special education resources, such as speech, physical, and occupational therapy. In children with learning difficulties, avoiding drug toxicity is important. Polytherapy and treatment with barbiturates and benzodiazepines should be avoided whenever possible.

School personnel working with the child should be informed of the child's condition and the treatment plan. Little is gained from trying to keep the diagnosis secret and epilepsy "off the record." Teachers can provide the physician with assessments regarding seizure frequency and drug side effects and can serve as advocates for the child. Because children with seizures may be the subject of ridicule by classmates, informed teachers can educate the class about the disorder and dispel many of the myths that accompany the diagnosis.

II. COUNSELING ISSUES FOR ADULTS

A. Pregnancy
See Chapter 13.

B. Risk of Epilepsy in First-degree Relatives
Patients with epilepsy often ask whether relatives (especially children) have an increased risk of epilepsy. The epilepsy syndromes are divided by etiology into symptomatic and idiopathic types (see Chapter 1). Little or no increased risk for epilepsy occurs in first-degree relatives of patients with symptomatic epilepsies. First-degree relatives of patients with idiopathic epilepsies have an increased risk (two- to threefold on average) of epilepsy. The increased risk of idiopathic epilepsy in relatives of patients with idiopathic epilepsy decreases with age; risk is not increased at age 35 or older.

C. Driving
The issue of driving privileges must balance the seizure risk to the patient and to the public against the other, considerable negative effects on the patient of the loss of driving privileges. Persons with active seizure disorders must be made known to the state registry of motor vehicles and have driving privileges suspended until their seizures are controlled.

In most states, it is the patient's responsibility to report an active seizure condition to the registry of motor vehicles. For the physician to make such a report is a breach of patient confidentiality. In a few states, the physician must report the patient to a state authority.

Adequate seizure control can be determined several ways. Most states require that a patient be seizure free on medication for a specified period (usually 3 to 12 months). The patient may then reapply for driving privileges. Such an application usually requires a letter from the patient's physician. Other states have a medical board that determines driving eligibility on an individual basis. Some states use a combination of the two methods.

Because state laws are variable and changing, physicians are best advised to contact state authorities in their states regarding current regulations. The Epilepsy Foundation maintains a list of regulations for each state on its Web site (www.epilepsyfoundation .org). The physician must advise the patient of current state regulations regarding driving. This advice should be given in writing to the patient as a form letter, and its distribution to the patient should be noted in the record. Regulations for operation of buses and large trucks usually are different and more restrictive than regulations for operation of a personal automobile.

Patients who cannot have driving privileges should be encouraged to make use of public transportation or car pools or to find a person (e.g., student, retiree) willing to serve as a driver.

D. Sudden Unexplained Death

Mortality rates are higher in people with epilepsy compared to the general population. The most common epilepsy-specific cause of death is sudden unexpected death in epilepsy (SUDEP). SUDEP is defined as: "The sudden unexpected, witnessed or unwitnessed, non-traumatic and non-drowning death in a patient with epilepsy, with or without evidence for a seizure and excluding convulsive status epilepticus in which post-mortem examination does not reveal a toxicological or anatomical cause of death." The risk is highest in studies of candidates for epilepsy surgery and epilepsy referral center (2.2 to 10 per 1000), intermediate in studies including patients with mental retardation (3.4 to 3.6 per 1000), and lowest in children (0 to 0.2 per 1000). Risk factors include an early age of onset of epilepsy, antiepileptic drug noncompliance, frequent generalized tonic-clonic seizures, and medical intractability. While the mechanism of SUDEP is unknown and currently can not be prevented, it is recommended that patients with high risk factors be told about the possibility of SUDEP. This is particularly important in patients who are noncompliant and are having generalized tonic-clonic seizures since improving compliance and seizure control is likely to reduce the risk of SUDEP.

E. Insurance
1. Health and Life
Some medical and life insurance companies either penalize persons with epilepsy or will not insure them at all. Many companies offer limited coverage, usually excluding preexisting epilepsy. The following advice is offered: (a) check any health or life insurance plan to be certain epilepsy-related events are covered; (b) keep in mind that employer group insurance plans tend to be less selective and more likely to cover preexisting epilepsy; (c) determine whether the patient is eligible for Medicare, Medicaid, or veterans' benefits or state-administered free medication programs; and (d) consult the state insurance regulatory agency where available.

2. *Driving*

Driving insurance may be difficult to obtain. Some states have a special pool providing driving insurance to persons perceived to be a greater risk.

F. Employment

The question of seizures may come up when a person with epilepsy seeks employment. The Americans with Disabilities Act (for private employers) and Federal Rehabilitation Act (for federal agencies and contractors) prohibit employers from discriminating against a person with a disability who could perform the job with "reasonable accommodations." Persons with epilepsy can perform most jobs and should be excluded only when having a seizure would pose a danger to the person or to co-workers (e.g., driving, operating dangerous machinery, working at heights). Persons with epilepsy should (a) learn about any job they are applying for before the interview; (b) complete the application process if they are qualified; and (c) take action if they are discriminated against. The Federal Department of Labor, state agencies for disabled persons, and the Epilepsy Foundation of America (EFA) are good resources for employment-related advice.

G. Income Assistance

Persons with reduced ability to work because of disability may qualify for Supplemental Security Income under the Social Security Administration or for veterans' benefits (health services, income, or both) under the Department of Veterans Affairs. The eligibility requirements are complex. Assistance may be obtained from (a) references at the end of this chapter; (b) social work agencies; (c) the Social Security Administration; (d) the Department of Veterans Affairs Assistance Hot Line [(800) 827-1000]; and (e) veterans' groups (e.g., Disabled American Veterans).

H. Alcohol and Marijuana Use

Consumption of one or two drinks per day probably does not increase seizure risk or alter antiepileptic drug metabolism. Consumption of larger amounts of alcohol may increase seizure risk, especially at times of decreasing alcohol levels. Although the data are incomplete, little evidence exists for a deleterious effect of marijuana on seizures. Use of either drug can lead to escalation of drug habits and noncompliance with antiepileptic drug regimens.

I. When All Else Fails

Local epilepsy groups, the EFA, and other advocacy groups often can lead the person with epilepsy to the right resource. Groups representing other disabilities (e.g., developmental disabilities, head injury) may have useful information. The state attorney general's office is responsible for protecting citizens' civil and consumer rights and can offer advice in these areas. Persons with epilepsy should ask forcefully for assistance and seek the resources they need.

REFERENCES

The Epilepsy Foundation (EF) has a number of booklets and videotapes for consumers that deal with general information on seizures, seizure first aid, children's issues, women's issues, driving, insurance, and benefits. These may be obtained from the EF by mail (4351 Garden City Drive, Landover, MD 20785), telephone [(301) 459-3700], or the World-wide Web (www.epilepsyfoundation.org). Many of these materials also are available through local chapters of the EF.

 1. Chadwick D. Driving restrictions and persons with epilepsy. *Neurology* 2001;57:1749–1750.
 2. Devinsky O, Westbrook LE. Quality of life with epilepsy. In: Wyllie E, ed. *The treatment of epilepsy: principles and practice.* Philadelphia: Lippincott Williams & Wilkins, 2001:1243–1250.
 3. Finucane AK. Legal aspects of epilepsy. In: Wyllie E, ed. *The treatment of epilepsy: principles and practice.* Philadelphia: Lippincott Williams & Wilkins, 2001:1251–1256.
 4. Gordon E, Devinsky O. Alcohol and marijuana use: effects on epilepsy and use by patients with epilepsy. *Epilepsia* 2001;42:1266–1272.
 5. Hermann BP, Seidenberg M, Bell B. The neurodevelopmental impact of childhood onset temporal lobe epilepsy on brain structure and function and the risk of progressive cognitive effects. *Prog Brain Res* 2002;135:429–438.
 6. Hitiris N, Suratman S, Kelly K, et al. Sudden unexpected death in epilepsy: a search for risk factors. *Epilepsy Behav* 2007:10: 138–141.
 7. Hoare P, Kerley S. Psychosocial adjustment of children with chronic epilepsy and their families. *Dev Med Child Neurol* 1991; 33:201–215.
 8. Hoare P, Mann H. Self-esteem and behavioural adjustment in children with epilepsy and children with diabetes. *J Psychosom Res* 1994;38:859–869.
 9. Krauss GL, Ampaw L, Krumholtz A. Individual state driving restrictions for people with epilepsy in the US. *Neurology* 2001; 57:1780–1785.
10. Meador KJ. Cognitive effects of epilepsy and antiepileptic medications. In: Wyllie E, ed. *The treatment of epilepsy: principles and practice* Philadelphia: Lippincott Williams & Wilkins, 2001:1215–1226.
11. Morrell MJ, Pedley TA. "The Scarlet E": epilepsy is still a burden. *Neurology* 2000;54:1882–1883.
12. Nashef L, Hindocha N, Makoff A. Risk factors in sudden death in epilepsy (SUDEP): the quest for mechanisms. *Epilepsia* 2007;48: 859–871.
13. Pedley TA, Hauser WA. Sudden death in epilepsy: a wake-up call for management. *Lancet* 2002;359:1790–1791.
14. Quirk JA, Fish DR, Smith SJ, et al. First seizures associated with playing electronic screen games: a community-based study in Great Britain. *Ann Neurol* 1995;37:733–737.

Subject Index

Page numbers followed by the letter "f" indicate figures; numbers followed by "t" indicate tables.

Phenytoin (Dilantin)
dosages of, 207
drug interactions with, 208
for eclampsia, 128
for elderly patients, 250
formulations of, 206–207
indications for, 206
for Lennox-Gastaut syn-
drome, 103
in neonates, 72
pharmacokinetics of, 206
in pregnancy, 208–209, 242
for seizures, 153–154
for status epilepticus, 231t,
232–233, 263
toxicity of, 207–208
Photosensitive seizures,
128–129
Plasma concentration. *See*
Drug-plasma concentra-
tion
Pneumonia, 35
Polypharmacy,
consequences of, 250
Polyspike-and-wave discharge,
113, 114f
Polytherapy, 151–152
Porphyria, safe and unsafe
drugs in, 126t
Positron emission tomography
(PET), 164–165
Posterior parietal seizures, 52
Postnatal infections, 69f
Postsynaptic potentials (PSPs),
13, 15f
Postural seizures, 26
Praxis-induced seizures, 130
Prednisone, for LKS, 106
Preeclampsia, 127–128
Pregabalin (Lyrica)
disease states and, 210
dosages of, 209
formulations of, 209
indications for, 209
mechanism of action of, 185t
pharmacokinetics of, 209
toxicity of, 209–210
Pregnancy
antiepileptic drugs and, 159,
243
complications of, 243
epilepsy and, 241–245
management of, 244–245
Primidone (Mysoline)
dosages of, 211
drug interactions with, 211
formulations of, 211
indications for, 211
mechanism of action of, 195t
pharmacokinetics of, 210
in pregnancy, 211

for seizures, 153–154, 155,
156t
toxicity of, 211
Progressive myoclonus
encephalopathies (PME)
electroencephalogram phe-
nomena, 107–108
features of, 107
management of, 108
prognosis of, 108
treatment of, 108
Progressive myoclonus epilepsies, 6t
Prolonged Q-T syndrome, 146
Proprioceptive input seizures,
130
Protein binding,
epilepsy and, 247
Proton magnetic resonance
spectroscopy, 166
Psychogenic seizures, 140–143,
142–143t
Psychosis, in complex partial
seizures, 32
Pulmonary edema, 35
Pykonolepsy, 98
Pyridoxine, 71–72

R
Rage attacks, 140, 141t
Rapid eye movement (REM)
sleep, 78, 87
Rasmussen's encephalitis, 51
Reading seizures, 130
Recreational drug-induced
seizures, 124–125
Reflex anoxic seizures,
145–146
Reflex epilepsies, 6t, 130
Reflex seizures
definition of, 128
induced by nonvisual stimuli,
129–130
management of, 131
with visual triggers,
128–129
Reproductive dysfunction, 245
Respiratory depression, 124
Responsiveness, defined, 24
Rhythmic ictal transformation
(RIT), 28
Rolandic epilepsy, 93–97

S
School, for children with
epilepsy, 261–262
Sedative-hypnotic drug-
withdrawal seizures,
125–127
Seizure activity
cessation of, 9–18, 18f